Student Learning Guide for

FUNDAMENTAL CONCEPTS AND SKILLS FOR NURSING

Susan C. deWit, MSN, RNCS
Formerly, Instructor of Nursing
El Centro College
Dallas, TX

W.B. Saunders Company
An Imprint of Elsevier Science
Philadelphia London New York St. Louis Sydney Toronto

W.B. SAUNDERS COMPANY
An Imprint of Elsevier Science
The Curtis Center
Independence Square West
Philadelphia, PA 19106-3399

NOTICE

Nursing is an ever-changing field. Standard safety precautions must be followed, but as new research and clinical experience broaden our knowledge, changes in treatment and drug therapy become necessary or appropriate. Readers are advised to check the product information currently provided by the manufacturer of each drug to be administered to verify the recommended dose, the method and duration of administration, and the contraindications. It is the responsibility of the licensed prescriber, relying on experience and knowledge of the patient, to determine dosages and the best treatment for the patient. Neither the publisher nor the editor assumes any responsibility for any injury and/or damage to persons or property.

The Publisher

Vice President, Nursing Editorial Director: Sally Schrefer
Senior Editor: Terri Wood
Senior Developmental Editor: Robin Levin Richman

Student Learning Guide for
FUNDAMENTAL CONCEPTS AND SKILLS FOR NURSING, First Edition ISBN 0-7216-6929-8

Printed in the United States of America

Last digit is the print number: 9 8 7 6 5 4

To the Student

The *Student Learning Guide for Fundamental Concepts and Skills for Nursing* is designed to help you achieve the objectives of each chapter and to provide reinforcement for the terms and concepts presented in the text. It will guide you in learning to set priorities, apply the nursing process, practice critical thinking, make good judgments and decisions, and increase your ability to communicate therapeutically.

STUDY HINTS

Ask Questions

There are no stupid questions. If you do not know something or are not sure, you need to find out. Other people may be wondering the same thing but may be too shy to ask. The answer could mean life or death to your patient! That is certainly more important than feeling embarrassed about asking a question.

Reading Hints

When reading each chapter in the textbook, look at the subject headings to learn what each section is about. Read first for the general meaning. Then reread parts you did not understand. It may help to read those parts aloud. Carefully read the information given in each table and study each figure and its caption. While studying, put difficult concepts into your own words to see if you understand them. Check this understanding with another student or the instructor.

Chapter Objectives

At the beginning of each chapter in the textbook are objectives that you should have mastered when you finished studying that chapter. Write these objectives in your notebook, leaving a blank space after each. Fill in the answers as you find them while reading the chapter. Review to make sure your answers are correct and complete. Use these answers when you study for tests. This should also be done for separate course objectives that your instructor has listed in your class syllabus.

Chapter Highlights

Use the Chapter Highlights at the end of each chapter in the textbook to help with review for exams.

Class Notes

When taking lecture notes in class, leave a large margin on the left side of each notebook page and write only on right-hand pages, leaving all left-hand pages blank. Look over your lecture notes soon after each class, while your memory is fresh. Fill in missing words, complete sentences and ideas, and underline key phrases, definitions, and concepts. At the top of each page, write the topic of that page. In the left margin, write the key word for that part of your notes. On the opposite left-hand page, write a summary or outline that combines material from both the textbook and the lecture. These can be your study notes for review.

Study Groups

Form a study group with some other students so you can help one another. Ask questions about material you are not sure about. Work together to find answers.

REFERENCES FOR IMPROVING STUDY SKILLS

Good study skills are essential for achieving your goals in nursing. Time management, efficient use of study time, and a consistent approach to studying are all beneficial. There are various study methods for reading a textbook and for taking class notes. Some methods that have proven helpful can be found in *Saunders' Student Nurse Planner: A Guide to Success in Nursing School* (Version 2). This book contains helpful information on test taking and preparing for clinical experiences. It includes an example of a "time map" for planning study time and a blank form that you can use to formulate a personal time map.

HELP FOR THE LIMITED ENGLISH PROFICIENCY STUDENT

The last portion of each chapter in the *Student Learning Guide*, "Steps Toward Better Communication," is designed to assist students with limited English proficiency to master the chapter content. Sections offer help in pronunciation, vocabulary building, points of grammar, and guidance in therapeutic communication. Although directed toward limited English proficiency students, this section is useful to all students. Because correct stress of syllables is the major determining factor in how easily you are understood, we have chosen to indicate stressed syllables in word and phrases rather than marking phonetic pronunciations, which are often difficult to understand. Two reference books that are helpful to students with limited English proficiency are (1) Gilbert, Judy B. (1993). *Clear Speech: Pronunciation and Listening Comprehension in North American English (2nd ed.), Student's Book.* New York: Cambridge University Press; and (2) the *Newbury House Dictionary of American English: An Essential Reference for Learners of American English and Culture*. (1996). Boston, MA: Heinle & Heinle Publishers.

I hope that you find the *Student Learning Guide* interesting and useful.

Susan C. deWit, MSN, RNCS

To the Instructor

The *Student Learning Guide for Fundamental Concepts and Skills for Nursing* is designed to provide reinforcement for the terms and concepts presented in the text. It will assist students to set priorities, apply the nursing process, practice critical thinking, make good judgments and decisions, increase ability to communicate therapeutically, practice critical thinking, and meet chapter objectives.

ORGANIZATION OF THE TEXT

Included is a wide variety of exercises, questions, and activities. Most chapters include Terminology; Short Answer; Multiple Choice; Critical Thinking Activities; Meeting Clinical Objectives; and a special section called Steps Toward Better Communication written by an English as a Second Language Specialist. Other sections that appear where appropriate are Completion; Sequencing; Identification; Review of Structure and Function; Setting Priorities; and Application of the Nursing Process.

Description of Exercises

The exercises are as follows:

- **Terminology**—matching or fill-in-the-blank questions to reinforce correct use of words from the chapter terms list
- **Short Answer**—list of brief answers to reinforce knowledge and assist students to meet the chapter objectives
- **Multiple Choice**—questions in NCLEX format, based on real-life situations, which require knowledge, synthesis, analysis, evaluation, and application
- **Critical Thinking Activities**—brief scenarios and questions to foster problem-solving skills in nursing care which may be practiced individually or in study groups
- **Meeting Clinical Objectives**—suggestions for practicing learned skills and obtaining experience in the clinical area. These exercises help students meet the clinical practice objectives and encourage focusing on the school's clinical objectives
- **Completion**—this exercise reinforces the chapter content with fill-in-the-blank questions
- **Sequencing**—the student practices decision making and problem solving by ordering the best way to carry out a task within the nursing process
- **Identification**—the student names appropriate steps in a process or procedure or verifies normal or abnormal laboratory values
- **Review of Structure and Function**—this is a reexamination of the anatomy and physiology of the body system pertinent to the text chapter
- **Setting Priorities**—students analyze information and make decisions to set priorities within tasks or clinical situations
- **Application of the Nursing Process**—critical thinking skills are used and the steps of the nursing process are applied to real-life patient care

All answers to the exercises are included on the *Instructor's Electronic Resource* (CD-ROM) *for Fundamental Concepts and Skills for Nursing*. The answers can be printed out and put on reserve in the library or posted so that students can check them should the instructor choose not to use the *Student Learning Guide* for class credit activities. In addition, a special feature for students, Mastering Skills and Steps, appears in the *Instructor's Electronic Resource*. It provides pointers for performing the skills and suggestions for student practice, and may be printed out for student use.

STUDENTS WITH LIMITED ENGLISH PROFICIENCY

Because so many students who are natives of other countries are entering nursing programs in the United States and Canada, we have enlisted the aid of an English as a Second Language specialist who has worked with many health care occupation students. She helped construct the exercises in the "Steps Toward Better Communication" within each chapter. Her letter to you follows. I hope you find this section helpful to your limited English proficiency students.

Susan C. deWit, MSN, RNCS

STEPS TOWARD BETTER COMMUNICATION

Imagine yourself back in nursing school—trying to read the texts and understand the lectures in Spanish or German. Students studying in a language that is not their native tongue face not only the challenge of learning the medical and physiological lessons that are required of all nursing students, but they must also decipher and use a language whose nuances and grammar are unfamiliar to them. In order to ease some of that burden, we attempted to simplify and regularize the language of *Fundamental Concepts and Skills for Nursing* and the *Student Learning Guide*, and to explain some of the colloquial uses of English that occur.

A major part of the nursing process could be described as "knowing your patient inside and out," and one key to that knowledge is being able to accurately and sensitively communicate with the patient and colleagues. To this end, after the regular exercises, we added a section for the ESL student entitled "Steps Toward Better Communication," which offers help in pronunciation, vocabulary building, and use of grammatical issues such as verb tense, and encourages asking for help and clarification. In addition, one section on understanding cultural nuances and mannerisms will help the student face real-life situations and clarify feelings; another offers facility in appropriately asking questions and carrying on conversations.

A note about pronunciation: we assume that the important medical terms will be used and modeled correctly by the instructor. In terms of conversation, intelligibility rather than native-like accuracy should be the goal. Correct stress is the major determining factor in how easily a person can be understood. Therefore we chose to indicate stressed syllables in words and phrases rather than giving phonetic pronunciations which students often find difficult to understand.

Description of Exercises

The following exercises appear in the Steps Toward Better Communication as appropriate:

- **Vocabulary Building Glossary** explains and defines idiomatic or unusual uses of nonmedical terms used in the chapter and indicates the stressed syllables by capitalizing them.
- **Completion** sentences offer opportunities to use the words presented in the Glossary, often in different contexts than they are used in the text, thereby offering yet another way to increase vocabulary.
- **Vocabulary Exercise** uses words from the chapter in various ways to increase facility of and ease of understanding.
- **Word Attack Skills** deal with word segments, suffixes, prefixes, and types of words, to help the student learn to decode new words and their usage.
- **Pronunciation Skills** offer practice in pronouncing difficult terms as well as phrases and sentences, with emphasis on stress and intonation.

- **Grammar Points** are made occasionally, especially when there is a recurring point raised by the chapter—such as the use of the past tense in taking case histories.
- **Communication Exercises** encourage communicative interchange, and writing and use of dialogues that might actually be used by a practicing nurse. The value of this section is enhanced if students can be paired in First and Second Language Speaker combinations, giving each the opportunity to experience the other's accent and offering the possibility for cross-cultural exchange. Answers to the Communication Exercise dialogue questions are found in the *Instructor's Electronic Resource*, and may be printed out for student use.
- **Cultural Points** present explanations and questions about issues and customs that may differ across the cultures represented in the class, and in the prospective patient community. They can explain the normative culture in which the individual will be working, while at the same time acknowledge and validate an individual's cultural difference.

In preparing these materials, I have drawn on my experience in teaching practicing and aspiring health care personnel. I have found them to be dedicated and eager to improve their own lives while helping others. I have learned much from them about hard work, perseverance, humor, and what they need in order to do a better job. My colleagues in teaching English and nurses with whom I have worked have been helpful with ideas for teaching projects, indicating language areas needing to be addressed, and offering suggestions and solutions for problems. However, any omissions and errors are my own.

I have been impressed with the similarity between learning language skills and nursing skills. Both require access to academic knowledge, but mastery occurs with hands-on practice and experience. The exercises are geared to provide this opportunity. Encourage your students to interact as often as possible. Look at each lesson with the question, "How can I structure this lesson so the students will have to generate their own language to complete the exercise?" Offer real-life challenges and tasks for speaking and communicative interaction with other students, colleagues, and patients whenever possible. An encouraging, open, and interactive classroom is the best setting for language learning and improvement. I wish you well in working with this special group of people.

Gail G. Boehme
English Language Instructor/Consultant
Santa Barbara City College
Continuing Education

Contents

Chapter 1	Nursing and the Health Care System	1
Chapter 2	Concepts of Health and Illness	7
Chapter 3	Legal and Ethical Aspects of Nursing	15
Chapter 4	Overview of the Nursing Process	23
Chapter 5	Assessment, Nursing Diagnosis, and Planning	29
Chapter 6	Implementation and Evaluation	35
Chapter 7	Communication and the Nurse–Patient Relationship	43
Chapter 8	Documentation of Nursing Care	53
Chapter 9	Patient Teaching	61
Chapter 10	Growth and Development: Infancy through Adolescence	69
Chapter 11	Adulthood and the Family	77
Chapter 12	Promoting Healthy Adaptation to Aging	87
Chapter 13	Cultural and Spiritual Aspects of Patient Care	93
Chapter 14	Loss, Grief, and the Dying Patient	103
Chapter 15	Infection, Protective Mechanisms, and Asepsis	111
Chapter 16	Infection Control in Hospital and Home	119
Chapter 17	Lifting, Moving, and Positioning Patients	129
Chapter 18	Assisting with Hygiene and Personal Care, Skin Care, and the Prevention of Pressure Ulcers	137
Chapter 19	Patient Environment and Safety	145
Chapter 20	Measuring Vital Signs	153
Chapter 21	Assessing Health Status	163
Chapter 22	Admitting, Transferring, and Discharging Patients	173
Chapter 23	Diagnostic Tests and Specimen Collection	181
Chapter 24	Fluid, Electrolyte, and Acid-Base Balance	189
Chapter 25	Concepts of Basic Nutrition and Cultural Considerations	197
Chapter 26	Diet Therapy and Assisted Feeding	207
Chapter 27	Assisting with Respiration and Oxygen Delivery	217
Chapter 28	Promoting Urinary Elimination	225
Chapter 29	Promoting Bowel Elimination	233
Chapter 30	Pain, Comfort, and Sleep	241
Chapter 31	Pharmacology and Preparation for Drug Administration	249
Chapter 32	Administering Oral, Topical, and Inhalant Medications	259
Chapter 33	Administering Intradermal, Subcutaneous, and Intramuscular Injections	267
Chapter 34	Administering Intravenous Solutions and Medications	277
Chapter 35	Care of the Surgical Patient	285
Chapter 36	Providing Wound Care and Treatment for Pressure Ulcers	295
Chapter 37	Promoting Musculoskeletal Function	305
Chapter 38	Common Physical Care Problems of the Elderly	315
Chapter 39	Common Psychosocial Care Problems of the Elderly	323
	Performance Checklists	333

ONE

Nursing and the Health Care System

TERMINOLOGY

Directions: Define and give an example of each of the following terms.

1. Apprenticeship Learning by doing—on-the-job training working in a hospital
2. Invasive procedure procedures that require entry into the body gallbladder surgery
3. Nursing process 1970's-1980's as an organized, deliberate systematic way to deliver nursing care. combines science + art of nursing.
4. Theory statement about relationships among concepts or facts, based on existing information. (humans, environment, health)

ACRONYMS

Directions: Write a brief answer for each question.

1. Describe how DRGs (diagnostic related groups) affect payment for health care. ______
2. Describe an HMO (health maintenance organization). ______
3. How does an HMO differ from a PPO (preferred provider organization)? ______

SHORT ANSWER

Directions: Write a brief answer for each question.

1. List four influences Florence Nightingale has had on nurses' training. Improved ventilation, sanitation and nutrician. Nursing should be taught by nurses, continuing education is needed for nurses, sick people need occupational and recreational therapy. Nurses should identify + meet patients personal needs + providing emotional support. importance of record keeping.

2. List two major influences on nursing education in the United States.
war
growth in population

3. Considering the functions of the practical nurse, describe four desirable attributes of the nurse.
   a. Only 1 yr. schooling
   b. can easily enter 2ND year RN Program
   c. Certification available for specializing
   d. more hands on care with clients

4. Compare the education and training of LPN/LVNs and registered nurses.

LPN/LVN	Registered Nurse
one year school	2 yr. school
greater number of Clinical Hours	can supervise care of many patients
less scientific knowledge	more scientific knowledge

5. The purpose of the Nurse Practice Act is to protect the public, & define legal scope of practice

MULTIPLE CHOICE

*Directions: Choose the **best** answer for each of the following questions.*

1. The first school of nursing was funded by
   1. physician payments for services rendered.
   2. contributions by Crimean war servicemen and their families
   3. the estate of Florence Nightingale.
   4. charges to patients for nursing care.

2. Nursing care during the Civil War was directed by
   1. Florence Nightingale.
   2. the Union government.
   3. Dorothea Dix.
   4. the Confederate government.

3. In the United States in the early schools of nursing, education was achieved through
   1. formal classes in anatomy and nursing.
   2. a set curriculum covering medical and surgical nursing.
   3. instruction by trained nurses in the hospital.
   4. working directly on the hospital units.

4. A nursing theory is
   1. a group of facts about a particular topic that has been proven by scientific method.
   2. a statement about relationships among concepts or facts that is not based on actual knowledge.
   3. a proven hypothesis based on gathered facts.
   4. a guess about what may happen in a particular situation.

5. The practice of nursing is governed by a nurse practice act and
   1. standards of nursing care.
   2. codes of ethics.
   3. institutional rules and regulations.
   4. licensure requirements.

6. Practical nursing arose to
   1. provide a stepping stone to becoming a registered nurse.
   2. provide more training than a nurse's aide receives.
   3. fill a gap left by nurses who enlisted in the military.
   4. provide less expensive employees to hospitals.

7. Under the DRG system, the hospital
   1. receives a set amount of money for each patient hospitalized with a particular diagnosis.
   2. must discharge patients within a set number of days.
   3. decides what care for a particular diagnosis will cost.
   4. is often overpaid for the care actually given a patient.

8. HMOs
   1. provide very high-quality care at a low price.
   2. enroll patients for a set fee per month.
   3. are very popular with physicians.
   4. have a preferred list of providers for health care.

9. A major effect of managed care is
   1. greater continuity of care for the patient.
   2. provision for the patient to stay with one primary physician.
   3. attention to delivery of cost-effective care.
   4. greater job satisfaction of health care providers.

10. A complaint of many health care professionals about managed care is the increased amount of
    1. documentation and paperwork necessary.
    2. trained personnel to staff hospital units.
    3. time required to care for each patient.
    4. accountability patients have for their own care.

CRITICAL THINKING ACTIVITIES

1. Within a small group of your fellow students, discuss your definition of nursing. Compare differences among the definitions of the various group members.
2. Identify some ways in which the *Standards of Nursing Care* are applied in the clinical setting.

MEETING CLINICAL OBJECTIVES

Directions: The following suggested activities will help you meet the stated clinical practice objectives for the chapter. Review your school's clinical objectives for the week and outline a plan of activities that will help you meet them. If unsure as to how to meet them, consult with your instructor at the beginning of the clinical day.

1. Talk with an LPN/LVN and an RN on your clinical unit and ask them what they see as differences in the roles of these two types of nurses.
2. Check within your clinical facility and in the local classified ads to determine what opportunities for employment as a LPN/LVN exist in your community.

STEPS TOWARD BETTER COMMUNICATION

VOCABULARY BUILDING GLOSSARY

Term	Pronunciation	Definition
active listening	AC tive LIS ten ing	to listen for the meaning of what a person is saying and repeat it back to them
attributes	AT tri butes	qualities, characteristics
ancillary	AN cil lar y	helping in a subordinate way
balanced ratio	BAL anced ratio	a correct proportion
charge out	CHARGE OUT	initiate a financial charge for something
collaborator	col LAB o ra tor	one who works together with others
contain (verb)	con TAIN	to limit
controversy	CON tro ver sy	disagreement
core curriculum	core cur RIC u lum	the basic set of what is taught
criteria	cri TER i a	rules or standards to judge by
Crusades	Cru SADES	religious wars made by European Christians against Muslims in the eastern Mediterranean in the 11th to 12th centuries
delegator	DEL e ga tor	one who tells others what to do
exacting	ex ACT ing	very careful with details
expertise	ex per TISE	a high level of experience
foster	FOS ter	encourage, promote
funded	FUN ded	provided with money for the support of something
funds	funds	money
gap	GAP	empty space in a line of things
implement	IM ple MENT	(verb) to do, to use
in other instances	in other IN stances	in other situations
inherent	in HER ent	naturally part of something, built into
lacking	LACK ing	absent
licensure	LI cens ure	giving licenses
midwife	MID wife	a woman who helps the birthing of a baby
nightmare	NIGHT mare	a very bad dream
phenomena	phe NOM e na	observable facts or events
pilgrims	PIL grims	people traveling on religious journeys
prior	PRI or	previous, coming before
regulatory body	REG u la tor y BOD y	a group that makes rules
scope	SCOPE	the range or limits of something
skyrocket	SKY rock et	to go up very quickly
sought (verb, past tense)	SOUGHT	desired, looked for (present = seek)

standards	STAN dards	the expected level, against which other things are measured (e.g., above or below standard
vigilant	VIG i lant	watchful, watching carefully

COMPLETION

Directions: Fill in the blanks with the correct term from the list to complete the sentence.

active listening	criteria	collaborator	gap
implement	prior	delegator	controversy
foster	skyrocket	sought	vigilant

1. The nurse gave instructions to the aides respectfully and is known as a good delegator.
2. A calm, unhurried attitude and display of concern will foster the formation of trust between nurse and patient.
3. The nurse went over every part of the patient's chart as he sought to gather all the pertinent information.
4. The type of treatment appropriate for that particular form of cancer is a matter of controvery.
5. After planning his work for the day, the nurse began to Implement the plan.
6. The nursing diagnosis of "Pain" was made based on the criteria listed for that diagnosis.
7. The patient had developed an allergy to penicillin during his prior respiratory infection.
8. The nurse must be vigilent in observing for side effects of medication.
9. The use of the latest technology for diagnostic testing is one factor that has made the cost of medical care Skyrocket.

VOCABULARY EXERCISE

Directions: Underline the correct definition of these words used in the Standards of Care.

1.	assessment:	test	evaluation
2.	diagnosis:	finding, conclusion	drawing
3.	outcome:	removal	result
4.	implementation:	carrying out	making equipment
5.	evaluation:	measurement	analysis
6.	collegiality:	education	relationship with other workers

WORD ATTACK SKILLS

Stress/Meaning change: Some words which are spelled the same change meaning when the stress is placed on a different syllable. Often, this shows the difference between the word as a noun and as a verb.

AT tri bute (noun) = a characteristic
at TRIB ute (verb) = to credit, to be the cause for
IM ple ment (noun) = a tool
IM ple MENT (verb) = to put into action, use

1. Underline the stressed syllables in these words in the following sentences:
   a. He attributed his success to his attributes of hard work and honesty.
   b. The use of the surgical implements was implemented with a training session.
2. If "ethics" means "a system of moral or correct behavior," then which of the following would be an "ethical manner" of behavior for the nurse?
   a. The nurse took some of the patient's medication because her sister needed it.
   b. The nurse contributed information during collaboration with the dietitian about the patient's food likes.
   c. The nurse told the visitor he could not tell her about the patient's prognosis, that she would need to ask the patient about that.

COMMUNICATION EXERCISE

Directions: Find a partner and practice your communication skills by doing one of the following:

1. Explain the difference between a licensed practical nurse/licensed vocational nurse and a registered nurse.
2. Explain the important role Florence Nightingale played in nursing.

CULTURAL POINTS

1. This chapter talks about the historical overview which shaped the nursing tradition in Europe and North America, and the bases for the art and science of nursing as currently practiced there. It also talks about the ways nurses are educated and the health care systems that operate today.
2. If you are from another country, think about the differences in nursing there. How are nurses trained there? Is the job of a nurse different? In what way? What is the health care system in your country? In what ways do you think it is better or worse than the system in North America? What are the traditions and history that have shaped the health care and nursing systems in your country? Share your answers with your peers.

Review the chapter highlights, answer the study questions, and complete the critical thinking activities at the end of the chapter in the textbook.

TWO

Concepts of Health and Illness

TERMINOLOGY

Directions: Match the terms in column I with the definitions in column II.

Column I		Column II
1. G	acute illness	a. Disease of body or mind
2. d	asymptomatic	b. Illness for which there is no cure
3. h	chronic illness	c. Unknown etiology
4. f	convalescence	d. Without symptoms
5. j	etiology	e. Tendency to maintain stability of the internal biologic environment
6. K	health	f. Recovery from illness
7. i	hierarchy	g. Illness that develops suddenly
8. e	homeostasis	h. Illness that persists for a long time
9. C	idiopathic	i. Arrangement of objects, elements, or values in order of importance
10. a	illness	j. Cause of disease
11. b	terminal illness	k. Absence of disease and complete physical, mental, and social well-being

SHORT ANSWER

Directions: Write a brief answer for each of the following.

1. Illness behaviors include how people
   a. how people monitor the body
   b. define & interpet symptoms
   c. seek health care
   d. follow advice & self-care measures to regain wellness

2. Rather than treating the illness itself, nursing is concerned with working with people to help them become more independent and better able to meet their own health care needs.

3. List three examples of health behavior.
   a. watching dietary intake
   b. regular excercise
   c. immunizations

4. A stressor can be helpful or harmful depending on the
   a. perception of the stressor
   b. Degree of health + Fitness
   c. previous life experiences and personality
   d. Social support system available
   e. personal coping mechanisms

COMPLETION

Directions: Fill in the blank(s) with the correct word(s) from the terms list in the chapter in the textbook to complete the sentence or idea.

1. The term high-level wellness was first used by Dunn to signify the ideal state of health in every dimension of a person's personality.
2. In Dunn's view, each person accepts responsibility for and takes an active part in improving and maintaining his or her own state of wellness.
3. With patients from so many different countries, cultural differences must be considered when planning nursing care.
4. Each patient must be dealt with as a(n) individual, whose concepts of health and illness and health care might be different from your own.
5. A holistic approach considers the biological, psychological, sociologic, and spiritual aspects of a person.
6. Maslow's hierarchy of needs consists of food needs, air needs, water needs, and rest needs.
7. Adaptability to a external environment is essential to stability and health.
8. When the equilibrium of the body is disturbed, stress occurs.
9. When the brain perceives a situation as threatening, the sympathatic nervous system stimulates the physiologic functions needed for fight or flight.
10. Hans Selye states that the body attempts to deal with stressors by the secretion of hormones.
11. Adjusting to or solving challenges is called coping.
12. Strategies that protect us from increasing anxiety are called Defense mechanisms.

MULTIPLE CHOICE

*Directions: Choose the **best** answer for each of the following questions.*

Situation: R.O. has had a flare-up of osteoarthritis in his knee. He is having difficulty walking.

1. You know that in the transition stage of illness the person may
 1. adopt a sick role.
 2. acknowledge that symptoms of illness are present.
 3. begin recovering from illness.
 4. withdraw from usual roles.

2. In planning care for R.O. you recall that Abraham Maslow states that
 1. people respond to needs as whole integrated beings.
 2. each person must take responsibility for improving his or her own state of wellness.
 3. stress plays a role in every disease process because of faulty adaptation by the body.
 4. humans are naturally inclined to be healthy.

3. Osteoarthritis is a chronic illness. A chronic illness differs from an acute illness in that the acute illness
 1. lasts a long time.
 2. cannot be cured.
 3. has no known cause.
 4. develops suddenly.

4. According to Maslow's hierarchy, which of the following would be the priority need?
 1. intimacy
 2. independence
 3. artistic expression
 4. psychological comfort

5. The general adaptation syndrome is said to occur in response to
 1. initial stress.
 2. short-term stress.
 3. any perceived stress.
 4. long term stress.

6. An example of the defense mechanism of rationalization would be
 1. forgetting the name of someone you intensely dislike.
 2. blaming the teacher for a poor grade on a test when you did not study sufficiently.
 3. kicking the dog when you are mad at your boss.
 4. praising someone whom you intensely dislike.

7. A disorder that is often stress-related is
 1. hypertension.
 2. appendicitis.
 3. influenza.
 4. multiple sclerosis.

MATCHING

Directions: Indicate with a check mark which of the following is a sympathetic nervous system action and which is a parasympathetic action.

Result of Action	Sympathetic	Parasympathetic
1. Dry mouth	✓	
2. Increased heart rate	✓	
3. Bronchial constriction		✓
4. Intestinal motility—diarrhea	✓	
5. Sweating	✓	
6. Pupil dilation	✓

CRITICAL THINKING ACTIVITIES

1. Identify ways in which holistic care can be practiced in the clinical area.
2. Describe ways in which your body attempts to maintain homeostasis when you contract a cold virus.
3. Identify the common signs of stress that you experience when approaching a major examination.
4. List four ways in which you think you might be able to decrease stress and anxiety for patients.

MEETING CLINICAL OBJECTIVES

Directions: The following suggested activities will help you meet the stated clinical practice objectives for the chapter. Review your school's clinical objectives for the week and outline a plan of activities that will help you meet them. If unsure as to how to meet them, consult with your instructor at the beginning of the clinical day.

1. Look for signs of stress from staff or patients on the nursing unit to which you are assigned.
2. Attempt to decrease stress or anxiety for at least one patient.

STEPS TOWARD BETTER COMMUNICATION

VOCABULARY BUILDING GLOSSARY

Term	Pronunciation	Definition
adverse	AD verse	not favorable
alters	AL ters	changes
atrophy	A troph y	to shrink, grow useless
condone	con DONE	to pardon or overlook wrongdoing
convey	con VEY	to communicate an idea
core	CORE	center
crucial	CRU cial	very important
deprivation	dep ri VA tion	a condition of want and need
detectable	de TECT able	something you can see or notice
deviation	de vi A tion	a difference, a move away from
dynamic	dy NAM ic	energetic, full of activity
emerge	e MERGE	appear, come out
esteem	es TEEM	respect
feedback	FEED back	information given in response
hierarchy	HI er ar chy	organization from high to low
hygiene	HY giene	health and cleanliness
integrated	in te GRA ted	combined

intervene	in ter VENE	to come between in order to change something
maladaptive	mal a DAP tive	giving the wrong reaction
merely	MERE ly	only
noncompliant	NON com PLI ant	not following the rules
perception	per CEP tion	seeing and understanding
prolong	pro LONG	to continue over a period of time
reimburse	RE im burse	pay back
resolves	re SOLVES	ends or concludes
reticular	re TIC u lar	like a net
susceptible	sus CEP ti ble	easily influenced or affected

COMPLETION

Directions: Fill in the blank(s) with the correct word(s) from the vocabulary building glossary to complete the sentence.

1. The patient suffered an *adverse* reaction from the drug; he broke out in a rash.
2. The patient did not have good *hygiene* practices and his teeth were in very poor condition.
3. The patient did not stick to the diet and was *noncompliant* with the exercise program as well.
4. Her *perception* of the situation after reviewing the data in the chart was that the patient was suffering from a serious infection.
5. Exposure to prolonged sunlight sometimes *alter* certain drugs, making them noneffective.
6. When signs of complications occur, the nurse can quickly *intervene* to have the treatment changed.
7. It is hoped that the patient will *emerge* from the chemotherapy treatments with no further signs of cancer.
8. His type of abdominal pain is a *deviation* from the classic signs and symptoms of appendicitis.
9. Crying all the time is a *dynamic* response to a crisis.
10. It is hoped that his pneumonia *resolves* without any permanent damage to the lungs.

VOCABULARY EXERCISE

This chapter discusses various aspects of a person and discusses assessing for factors within those various aspects. The various aspects are:

biologic	refers to	the body
psychologic	refers to	the mind and emotions
sociologic	refers to	culture, environment, life roles
spiritual	refers to	religion, soul

Directions: Match the word to a corresponding action or response, then give another example.

1. f biologic
   ____
   ____
2. c psychosocial
   ____
   ____
3. e spiritual
   ____
   ____

a. refusing to see a doctor
b. running a fever
c. joining a group
d. meditating each day
e. praying before meals
f. feeling sharp pains in the chest

WORD ATTACK SKILLS

A. OPPOSITES

Directions: Give the opposite for these words from the textbook. Use words from the vocabulary building glossary above when possible.

Term	Pronunciation	Definition
1. optimum	OP ti mum	at the highest or best level
2. monitor	MON i tor	watch over a period of time
3. vague	VAGUE	not clear or specific
4. passive	PAS sive	not active
5. thrive	THRIVE	grow strong and healthy
6. adversity	ad VER si ty	bad luck
7. under react	UN der re ACT	not enough response
8. malaise	ma LAISE	general feeling of illness, unhappiness

B. MEANINGS OF NOUNS AND VERBS

Directions: Note how these words from the chapter change, depending on whether they are used as a verb or a noun.

Verb	Noun
intervene	intervention
motivate	motivation
ambulate	ambulation
validate	validation
deprive	deprivation
clarify	clarification
deviate	deviation
adapt	adaptation

COMMUNICATION EXERCISE

1. Considering Figure 2-2 in the textbook, consider the variables in health and illness. Give an example from your life (or that of a friend) for each of these variables:
   a. Culture ______________________
   b. Religion ______________________
   c. Standard of living ______________________
   d. Support system ______________________
   e. Genetic influence ______________________
2. Referring to table 2-7 in the textbook, consider what illness prevention measures should be used by the following age groups. Verbalize your thoughts to a peer.
   a. Teenagers don't smoke
   b. Elders excercise
   c. Pregnant women eat good
3. Look at the list of stressful situations below. Numerically rank them according to which are most stressful to you, with the most stressful being #1, the next #2, and so forth. Then compare your list with the lists of some of your peers.

4 Not having enough time to study
2 Not having enough money
5 Concern over how you look
3 Lack of sleep
1 Worry about family
6 A dirty room
4 Feeling like you didn't do a good job
5 Worry over not enough quality time with loved ones

4. List things that are stressful to you, such as:

unmade bed

sink full of dirty dishes

unmowed lawn

clutter

unfinisled laundry

clothes unorganized

beds sleets need to be changed

CULTURAL POINTS

1. What things about being with a group of people from a different culture do you find stressful? How do you cope with these stresses?
2. If you are from a different country, do you think there is a different level of stress in your native country than here? Is it higher or lower? Why?
3. What are some ways people in your culture deal with stress?

Review the chapter highlights, answer the study questions, and complete the critical thinking activities at the end of the chapter in the textbook.

THREE

Legal and Ethical Aspects of Nursing

TERMINOLOGY

Directions: Define and give an example of each of the following terms:

1. standard of care participation in attending workshops, giving proper meds. at proper time
2. negligence failure to report physical change of pt.
3. malpractice when a student nurse performs a procedure incorrectly / when nurse didn't check vitals on surgical patient + died
4. confidential telling a neighbor about a patients diagnosis
5. libel a newspaper article stating a nurse is incompetent
6. invasion of privacy not closing a curtain when giving pt a bath
7. slander talking badly about a physician to another person
8. assault and battery threatening a pt. to take an injection—then holding patient + administering
9. accountability when a student nurse asks instructor about a procedure
10. prudent making sure an immobile patient is turned every 2 hrs. to prevent ulcers

SHORT ANSWER

Directions: Read the Code for Nurses and the Code of Ethics for the Licensed Practical Nurse in the chapter of the textbook. When you have completed your study of the two codes, fill in the blanks.

1. Ethics is a code of guidelines (rules) that represents moral conduct for a particular patient (profession)
2. A violation of ethical behavior may result in discipline by temporary suspension or loss of liscensure.
3. Ways in which nurses can prevent patient lawsuits against themselves or the hospital include:
   maintain competence, document fully, establish Rapport and communicate effectively

4. The consequences of violating the nurse practice act could be: potential lawsuits for malpractice and negligence, loss of liscensure and temporary suspense, imprisionment

5. The purpose of the *Standards of Nursing Practice* is to set forth job description and duties, liscensure, give professional accountability, standards of care, professional discipline

and to continue education

MULTIPLE CHOICE

*Directions: Choose the **best** answer for each of the following questions.*

1. Although both a statute and a tort are laws, a tort is a
   1. civil or criminal law.
   2. wrong against the public.
   3. violation of civil law.
   4. felony crime.

2. The scope of practice for nurses is set forth in the
   1. *Standards of Practice.*
   2. code of ethics.
   3. laws of the state.
   4. nurse practice act.

3. You decide to delegate frequent vital sign measurements on your postoperative patient to the nursing assistant. When delegating nursing tasks to others, you are responsible for
   1. knowing whether the task can be legally delegated.
   2. training the person to do the task.
   3. observing the person performing the task.
   4. supervising the person's charting of the task performed.

4. Two of your colleagues ask you if you wish to join them at a seminar on current neurological care. Continuing education for nurses is important because
   1. self-esteem is dependent on continued learning.
   2. there are constant changes in health care practice.
   3. pay raises depend on continuing education activities.
   4. the up-to-date nurse is respected by colleagues.

5. One nurse says to another, "Well, did you make it with Dr. S. last night?" Making sexual comments on the nursing unit is considered sexual harassment, and is illegal when it
   1. is offensive to the people in the vicinity of the speaker.
   2. is concerned with some aspect of patient care.
   3. interferes with someone's job performance.
   4. is directed from supervisors to employees.

6. L.C. is brought to the emergency room after an automobile accident. She is seriously injured and needs immediate surgery. No next of kin can be quickly located. A signed informed consent is not necessary since L.C.
   1. is unconscious and unable to communicate.
   2. is to undergo a lengthy exploratory surgical procedure.
   3. was admitted through the emergency room.
   4. has been very seriously injured.

7. Which consent form is used to show the patient has consented to have blood drawn for laboratory tests, treatments by the nurses such as dressing a wound or catheterization, and treatment by the physical or respiratory therapist?
   1. consent for surgery
   2. "informed consent"
   3. conditions of admission
   4. consent for special procedures

8. Which one of the following is NOT considered an incident and does not need to be reported on an incident or occurrence form?
   1. a fall to the floor while getting out of bed
   2. a hole burned into the mattress by a smoldering cigarette butt
   3. giving the patient the wrong medication
   4. the patient's having developed a pressure area on the sacrum

ETHICAL SITUATIONS

SITUATION A

A young girl has been brought by ambulance to the emergency room. You are the admitting nurse and note that she has swallowed an overdose of sedatives and is now having her stomach emptied of its contents. Since this was an attempted suicide, the police reporters were in the hallway. When you go to lunch, your friends from other units want to know how old the girl is, and why she was brought in. You were the person who recorded the emergency room notes into her chart and so you have some information.

1. When asked if the girl took an overdose, you might answer:
   a. "Yes, but she's O.K."
   b. "She must have had a desire to die."
   c. "This information is confidential."

2. In this situation, to discuss the patient not only violates her right to privacy, but could result in a lawsuit ____ and possibly terminate ____ employment.

SITUATION B

H.G., in the suite at the end of the hall, orders his meals from the hospital's special gourmet menu. At noon on Sunday he did not touch any of the food, although the meal was excellent. The chef's salad and strawberry pie looked very good. You pick up his tray from his room.

3. Thinking that it is a shame to waste such food, you
   a. give it to the housekeeping staff.
   b. send it back to the kitchen.
   c. offer it to the entire unit staff.
   d. eat it yourself.

SITUATION C

A unit secretary is very tense about her new job on the cardiac telemetry unit. Her doctor has prescribed a mild tranquilizer for her. She knows that when clients go home, the medications are often left behind and returned to the pharmacy. She asks the nurses if they could give her the tranquilizers that are left upon a patient's discharge, saving her the expense of having the prescription filled.

4. This is a distinct breach of contract ____ on her part.

5. If the nurses grant her request, they are prescribing or dispensing medicine without a license and this is a Criminal offense.

SITUATION D

You have been M.J.'s nurse for her entire stay in the hospital. She has come to rely on you and when she is ready to go home, she wants to give you a sum of money in appreciation for the "lovely things you have done for her."

6. In this situation you should
   a. explain to her that the service is part of her care.
   b. accept the money because although you receive a salary from the hospital, clients should pay for the service you render them individually.
   c. accept the gift of money and tell nobody so that no one else will feel hurt that she selected only you.
   d. suggest she give the money to the nursing assistant who needs it more than you do.

7. M.J. insists that you take the money or you will hurt her feelings. Therefore you
   a. tell her of some specific need the hospital has to which she could make a contribution.
   b. suggest a fund in her name with suitable recognition.
   c. accept the gift so that there are no hurt feelings in the situation.
   d. tell her to give it to the nursing assistant since she needs the money more than you do.

CRITICAL THINKING ACTIVITIES

1. You overhear a nurse say to a patient, "If you won't stay in your bed, I will have to find a way to keep you there." Is this a breach of legal or ethical conduct? How would you handle the situation?
2. How would you tactfully explain the process of placing "advance directives" on file in the chart?
3. As a student, explain the rules that govern the care you give while in the clinical setting.

MEETING CLINICAL OBJECTIVES

Directions: The following suggested activities will help you meet the stated clinical practice objectives for the chapter. Review your school's clinical objectives for the week and outline a plan of activities that will help you meet them. If unsure as to how to meet them, consult with your instructor at the beginning of the clinical day.

1. Review the documentation in the nurse's notes for one of your assigned patients from the previous 24 hours. Determine if it meets the guidelines for legally sound charting. Look at legibility, judgmental statements, objectivity, thoroughness, and correction of any errors. Are there any problems noted for which interventions do not seem to have been done? Think about how you might have charted differently.
2. During a clinical day, observe for ways in which patient's rights are being observed. Were there any instances of when patient's rights were violated? Discuss these in your clinical group.
3. Properly obtain a signature on an informed consent form.

STEPS TOWARD BETTER COMMUNICATION

VOCABULARY BUILDING GLOSSARY

Term	Pronunciation	Definition
access	AC cess	able to get to or see something
bound	BOUND	required
breach	BREACH	a break or neglect of a rule; a violation
contrary	CON trar y	opposite
disciplines	DIS ci plines	areas of interest or experience
emancipated minor	e MAN ci PA ted MI nor	a person who is normally under the legal age to take action for him- or herself, but has been declared by law to be able to make legal decisions for him- or herself
escalated	ES ca la ted	raised the level, increased
explicit	ex PLIC it	clear and definite
gravely	GRAVE ly	severely, seriously
harass	ha RASS	to trouble and annoy continually
inservice classes	IN service classes	classes offered at the place of employment
jeopardize	JEOP ar dize	to put in danger
likelihood	LIKE li hood	probability
means	MEANS	way, ability
pertinent	PER tin ent	directly related to what is being talked about
precedent	PREC e dent	an example that sets a standard for future action
prescribed (adj)	pre SCRIBed	as directed
proxy	PROX y	acting for someone else on his or her behalf either in person, or by document
rapport	rap PORT (silent t)	a friendly, sympathetic relationship
resuscitated	re SUS ci ta ted	brought back to life or consciousness
scope	SCOPE	the extent or limits of something
seemingly	SEEM ing ly	appears true on the surface, but may not be
suggestive	sug GES tive	indicating an indecent or sexually improper meaning
surrogate	SUR ro gate	a substitute, a person who acts in place of another
whistle blowing	WHIS tle BLOW ing	telling about someone's wrong or illegal activity to the authorities
witnessed	WIT nessed	observed

COMPLETION

Directions: Fill in the blank(s) with the correct word(s) to complete the sentence.

1. Use the correct verb in the following sentences (*jeopardize, witness, resuscitate, escalate*).
   a. That type of action can jeopardize a nurse's license.
   b. The argument was heated, and her remarks made the situation escalate.
   c. The nurse was asked to witness the signing of the consent form.
   d. When a patient's heart stops, it is mandatory to try to resuscitate him.
2. Use the correct adjective in these sentences (*prescribed, suggestive, pertinent*).
   a. He took all of the prescribed medication but was not well.
   b. The physician wanted only the pertinent facts such as the vital signs and intake and output amounts.
   c. The abdominal pain and nausea were suggestive signs of appendicitis.
3. Use the correct noun in these sentences (*precedent, scope, access, proxy, means*).
   a. At the end of the first semester of nursing school, the nursing student's scope of knowledge of nursing is very small.
   b. Since he was incapacitated, his proxy in the legal matter was his brother.
   c. The consulting physician needed access to the patient record in order to gather data needed for a diagnosis.
   d. The patient did not have the means with which to obtain his prescribed medications.
   e. Allowing a family member to visit after visiting hours were over set a precedent in the unit.
4. Use the correct adverb in these sentences (*seemingly, gravely*).
   a. The patient was seemingly more cheerful after his family visited.
   b. After reviewing the diagnostic tests, the doctor became gravely concerned about his patient's condition.

VOCABULARY EXERCISE

Reasonable can be defined as being within the bounds of common sense. *Prudent* means careful in conduct and exercising good judgment or common sense.

Write a definition of ethics: rules of conduct that have been agreed to by a particular group. Believed to be morally right or proper for that group.

WORD ATTACK SKILLS

The verb *prescribe* means to:

1. advise the use of something (medicine).
2. set a rule to be followed.

The noun *prescription* means a:

1. doctor's written instruction for medicine.
2. rule or suggestion to follow.

Directions: Write sentences for the above words.

1. prescribe: The doctor prescribed a stronger medication for his abating infection.
2. prescription: The prescription is widely used for combating for allergies.

PRONUNCIATION PRACTICE

Directions: Underline the accented syllable on the following words and practice pronouncing them with a partner or to yourself.

accountability	competent	consent	defamation	delegation
liable	libel	malpractice	negligence	reciprocity

COMMUNICATION EXERCISE

Directions: If there is some part of the chapter you do not understand, ask your teacher or another student to explain it to you. Clarify your understanding by repeating points, restating in your own words, and asking clarifying questions.

1. Read and practice the following dialogue.

Mary and Jim prepare to move a patient up in bed. N.T. is Jim's patient. Mary goes to the far side of the bed.

Jim: "We are going to move you up in bed, Ms. T."

Mary : "Let me move your pillow to the top of the bed."
Jim crouches down in preparation for moving Ms. T.

Mary : "Jim, I find it easier to raise the bed up before trying to move my patients. Could we do that?"

Jim: "The control is on your side; I'm sorry, I just got to thinking about Ms. T.'s dressing change and wasn't paying close attention."

Mary : "That's O.K., sometimes I forget too."

2. Read and practice the following dialogue.

Ms. H.: "I'm feeling like I don't want this surgery now that I signed the consent."

Nurse: "You've changed your mind? Are you feeling better than you were?"

Ms. H.: "It just seems like such an inconvenient time right now with my husband having to leave town for two weeks on business."

Nurse: "Oh, it isn't because the pain has suddenly disappeared?"

Ms. H.: "Oh no, the pain is still there, but I seem to be more used to it now."

Nurse: "Didn't you tell me that this was your third attack of severe pain from your gallbladder?"

Ms. H.:	"Yes, it is the third time it has happened, but it has been over a period of two years."
Nurse:	"I know it will be difficult recovering while your husband is out of town, but you have a very large gallstone according to your ultrasound report and that could cause a problem with bile flow that can affect your whole body. It really would be best to attend to the problem now."
Ms. H.:	"Oh, I know, I'm just not looking forward to being put to sleep."
Nurse:	"Does anesthesia scare you?"
Ms. H.:	"When I had it once before I was really terribly sick afterwards."
Nurse:	"How long ago was that?"
Ms. H.:	"About 22 years ago."
Nurse:	"There are newer types of anesthesia that don't tend to cause as much nausea. Talk to the anesthesiologist about that."
Ms. H.:	"O.K., I'll do that."

3. Write a dialogue where a patient refuses to have a nasogastric tube inserted even though she is vomiting. Share your dialogue with a peer by reading it to him or her.

CULTURAL POINTS

1. Many industries in the United States are heavily regulated by state and federal laws. The medical and health professions are regulated by laws and by professional guidelines and licensing. This is done for the protection of the patients and the health care professionals. Is this done in your country? To what extent? Do you think it is a good idea or not? Why? Discuss this with your classmates from other countries.
2. What are the ethical standards for nurses in your country?

Review the chapter highlights, answer the study questions, and complete the critical thinking activities at the end of the chapter in the textbook.

FOUR

Overview of the Nursing Process

TERMINOLOGY

Directions: Match the terms in column I with the definitions in column II.

Column I	Column II
1. __b__ critical thinking	a. Step-by-step process used by scientists to solve problems.
2. __e__ decision making	b. Directed, purposeful mental activity by which ideas are created and evaluated, plans are constructed, and desired outcomes are decided.
3. __c__ priority	c. Something taking precedence over other things at a particular time because of greater importance.
4. __d.__ nursing process	d. Way of thinking and acting based on the scientific method.
5. __a__ scientific method	e. Choosing actions to meet a desired goal.

SHORT ANSWER

Directions: Write a brief answer for each question.

1. List the components of the nursing process in order.
   a. assessment
   b. diagnosis
   c. Plan
   d. Implementation
   e. Evaluation

2. In order to solve a problem, one should use the following steps:
   a. define the problem clearly
   b. consider all possible outcomes
   c. consider possible outcomes for each Alternative
   d. predict the likelihood of each outcome occuring
   e. choose the Alternative with the best chance of success that has the fewest undesirable outcomes.

3. Explain how critical thinking differs from ordinary thinking.
effective reading, effective writing, attentive listening, and effective communication.

4 How could you have a peer help you learn to listen attentively?
repeat back the main ideas of what was stated confirm with what speaker said

5. How might you improve your critical thinking skills?
practicing careful considerations of problems and purposeful thinking, rather than random thinking.

6. How are patient problems usually prioritized?
using maslow's hierchy, Phsiological needs come first, Lungs - considered priorty then circulation

7. When prioritizing nursing tasks, you should consider:
phsiological needs first - Life-threatening problems 1st medium priortys - health threatening problems & coping low priorty

8. To maintain organization with a shift workload, you must be flexible and frequently reorder tasks as needed.

MULTIPLE CHOICE

*Directions: Choose the **best** answer for each of the following questions.*

1. The nursing process
   1. ensures high-quality nursing care.
   2. is essential for the provision of nursing care.
   3. provides a framework for planning, implementing, and evaluating nursing care.
   4. guarantees expected outcomes will be met.

2. The development of clinical judgment requires
   1. dedication to studying and learning.
   2. critical thinking skills.
   3. ability to delegate to others.
   4. ability to communicate clearly.

3. Attentive listening requires
   1. focusing on the topic of discussion.
   2. listening while conversing with another.
   3. watching the speaker's face.
   4. thinking of a response while listening.

4. When setting priorities for nursing care, problems that threaten health are considered
   1. high priority.
   2. not a priority.
   3. low priority.
   4. medium priority.

5. When all tasks have relatively high priority and it is not possible to accomplish them all, you must
   1. postpone some of the tasks to the next shift.
   2. rush through care for other patients to provide extra time.
   3. delegate some tasks to others to complete.
   4. apologize to the patient for what cannot be done.

CRITICAL THINKING ACTIVITIES

Directions: Consider the following situation and determine what needs to be done. Then, using the problem solving/decision making process, prioritize what needs to be done.

You are a single mother and you have become a new nursing student. On the first day of classes you arrive at the college at 8:15 A.M. (0800). You must buy your books, find your classrooms, and buy a parking permit for the campus, as well as attend two classes at 9:00 A.M. (0900) and 11:00 A.M. (1100). Your daughter has had an earache and you need to call the doctor's office to obtain an afternoon appointment time for her. Your son needs some school supplies before tomorrow. You must grocery shop for food to fix dinner and the rest of the week's meals.

Priority Rating	What Needs to Be Done
________	________________________________
________	________________________________
________	________________________________
________	________________________________
________	________________________________
________	________________________________
________	________________________________
________	________________________________

MEETING CLINICAL OBJECTIVES

Directions: The following suggested activities will help you meet the stated clinical practice objectives for the chapter. Review your school's clinical objectives for the week and outline a plan of activities that will help you meet them. If unsure as to how to meet them, consult with your instructor at the beginning of the clinical day.

1. Ask several nurses in the clinical area how they organize their work for the shift.
2. Devise a personalized work organization form.
3. Practice attentive listening with different patients.
4. Think about the steps (components) of the nursing process as you carry out tasks on the unit. Decide what part of the process you are using for each task you perform.

STEPS TOWARD BETTER COMMUNICATION

VOCABULARY BUILDING GLOSSARY

Term	Pronunciation	Definition
attribute	AT tri bute	characteristic
coherent	co HER ent	fits together, connects logically
concisely	con CISE ly	briefly, in a few words
delegate	del e GATE (v)	to appoint another person to do something
dynamic	dy NAM ic	energetic, active
enhance	en HANCE	to make better, more complete

implement (v)	IM ple ment	use, put into action
input	IN put	information or advice from someone
overlapping	O' ver LAP ping	partly covering another thing or time
prognosis	prog NO sis	the expected outcome
unforeseen	UN fore seen	not expected

VOCABULARY SIMILARITIES EXERCISE

These words have different meanings depending on the pronunciation:

AT tri bute (n)—a characteristic; a TRI' bute (v)—to give credit to, or reason for
DEL e gate (n)—someone given responsibility; del e GATE (v)—to give responsibility to another

Directions: The following definitions for the individual words are all correct meanings. Check the ones that give the correct meaning for this phrase: "sound conclusions" (con CLU' sions).

sound: _✓_ correct _✓_ noise _✓_ healthy
conclusion: _✓_ an ending ___ an opinion

1. The phrase "sound conclusions" means correct ending.

COMPLETION

Directions: Fill in the blank(s) with the correct word(s) from the vocabulary building glossary to complete the sentence.

1. Performing a thorough patient assessment helps prevent unforeseen problems while giving care.
2. Once the nursing care plan is written, the nurse can implement the individual actions.
3. Characteristics of effective writing are expressing thoughts coherently and concisely.
4. The steps of assessment and evaluation of the nursing process are overlapping, in that assessment occurs during the evaluation phase to determine the effectiveness of actions.
5. Obtaining a complete patient history often requires input from the family.
6. Reading articles from the chapter bibliography will enhance learning.
7. The nursing care plan must be written in a coherant manner so that all caregivers know exactly what the goals are and what actions to carry out.
8. Before explaining treatment plans to a patient, the physician should tell the patient the prognosis.

COMMUNICATION EXERCISE

1. You have prioritized care for your patients and attend to the man with chest pain before treating the boy with a cut arm. Your instructor asks, "Why did you decide to attend to the man with the chest pain first?"

   You respond: The percentage rate for mortallity of man with chest pain was lower than the boy with a cut arm.

2. Reread Critical Thinking Activity #2 in the chapter in the textbook. A nursing assistant has the only portable sphygmomanometer. What would you say to her to solve your problem?

   I need to use this sphygmomanometer quickly, I'll return it as soon as I'm done for I have a client who needs his vitals taken immediately.

ATTENTIVE LISTENING EXAMPLE

Directions: Practice the following dialogue with a partner.

You wish to delegate ambulating M.S. to the nursing assistant. You approach the aide to discuss this.

You: "I would like you to ambulate M.S. in room 232, bed 2, once this morning and again after lunch. She is recovering from pneumonia and is still quite weak. Please use a gait belt."

Aide: "I already have three baths to give and vital signs to take for eight patients. I don't know that I can fit ambulating her into my schedule."

You: "You have already been assigned to do eight sets of vital signs and three full baths?"

Aide: "Well, I'm to do the vital signs and set up the three patients for their baths, not give full bed baths."

You: "It seems like you will have time to do the ambulation. Let me check with you at 10:00 A.M. to see how things are going. If there is a problem, then I will have to find another way to ambulate her."

Review the chapter highlights, answer the study questions, and complete the critical thinking activities at the end of the chapter in the textbook.

FIVE

Assessment, Nursing Diagnosis, and Planning

TERMINOLOGY

Directions: Match the terms in column I with the definitions in column II.

Column I

1. __h__ cues
2. __a__ data
3. __G__ goal
4. __e__ signs
5. __f__ symptoms
6. __c__ interview
7. __b__ database
8. __d__ inferences

Column II

a. Pieces of information on a specific topic.
b. All the information gathered about a patient.
c. Conversation from which facts are obtained.
d. Conclusions made based on observed data.
e. Abnormalities objectively verifiable by repeat examination.
f. Data the patient says are occurring, but not verifiable by objective means.
g. Broad idea of what is to be achieved through nursing intervention.
h. Pieces of information that influence decisions.

COMPLETION

Directions: Fill in the blank(s) with the correct word(s) to complete the sentence.

1. Assessment consists of gathering information about patients and their __needs__ using __a variety of methods__.
2. Assessment is an __on-going__ process.
3. Defining characteristics are the specific __signs__ and __symptoms__ attached to the nursing diagnosis that indicate the data from which the diagnosis was derived.
4. Etiological factors are those factors that indicate the __causes__ of the patient's problem.
5. A nursing diagnosis is a statement that indicates the patient's __actual health__ status or the risk of a __problem developing__, the causative or related factors, and the specific __signs and symptoms. (defining charectoristics)__

6. In order to perform even the simplest nursing skill you need to critally think how to do it.

7. Whenever nursing care is performed, it is essential to consider the physocial needs of the patient.

√ 8. A nursing database is compiled by using the nursing process.

√ 9. The nursing problems present for a patient are determined by clustering the assessment data.

10. In many agencies, problems of the patient are stated as nursing diagnosis.

√ 11. Nursing care is delivered by considering the order of importance of the patient's needs or problems.

√ 12. Expected outcome statements should be written so that it is easy to evaluate (obtain measurable criteria) whether they have been achieved or not.

13. When formulating a nursing care plan, the nurse chooses interventions that are most likely to achieve the expected outcomes.

14. In order to function effectively, the nurse must use a method of priorization.

15. Sources of data used for the formulation of a patient database are:
objective data
subjective data

16. Methods used to gather a patient database are:
a. interview
√ b. physical examination
c. analysis of

CORRELATION

Directions: For each of the following patient problems, choose the most appropriate nursing diagnosis from the NANDA list in your textbook.

1. B.A. is admitted with severe abdominal pain.
chronic PAIN

2. L.H. has fallen and fractured his hip.
physical mobility impaired

3. J.T. is admitted with burns on his chest.
tissue perfusion altered-cardiopulmonary
risk for perioperative positioning injury

4. Although recovering, T.P. suffered a stroke that has paralyzed his right extremities. He is right-handed.
physical mobility impaired

5. V.T. has emphysema and becomes very short of breath whenever she tries to perform a task.
Breathing pattern, ineffective
? DVWR (Dysfunctional Ventilatory weaning response) ?

MULTIPLE CHOICE

*Directions: Choose the **best** answer for each of the following questions.*

1. An example of objective data is
   1. blood pressure.
   2. pain.
   3. nausea.
   4. itching.

2. Subjective data
   1. can be verified by laboratory or diagnostic tests.
   2. are data that the patient states.
   3. can be observed by the senses or use of equipment.
   4. can be verified by physical assessment of the patient.

3. Analysis of the database is necessary for the formulation of
   1. expected outcomes/goals.
   2. nursing interventions.
   3. nursing diagnoses.
   4. evaluation statements.

4. Which one of the following is a NANDA accepted nursing diagnosis?
   1. Gall stones
   2. Shortness of breath
   3. Impaired gas exchange
   4. Itching

5. The difference between a medical diagnosis and a nursing diagnosis is that a nursing diagnosis
   1. labels the illness.
   2. defines the patient's response to illness.
   3. indicates the priority of the problem.
   4. is made by the physician and nurse together.

6. When considering the order of priority of patient problems according to Maslow
   1. pain takes precedence over elimination needs.
   2. sleep is more important than food.
   3. safety and security needs take precedence.
   4. physiological needs take precedence.

7. Short-term nursing goals are those that
   1. are accomplished before discharge from the hospital.
   2. take many weeks or months to accomplish.
   3. are achievable within 7–10 days.
   4. are achieved through medical intervention.

8. An expected outcome
   1. is a short-term goal.
   2. is data gathered after nursing intervention.
   3. is a broad, long-term goal statement.
   4. should contain measurable criteria.

9. The primary objective of choosing nursing interventions is to
   1. keep the patient safe and comfortable.
   2. help the patient meet the expected outcomes.
   3. carry out the physician's orders.
   4. organize the nurse's work for the shift.

10. The practical/vocational nurse's role in nursing care planning is to
    1. assist with the writing of the nursing care plan.
    2. evaluate the plan written by the registered nurse.
    3. perform the initial physical assessment of the patient.
    4. enter the care plan into the computer.

CRITICAL THINKING ACTIVITIES

1. Analyze the following assessment data obtained about a patient and determine the patient's needs. Then place the needs in order of priority.

   O.N., a 78-year-old female, is admitted with pain in the left hip after a fall. She is unable to move her left leg without severe pain. She is apprehensive and scared. There is a bruise on her left forearm. She cries out when she tries to move her left leg.

2. Choose appropriate nursing diagnoses from the NANDA list for the above patient's needs. Write expected outcomes for each nursing diagnosis chosen.

3. Determine which of the data from the above situation are objective and which are subjective. Write an "S" or "O" beside each one to indicate your choice.

   a. __O__ Blood pressure is 132/84.
   b. __S__ Cries out when leg is moved.
   c. __O__ Has a bruise on left forearm.
   d. __S__ Is apprehensive and scared.
   e. __O__ Pulse is 92.
   f. __S__ Winces when left leg is moved.
   g. __S__ States that leg really hurts.
   h. __O__ Respirations are 18.

MEETING CLINICAL OBJECTIVES

Directions: The following suggested activities will help you meet the stated clinical practice objectives for the chapter. Review your school's clinical objectives for the week and outline a plan of activities that will help you meet them. If unsure as to how to meet them, consult with your instructor at the beginning of the clinical day.

1. Before your first clinical patient assignment, perform an assessment on a classmate, friend, or family member.
2. Review the nursing assessment and history form on your assigned patient's chart. Note the types of information and the nursing comments it contains.
3. Find the physician's history and physical on your assigned patient's chart. Read it. Look up any unfamiliar terms.
4. Perform an assessment on your assigned patient. Now find the nursing care plan in the patient's chart. Determine if the nursing diagnoses designated for this patient are appropriate by determining if the data you collected supports them. Are there other appropriate nursing diagnoses that seem to be missing?

STEPS TOWARD BETTER COMMUNICATION

VOCABULARY BUILDING GLOSSARY

Term	Pronunciation	Definition
affect	AFF ect	emotional feeling or expression
alleviate	al LEV i ate	to relieve, make less painful

concurrent conditions	con CUR rent con DI tions	conditions happening at the same time
correlate	corr e LATE	to show how one thing relates meaningfully to another
deviate	DE vi ATE	to be different, or move away from
differentiate	diff er EN tiate	to show differences between several things
elicit	e LI cit	to get, bring out (usually information)
formulate	FORM u late	to put together, organize
infer	in FER	to guess, or figure out from the information given
next of kin	NEXT of kin	closest relative
over-the-counter	O ver the coun ter	medications available without prescription
pertinent	PER ti nent	directly relating to a situation
prosthesis	pros THE sis	an artificial limb (hand, arm, leg, etc.)
rapport	ra POR (t is silent)	a sympathetic relationship between people
scan	sCAN	to look over quickly
significant other	sig NIF i cant other	someone important to the patient, usually a spouse or close loved one—not a blood relative

COMPLETION

Directions: Fill in the blank(s) with the correct word(s) from the vocabulary buidling glossary to complete the sentence.

1. Jan is Tom's significant other and has lived with him for eight years.
2. It is not a good idea to deviate from the accepted procedure when administering medications.
3. Sometimes it is difficult to correlate between symptoms of a minor illness and a major illness in the beginning stages.
4. Ibuprofen is a commonly used over-the-counter medication.
5. Whether a patient is experiencing side effects of medication is pertinent information to have before giving another dose of the medication.
6. Heat is sometimes used to alleviate pain.
7. Once all the assessment data are gathered, the nurse will formulate the nursing care plan.
8. When unexpectedly assigned a new patient, it is good to scan the chart for the current diagnostic test results.
9. Nurses learn to differentiate laboratory data with the signs and symptoms the patient has.
10. Diabetes is often a concurrent for a patient who is hospitalized for renal failure.
11. When the lower leg is amputated, the patient will be fitted with a prosthesis.

12. When the blank on the admission form for "religion" lists "none," one can ___Infer___ that the patient does not belong to an organized religious group.

WORD ATTACK SKILLS

Directions: Pronounce these word pairs, and tell the difference in the definition of the noun and the verb or adjective.

1. rapport (n) ____________________

   report (n) ____________________

2. elicit (v) ____________________

   illicit (adj) ____________________

3. affect (v) ____________________

   effect (n) ____________________

Usage note: the verb "affect" means to have an influence or cause a change. The noun "affect" means the general feeling or emotion felt by a person. *Her diet affected her health. Her affect reflected how poorly she was feeling.*

COMMUNICATION EXERCISE

Directions: You need to assess Ms. N. for pain. Here is an example of such a communication interaction. Practice the dialog with a peer, taking turns being the nurse and the patient.

Nurse: "Are you having much pain this morning?"

Ms. N.: "Yes, I'm hurting quite a bit."

Nurse: "Can you show me where it seems to be hurting the most?"

Ms. N.: (Points to the area of her incision over the hip.) "It's mostly right here, but it does go down this leg muscle."

Nurse: "Can you describe the type of pain you are experiencing?"

Ms. N.: "It is a dull ache with throbbing in the incision area. When I move, I get a stabbing pain here in my thigh."

Nurse: "How would you rate it on a scale of 1–10 with 1 being the least pain and 10 being the most pain?"

Ms. N.: "I guess I would rate it at about 8."

Nurse: "O.K., I think it is probably time for some more pain medication now. I'll check to see when you last had it."

Other terms that might be used to describe pain are: *sharp, dull, burning, knife-like, radiating, searing, needle-like.*

Review the chapter highlights, answer the study questions, and complete the critical thinking activities at the end of the chapter in the textbook.

SIX

Implementation and Evaluation

TERMINOLOGY

Directions: Match the terms in column I with the definitions in column II.

Column I

1. __d__ implement
2. __L__ interventions
3. __k__ documentation
4. __i__ evaluation
5. __b__ critical pathway
6. __C__ quality management
7. __h__ nursing audit
8. __f__ independent nursing action
9. __G__ dependent nursing action
10. __J__ interdependent
11. __a__ time-flexible action
12. __e__ time-fixed action

Column II

a. Can be done at any time
b. Step-by-step approach to total care of the patient
c. Manage the quality of performance
d. Carry out nursing interventions
e. Must be done at a set time
f. Nursing action based on nursing judgment that does not require an order
g. Action requiring a health care provider's order
h. Examination of patient records to see if care meets accepted standards
i. Assessment of effectiveness of nursing actions in meeting expected outcomes.
j. Actions that come from collaborative care planning
k. Recording of pertinent data on the clinical record
l. Actions involving more than one health care professional

SHORT ANSWER

A.

Directions: Recalling information from Chapters 4 and 5, complete the following exercise. For each nursing action on the left, give the name of the step of the nursing process in which the action occurs (assessment, nursing diagnosis, planning, implementation, evaluation).

1. Interviewing the patient to obtain a history. __assessment__
2. Setting a goal for improved mobility. __planning__

3. Assisting the patient to turn, cough, and deep breathe after surgery. implementation
4. Auscultating for bowel sounds. assessment
5. Checking a lab report to see if there are abnormalities in the patient's urine. assessment, evaluation
6. Teaching a patient to take his or her own blood pressure. Implementation
7. Reaching the conclusion that the patient has a fluid volume deficit. evaluation
8. Gathering data to determine if expected outcomes have been met. evaluation
9. Writing "Activity Intolerance related to decreased oxygenation" on the nursing care plan. nursing diagnosis
10. Checking the intake and output record to see if the patient is taking in 1500 mL of fluid a day as planned. evaluation
11. Writing "Pain will be controlled by analgesia within 8 hours" on the nursing care plan. planning
12. Writing on the nursing care plan "Encourage family to bring in ethnic foods allowed on therapeutic diet." implementation

B.

Directions: Write a short answer or fill in the blanks for each of the following questions.

1. The first step in organizing actions for implementation is to set priorities of tasks.
2. Clues for imminent deadlines for certain tasks can be found in the change-of-shift report.
3. When planning time for uninterrupted care, consider:
   a. if visitors will be coming
   b. when diagnostic tests are scheduled
   c. what time physician may come to see the patient
   d. medication administration schedules
4. Before carrying out a planned nursing action, besides knowing the reason for the intervention, the expected outcome, and the usual standard of care, it is necessary to consider the reason.
5. The critical pathway is a step-by-step approach to patient care and is an outgrowth of managed care.
6. The designated standard of care for performing a procedure can be found in the ANA-Standards. of clinical practice

7. After implementing patient care, documentation must be done.
8. You will know goals have been met when expected outcomes have been reached.
9. Evaluation is a(n) continuous process.
10. Nursing care plans are usually revised every 24 hrs.

SETTING PRIORITIES

Directions: Considering the Standard Steps used when performing a nursing procedure, prioritize the following with #1 being highest priority and #7 being lowest..

1. 5 Clean and dispose of used supplies.
2. 7 Document.
3. 3 Prepare the patient.
4. 2 Explain the procedure.
5. 1 Wash your hands.
6. 4 Perform the procedure.
7. 6 Restore the unit and make the patient comfortable.

MULTIPLE CHOICE

Directions: These questions require use of prior knowledge from preceding chapters. Choose the ***best*** *answer for each of the following questions.*

1. A part of the assessment step of the nursing process is
   1. setting goals to be accomplished.
   2. gathering data about the patient's condition.
   3. choosing nursing interventions to solve problems.
   4. carrying out nursing interventions to meet the goals.

2. Nursing diagnosis is a way of
   1. stating patient problems.
   2. labeling the patient's medical problem.
   3. devising a nursing care plan.
   4. analyzing assessment data.

3. Which one of the following is a correctly written expected outcome for the nursing diagnosis "Pain related to abdominal incision"?
   1. Pain will be relieved by giving analgesia.
   2. Analgesia will be given for pain relief.
   3. Pain will be relieved before discharge.
   4. Pain will be controlled by analgesia for at least three hours.

4. When implementing nursing orders on the care plan, it is *most* important to consider
   1. the safety of the patient.
   2. convenience for the patient.
   3. the degree of importance of the task.
   4. whether a procedure will be interrupted.

5. When evaluating whether the expected outcome "Wound infection will subside within seven days" has been met, you would gather which of the following data?
   1. evidence that the antibiotic doses were given
   2. appearance and characteristics of the wound
   3. evidence that the patient is taking decreasing amounts of pain medication
   4. observations that the patient is able to perform self-care

6. Which one of the following would be an independent nursing action?
   1. giving a medication
   2. applying a heating pad
   3. assisting a patient with speech therapy exercises
   4. teaching about the side effects of a medication

7. Which of the following is true regarding a critical pathway?
   1. It is devised by the physician and the nurse.
   2. All disciplines involved in the patient's care provide input.
   3. It addresses only the critical problems of the patient.
   4. It is a standardized plan of care used for each patient.

8. Efficiently implementing patient care requires
   1. following the procedure manual's standards of care.
   2. following a work organization plan exactly.
   3. prioritizing and combining tasks.
   4. enlisting the help of a nurse's aide.

9. Evaluation as a step of the nursing process is a method of determining
   1. whether actions are effective in helping the patient reach expected outcomes.
   2. how expected outcomes should be written on the nursing care plan.
   3. which patient problems need to be addressed first.
   4. whether the nursing diagnosis was chosen correctly.

10. The goal of a continuous quality management program is to
    1. make nurses evaluate the care they give.
    2. identify care that is not up to the standard.
    3. determine if nurses are documenting care accurately.
    4. improve nursing practice within an agency.

11. O.T. has had a hip replacement. When you go to check on him, he is grimacing and says he needs pain medication. When asked, he states that his pain is at a 7 on a scale of 1–10. You check the orders and give him his narcotic analgesic. This action is a(n) _______________ nursing action.
    1. independent
    2. dependent
    3. collaborative
    4. interdependent

12. An expected outcome for O.T.'s nursing diagnosis of "Pain related to surgical procedure" is "Pain will be relieved for at least three hours with medication." An important part of writing an expected outcome is that it must be
    1. subjective
    2. relevant
    3. measurable
    4. patient-oriented

13. The evaluation step of the nursing process determines
    1. if all the actions on the plan were implemented.
    2. whether the expected outcomes are measurable.
    3. the patient's response to medical treatment.
    4. if actions have helped the patient meet the expected outcomes.

14. When evaluation shows that the expected outcomes are not being met, you would
    1. consider different actions to assist the patient to meet the outcomes.
    2. revise the nursing diagnosis.
    3. rewrite the expected outcomes.
    4. reassess the patient's status and rewrite the entire nursing care plan.

15. The difference between a goal and an expected outcome is that a goal is
    1. more specific.
    2. patient-oriented.
    3. broader.
    4. long term.

CRITICAL THINKING ACTIVITIES

1. What factors will you consider when planning your work for a shift?
2. Identify the positive aspects of a quality management program for nursing.
3. L.R. was injured in an automobile accident. You are assigned to care for him. Consider the following information and then construct a nursing care plan for this patient.

   L.R. had surgery two days ago for removal of a ruptured spleen. He has an abdominal incision that is oozing slightly onto the dressing. He has a badly swollen right knee and bruises on the right extremities. He cannot walk without pain. He states that he is very sore and that his incisional area is hurting. He states that the pain is a 6 on a scale of 1–10. His orders read "Daily dressing change; Vicodin q 4h prn pain; right leg elevated; BRP with assistance."

   How would you evaluate the success of your care plan?

MEETING CLINICAL OBJECTIVES

Directions: The following suggested activities will help you meet the stated clinical practice objectives for the chapter. Review your school's clinical objectives for the week and outline a plan of activities that will help you meet them. If unsure as to how to meet them, consult with your instructor at the beginning of the clinical day.

1. Devise your own work organization form/tool.
2. Study how unit nurses perform procedures. Are they carrying out the "standard steps"?
3. Construct a nursing care plan for an assigned patient.
4. Revise the above-constructed nursing care plan at the end of the shift.

STEPS TOWARD BETTER COMMUNICATION

VOCABULARY BUILDING GLOSSARY

Term	Pronunciation	Definition
accreditation	a ccred i TA tion	approval to a set of standards
adept	a DEPT	skillful; clever
agency-wide	A gen cy wide	through all departments or people in an agency
blame	blAMe	to accuse; say someone is responsible for something bad
buckling	BUCK ling	fastening with a buckle

clue	CLUE	information that helps provide an answer
collaborative	col LAB bo ra tive	working together with others
deadline	DEAD line	the time or date when something must be completed
imminent	IM mi nent	immediate, ready to happen soon
impairment	im PAIR ment	weakness or damage
incorporated into	in COR por a ted into	made a part of; included in
intervening	in ter VEN ing	coming between
latter	LA tter	the last of two things mentioned
process evaluation	PRO cess e val u A tion	looking at how well a process is working
rationale	ra tion ALE	the reasons behind a decision
refresh your memory	re FRESH your MEM o ry	to go back and think about something again
sequence	SE quence	a connected series of acts; an order
strive	strIve	to try hard

COMPLETION

Directions: Fill in the blank(s) with the correct word(s) from the vocabulary building glossary to complete the sentence.

1. The ___deadline___ for the assignment to be turned in was Friday.
2. It is important to master skills quickly as the first clinical day is ___imminent___.
3. Nursing care planning is a ___collaborative___ process between nurses and other health professionals.
4. Each student should ___strive___ to be well-prepared for each clinical day.
5. The stroke left the patient with left-sided ___impairment___.
6. That nurse is ___adept___ at eliciting information quickly from patients.
7. The patient fell in the hall, but did not ___blame___ the nurse for his fall.
8. Having clinical days on Tuesday and Thursday is difficult because of the ___latter___ lecture day. ✓
9. The fine rash provided a ___clue___ about what might be wrong with the patient.
10. Nurse's notes must be written in the ___sequence___ in which events occur.
11. Patient teaching is often ___incorporated___ into providing patient care.
12. An instructor will often ask for the ___sequence___ of a step of a nursing procedure.
refresh your memory

WORD ATTACK SKILLS

Some words and phrases have equal meaning (synonyms):

write = note = jot down

critical pathway = care path = care map

Equivalent words with different meanings and pronunciations depending upon how they are used.

Verbs	Nouns	Nouns
note	note	no TA tion
im ple MENT	IM ple ment	im ple men TA tion
doc u MENT	DOC u ment	doc u men TA tion
in ter VENE		in ter VEN tion
pri OR i tize	pri OR i TY	pri or i ti ZA tion

The suffix "-ation/tion" means an action or a process, or something connected with an action or a process: *Intervention is the act, or result, of intervening.*

ABBREVIATIONS

Directions: Give the meaning for each abbreviation.

1. ST short term
2. LT Long term
3. q every
4. 4h 4 hours
5. ROM range of motion
6. PT physical therapist
7. CVA cerebrovascular accident
8. r/t related/to
9. UA urinalysis
10. CQM Continuous Quality Management

COMMUNICATION EXERCISE

1. Make a list of questions you would like to ask a unit nurse about performing a patient assessment. Make brief notes of the answers you receive and later rewrite them into complete sentences.
2. Make a list of points to consider when you are making a work organization plan for giving patient care. Remember to include visiting time, diagnostic tests, doctors' rounds, and so forth.

CULTURAL POINTS

1. Some questions and procedures may seem very personal and even objectionable to some people of different ages and cultures. For example, an older woman of any culture may feel uncomfortable having a male nurse doing peri-care, or a man may feel uncomfortable being catheterized by a female nurse. In some cultures where the women dress very modestly and may not even have much social contact with men outside the family (as in some Muslim groups), having a male nurse or even a male doctor examine them and observe or touch their unclothed bodies could make them uncomfortable or be considered sinful.

2. Southeast Asian immigrants may believe that the spirit might leave the body on risky occasions, so they tie a string around the wrist of the patient to bind the spirit to the body. Nurses may be tempted to remove these strings before transporting the patient to the operating room, but this is very traumatic for the patient, and there is an emotional value in leaving on the strings. If the nurse is from such a culture or of an older generation, he or she may find it difficult or uncomfortable to perform some of these required procedures.

3. Remember that what is required is done for the good of the patient and is necessary for the success of the diagnosis and treatment. Such questions and procedures must be handled in a matter-of-fact and straightforward manner.

4. Nursing care plans need to take into account the needs and beliefs of patients of different ethnic backgrounds, and those of their families. Food preferences should be accommodated for as much as possible within the prescribed diet and capabilities of the dietary department.

Review the chapter highlights, answer the study questions, and complete the critical thinking activities at the end of the chapter in the textbook.

SEVEN

Communication and the Nurse–Patient Relationship

TERMINOLOGY

A. MATCHING

Directions: Match the terms in column I with the definitions in column II.

Column I		Column II	
1. g	aphasic	a.	communication in words
2. f	congruent	b.	return of information and how it was interpreted
3. e	empathy	c.	relationship of mutual trust or affinity
4. b	feedback	d.	communication without words
5. h	input	e.	ability to understand by seeing the situation from another's perspective
6. d	nonverbal	f.	in agreement
7. c	rapport	g.	difficulty expressing or understanding language
8. a	verbal	h.	information given or put in

B. COMPLETION

Directions: Fill in the blank(s) with the correct word(s) to complete the sentence.

active listening	confidentiality
body language	shift report
communication	therapeutic

1. The essential communication regarding patients that takes place between nurses going off a shift and those coming on the next shift is termed shift report.
2. A patient may express pain by using body language rather than explicitly telling a nurse.
3. Communication of messages is a continuous, circular process occurring both verbally and nonverbally.
4. therapeutic communication promotes understanding between the sender and the receiver.

5. Concentration and focusing on what is being said by the other person is essential for active listening.

6. Confidentiality must be kept for all communication between the patient and the nurse.

SHORT ANSWER

Directions: Write a brief answer for each question.

1. Necessary components of the communication process are:
when person sends message + another peron who recieve it, processes it and indicated the message has been interpreted.

2. Factors that influence communication are:
   a. cultural differences
   b. past experience
   c. emotions and mood
   d. attitude

3. When conducting an admission interview, both closed-ended questions and open-ended questions are used. List three types of information for which you would want to ask a closed-ended question:
   a. what medications did you take today
   b. Do you have allergies
   c. Do you have pain

4. An example of an open-ended question that might be asked during an admission interview would be ask patient how he feels about the hospitalization

5. Identify four ways to delegate effectively:
   a. active listening
   b. interpreting verbal messages
   c. focusing
   d. obtaining feed back

6. Three key factors in the nurse-patient relationship are that this relationship:
   a. helper role rather than social - focus on goals
   b. focuses on patient
   c. defined by specific boundaries

7. In a therapeutic relationship, interaction between the nurse and the patient should build trust.

8. Four characteristics of the nurse that facilitate a therapeutic nurse-patient relationship are:
   a. Silence — empathy
   b. re-stating good communication - Non-judgemental
   c. touch confidentiality maintaining hope
   d. offering of self

9. When calling a physician regarding a patient, you should assess the patient before the call. What data should you have on hand in case the physician asks for it?
have current data on - updated

10. List three tasks you as a nurse might have to perform by computer during a shift.
    a. medications orders entered
    b. Supplies that a patient needs have to be ordered
    c. nurse care plans -

11. To communicate more successfully with the elderly patient, it is best to:
    a. Wait for an answer to one question before asking another
    b. Eliminate outside distractions
    c. Introduce one idea at a time
    d. Do not rush a person - may cause confusion

12. When communicating with a young child, the best techniques are to:
    approach them at eye level & use a calm, quiet, friendly voice when communicating. Be honest & tell the child what to expect

13. Three specific actions to increase success when trying to communicate with an aphasic person are:
    a. get an interpretator
    b. get a white erasable board
    c. speech therapists

14. When communicating with a hearing-impaired patient, four specific actions that enhance success are:
    a. speak distinctly
    b. Keep voice pitch at mid range - speak slowly
    c. Face person eye-level (about 2.5'-4 ft)
    d. Be aware of non-verbal gestures
    ask for rephrasing

MULTIPLE CHOICE

*Directions: Choose the **best** answer for each of the following questions.*

1. Within the communication process, active listening is very important. However, in order for the initiator of the communication to know that the message was received,
   1. an answer must be given.
   2. feedback must be received.
   3. words must be spoken by each person.
   4. the listener's expression must indicate comprehension.

2. Greater comprehension of what a person is saying will occur if the nurse also pays attention to the
   1. timbre of the voice.
   2. level of the vocabulary used.
   3. body language displayed.
   4. degree of enthusiasm expressed.

3. The "active listener" does **not**
   1. establish eye contact.
   2. give cues showing interest.
   3. maintain open body posture.
   4. show impatience.

4. The use of silence in therapeutic communication is to encourage
   1. verbalization of feelings or thoughts.
   2. a nonthreatening atmosphere.
   3. expression of concerns.
   4. expression of innermost thoughts.

5. Nurses do a lot of patient teaching, but giving advice is considered
   1. a routine part of nursing care.
   2. essential for recovery and healing.
   3. a tool for encouraging communication.
   4. a block to therapeutic communication.

6. A nonjudgmental attitude is essential for
   1. effective communication.
   2. a therapeutic nurse-patient relationship.
   3. adequate comprehension of patient teaching.
   4. collaboration regarding patient care.

7. Giving a shift report is a daily nursing task. A thorough report on an average patient should take about
   1. 3–5 minutes.
   2. 30–60 seconds.
   3. 1–3 minutes.
   4. 1 1/2–2 minutes.

8. Touch can be therapeutic and must be used judiciously. It may be used to signify
   1. agreement with what is being said.
   2. caring and comfort.
   3. the need to listen closely.
   4. the need to gain the person's attention.

9. The best way to encourage elaboration when interacting with a patient is to say,
   1. "I'm not certain that I follow what you mean."
   2. "The treatment caused pain?"
   3. "I'll listen if you will tell me more."
   4. "We'll continue after the doctor checks you over."

10. An example of offering false reassurance would be to say,
    1. "We'll have the report back in three days."
    2. "The pathologist is very good."
    3. "The results only take 24–48 hours."
    4. "I'm sure the pathology report will be just fine."

11. Empathy is
    1. feeling concerned about how another is feeling.
    2. showing you care about the other person.
    3. placing oneself in another's position to understand how she or he feels.
    4. making sympathetic statements to someone who has had a loss.

12. When communicating with an elderly person who is slightly hard of hearing it is important to
    1. speak very slowly.
    2. eliminate other noise in the room.
    3. speak in low tones.
    4. speak as loud as possible.

13. One action that enhances communication success with a hearing-impaired person is to
    1. sit within five feet of the person.
    2. be sure the area is well lit.
    3. be certain to face the person when speaking.
    4. use higher tones when speaking.

14. Which one of the following is a nonverbal communication?
    1. a giggle
    2. shouting
    3. smiling
    4. "yes"

15. When obtaining a history from an elderly patient, you should
    1. allow sufficient time to answer a question.
    2. anticipate the person's answers and fill in for him or her.
    3. quickly ask another question to keep him or her on topic.
    4. tell the person, "Just answer the question."

MATCHING

Directions: Match the therapeutic technique in column II with the statement/question in column I.

Column I		Column II	
1. i	"…won't do it?"	a.	offering self
2. h	"…go on…"	b.	clarifying
3. d	"He said you couldn't go home until Saturday."	c.	restatement
4. a	"I'll come quickly if you call."	d.	summarizing
5. c	"So you have pain when you move, but it isn't very bad."	e.	using silence
6. e	Leaning forward, nodding head…	f.	giving information
7. h	"How do you feel about that?"	g.	open-ended question
8. j	"Tell me what the doctor said."	h.	general lead
9. b.	"You think it was the coffee that kept you awake?"	i.	reflection
10. f	"Your surgery is scheduled for 10:00 AM."	j.	seeking information

APPLICATION OF COMMUNICATION TECHNIQUES

Directions: For each of the following communication exchanges, indicate the technique being used. Label the exchange "therapeutic" or "nontherapeutic." If the exchange is nontherapeutic, give an alternative statement that would have been more therapeutic.

1. Patient: "I can't believe what that doctor said to me!"
   Nurse: "He didn't mean it the way it sounded."
   offering false reassurance — non-therapeutic – You sound upset – can you tell me more about it?

2. Patient: "I'm really scared about this surgery."
   Nurse: "Is it the idea of anesthesia that bothers you?"
   reflection — therapeutic

3. Patient: "It's so hard to watch him die."
   Nurse: "It's time to do your exercises now."
   changing the subject — non-therapeutic – silence

4. Patient: "It's been a really rough year for me."
   Nurse: "I'd like to hear more about that."
   encouraging elaboration — therapeutic

5. Patient: "I wonder if the chemotherapy will work."
   Nurse: "I'm sure it will and you'll be fine."
   non-theapeutic – silence

6. Patient: "I had a really hard time with the medication last time."

   Nurse: "Tell me more about that experience."

   open-ended question — therapeutic

7. Patient: "I'm trying to decide if I should have the colonoscopy."

   Nurse: "If I were you, I would have it done."

   Giving advice — non-therapeutic — present alternatives + options

8. Patient: "Then he started shouting at me."

   Nurse: "Ummmmm…"

   General Lead — therapeutic

9. Patient: "I know the bone marrow aspiration is going to really hurt."

   Nurse: "It won't hurt for long."

   offering false reassurance — non-therapeutic — give information

10. Patient: "I really tossed and turned last night."

    Nurse: "You had a really hard time sleeping."

    restatement — therapeutic

CRITICAL THINKING ACTIVITIES

1. List three instances in which communication would be important to the collaborative process (with other health care workers).
2. From the following scenario, underline the information that should be included in the end-of-shift report.

   B.F., room 328, states he is in pain and wants his medication. At 8:30 AM he is given a Vicodin. The pain is relieved by 9:15. He is interrupted by three phone calls during his assisted bath. His IV site is clean and dry; the doctor discontinues the IV when he makes afternoon rounds. The dressing over the abdominal incision is clean and dry. His wife comes to visit at noon. He is cooperative with his coughing and deep-breathing exercises. He walks in the hall three times. He has been taking fluids and a clear liquid diet without signs of nausea.

MEETING CLINICAL OBJECTIVES

Directions: The following suggested activities will help you meet the stated clinical practice objectives for the chapter. Review your school's clinical objectives for the week and outline a plan of activities that will help you meet them. If unsure as to how to meet them, consult with your instructor at the beginning of the clinical day.

1. Listen carefully to various nurses give report. Determine which one gives the best report and try and figure out why you feel this report is the best.
2. When you come home from your clinical experience, take the information you have on your worksheet for the patients you cared for and using a tape recorder, practice giving report.

3. Plan a specific interaction with a patient or family member and practice using therapeutic communication techniques.
4. During lunch, practice "attentive" listening with a classmate.
5. Interview a patient and compile an admission assessment.
6. Seek assignment to a hearing-impaired person for practice in communication with such a person.
7. Review your interactions with patients on the way home at the end of the clinical day. Pick out any instances where you felt your communication was ineffective and by using therapeutic techniques, see what you could have said that might have made the outcome of the interaction better.

STEPS TOWARD BETTER COMMUNICATION

VOCABULARY BUILDING GLOSSARY

Term	Pronunciation	Definition
A. Individual Terms		
abrupt	a BRUPT	sudden, quick, short
ambivalent	am BIV a lent	uncertain, especially between two choices
closure	CLO sure	a satisfactory ending or conclusion
concisely	con CISE ly	in a few words, briefly
conveyed	con VEYed	to make known, to communicate something; carried or transferred from one place to another
discount (verb)	dis COUNT	to not pay attention to, to disregard; to not consider valuable
elaborating	e LAB or a ting	explaining in more detail
elicit	e LI cit	bring out
format	FOR mat	an arrangement or order
gesture	GES ture	a movement, especially of the hands or arms
hunched	HUNCHed	shoulders pulled forward and down, forming a hump with the back
intonation	in to NA tion	rising and falling level of the voice in speech
judiciously	ju DI cious ly	carefully; in small amounts
lead (noun)	LEAD	something to get you started
mood	MOOD	an emotional state or feeling that lasts for a period of time
optimal	OP ti mal	the best possible
pry	PRY	to force by continual pressure
ramble	RAM ble	to go around in different directions without making connections; off of the point
refrain	re FRAIN	to stop oneself, to avoid doing something

side-tracked	SIDE-tracked	get away from the main track or issue
strive	strive	try
transpired	tran SPIR ed	occurred
verify	VER i FY	make sure
wincing	WIN cing	a facial expression of pain

B. Phrases and Idioms

all walks of life	all walks of life	all levels and conditions of society
being defensive	BE ING de FEN sive	defending oneself against criticism, some times where none is intended
closed body stance	closed BOD y stance	a way a person holds his or her body with arms close to the body or crossed over the chest, legs crossed or pulled up, in a protective way May even turn away from others.
issue at hand	IS sue at HAND	the topic being discussed
nonjudgmental attitude	NON judge men tal AT ti tude	accepting, not criticizing
open ended	O pen END ed	something for which there is no definite answer or decision
personal space	PER son al SPACE	the amount of space around a person that feels comfortable in communication with others, such as the distance between speakers or people in an elevator
put oneself in another's shoes	put ONE self in an O ther's shoes	to think about how another person would feel in this situation
seen through their eyes	seen through their eyes	see things as the other person would, with his or her beliefs and circumstances
take personally	take PER son ally	interpret that another's emotions, words, or actions (especially negative ones) are directed toward or caused by oneself

COMPLETION

Directions: Fill in the blank(s) with the correct word(s) from the vocabulary building glossary to complete the sentence.

1. The patient was conveyed from his room to the O.R. on a stretcher.
2. While she was elaborating about the care needed for the wound, the patient took notes on the steps involved.
3. When surgery is performed, all concerned hope for an optmal outcome.
4. Never discount the family's input as it is often very valuable.
5. The medication is to be used judiciously on the skin lesions; a little bit is better than a lot.
6. The nurse checks the patient's armband when administering medications to verify the patient's identity.

7. The fact that the patient worked in a metal foundry gave the nurse a elicit ______________ regarding the possible cause of his symptoms.
8. Each nurse must strive ______________ to do the best job possible for every patient.

VOCABULARY DIFFERENCES

Directions: Note the difference in the following similar words.

elicit vs. illicit

> *Elicit* means to bring out information from another person.
> *Illicit* means something is illegal.

Consider the difference between two meanings of *discount.*

> DIS count (noun)—means an amount of money taken off the full price.
> dis COUNT (verb)—means to disregard; to not consider valuable.

COMMUNICATION EXERCISE

Certain expressions used in English show the other person that you are listening and that you want him or her to continue to talk. Some of these expressions (from the informal to the more formal) are:

> Yeah. Mmmmm. Uh-huh. Right. Go on. Yes. I see.

Nonverbal behavior is another important way to show you are listening. Looking the speaker in the eye is a way of showing you are paying attention. Leaning forward in a chair toward the person indicates that you are really interested in what is being said. Nodding your head up and down and changing the expression on your face according to what is being said also show attention and interest. The following is an example of delegating a task to a nurse's aide.

Directions: After studying the example, write out a conversation on a separate sheet of paper where you delegate taking vital signs for several patients to the aide.

Nurse: "Jim, I want you to shower Ms. B. and change her bed. After you are finished showering and performing her hygiene care, take her for a walk in the hall down to the solarium and back."

Jim: "Does she have any special problems I need to know about?"

Nurse: "She does have a PRN lock in place and that needs to be covered with plastic before showering like I have shown you. She has dentures that need to be cleaned and she may need help with the adhesive. She uses a cane for ambulation. Check her skin before helping her dress and let me know if there are any new lesions. She has a reddened area on the sacrum."

Jim: "O.K."

Nurse: "Jim, what do you understand that you are to do?"

Jim: "I'm to shower Ms. B. and make her bed. I help her with her hygiene care and then take her for a walk to the solarium and back."

Nurse: "Yes that is right. And, please check her skin and let me know if there are any new lesions. Be sure to have her use her cane for walking."

Jim: "I've got it."

CULTURAL POINTS

1. The chapter points out that it is considered impolite in some cultures to maintain eye contact when speaking to a person. If this is true in your culture, can you explain to your peers the rationale and how another person knows you are paying attention to what he or she is saying when eye contact is not maintained?
2. With your classmates or a partner, discuss personal space. How much space do you need around you to feel comfortable when talking to others, or in an elevator? Americans generally prefer not to be touched in such situations, and will apologize if they touch or bump another, but other cultures take touching as normal. What differences have you noticed about touch within various cultures?
3. What about intentional touching, such as shaking hands or holding hands, or patting someone on the shoulder, or hugging another person? Are these the same or different in your country, and how do these instances of touching make you feel?
4. Do people in your culture have difficulty taking orders from someone younger or someone of the opposite sex? Give an example of a situation in which you might feel uncomfortable acting as a nurse for another person.

Review the chapter highlights, answer the study questions, and complete the critical thinking activities at the end of the chapter in the textbook.

EIGHT

Documentation of Nursing Care

TERMINOLOGY

Directions: Match the charting acronym in column I with the correct meaning in column II.

	Column I			Column II
1.	d	POMR	a.	Data, action, response
2.	c	MAR	b.	Subjective data, objective data, assessment, plan
3.	e	PIE	c.	Medication administration record
4.	b	SOAP	d.	Problem-oriented medical record
5.	f	SOAPIE	e.	Plan, implementation, evaluation
6.	a	DAR	f.	Subjective data, objective data, assessment, plan, implementation, evaluation

VOCABULARY

Directions: Using the textbook glossary or your dictionary, match up the term in column I that is useful in documentation with its meaning in column II.

	Column I			Column II
1.	d	radiates	a.	Difficulty breathing
2.	______	productive cough	b.	Large amount
3.	b	copious	c.	Coughing up material
4.	h	serosanguineous	d.	Spreads to other areas
5.	J	spasm	e.	Situated close together
6.	a	dyspnea	f.	Empty the bladder
7.	m.	paresthesia	g.	Containing an excess of fluid
8.	e	paroxysmal	h.	Mixed blood and serum
9.	k	distended	i.	Sudden attacks
10.	f	void	j.	Localized muscle contraction
11.	g	edematous	k.	Enlarged; stretched out
12.	o	exudate	l.	Itching
13.	______	approximated	m.	Numbness and tingling
14.	n	intact	n.	Undisturbed, uninjured
15.	L	pruritus	o.	Fluid with cellular debris

SHORT ANSWER

Directions: Write a brief answer for each question.

1. Three purposes of documentation are:
   a. provides written record of history, treatment, care & response of patient
   b. acts as a guide for reimbursement of costs of care (INS)
   c. serves as evidence of care in a court of law

2. The medical record is a legal document and for that reason nurses must adhere to the following rules:
   a. Each pg. should have an imprint of the pt's name & hospital number
   b. Preferably use black Ink
   c. Place date at Beginning of day's entries & time each entry
   d. chart the initial assessment at beginning of shift
   e. Charting is done only by person who made observation or performed
   f. Write legally & Print (use acronyms, ABBR)
   g. sign with 1 initial plus last name & title (J. Jones, LPN; m. white, SVN)
   h. Chart objective data after completing task (NEVER BEFORE)
   i. A horizontal line is drawn thru center of empty line or part of line

   j. If late entry, circle it, write "Late entry" & your initials above

3. Briefly correlate the nursing process to the process of charting.
   Nurse writes down observations made about the patient's condition notes the care & treatment that was delivered and adds the patient's response. Documentation shows progress toward expected outcomes. Useful for supervisory purposes to determine how staff is performing.

4. The six main methods of charting are:
   a. Source-oriented or narrative style - focuses on patients disease
   b. problem oriented medical Records (POMR) focus on problems experienced by pt.
   c. Focus charting - centers on pt. from a positive perspective
   d. Charting by exception - focuses on deviance, using preset protocols
   e. Computer-assisted charting - where data is input to the computer
   f. case-management system charting - tracks variances from critical pathway

COMPLETION

Directions: Fill in the blank(s) with the correct word(s) to correctly complete the sentence.

1. Insurance companies rely on documentation to estimate reimbursement of expenses for care given.

2. Documentation is used to track the application of the nursing process.

3. Documentation should show progress toward expected outcomes listed on the nursing care plan.

4. Only health care professionals caring for the patient, or those involved in legitimate research or teaching, should have access to the chart.

5. The chart is the property of the health facility or agency.

6. Narrative charting requires the documentation of care in chronological order.

7. An advantage of source-oriented—or narrative—charting is that it indicates the patient's baseline condition for each shift.

8. POMR methods of charting are said to improve continuity of care and communication by keeping relative data related to a problem all in one place.

9. Focus charting is directed at a nursing diagnosis, a patient problem (pressure sore), a concern, a sign , a symptom, or a(n) event (return from surgery)

10. An advantage of the FOCUS charting method is that it shortens charting time by using many flowsheets and checklists.

11. Charting by exception is based on the assumption that all standards of practice are carried out and met with a normal or expected response unless otherwise documented

12. The heart of the charting by exception method is unit-specific protocols and standards of nursing care.

13. An advantage of the charting by exception method of documentation is that it highlights abnormal data and patient trends.

14. An advantage of some computer-assisted charting is that documentation is done as interventions are performed.

15. To protect patient confidentiality when using computer-assisted charting, each nurse must have a password in order to access the computerized chart.

16. A major advantage of computer documentation is that notes are always legible + easy to read

17. When a case management system is used, documentation of variances is placed on the back of the critical pathway sheets.

18. When documenting, the patient's needs, problems, and activities should be presented in terms of behavior.

19. A Kardex is a quick reference for current information about the patient and ordered treatments

20. Home care charting must particularly note safety factors in place and the need for continued care.

ABBREVIATIONS

Directions: Consult Appendix 5 and list the abbreviation for each of the following terms that are often used when charting.

1. activities of daily living adL
2. as desired ad lib
3. estrogen replacement therapy ert
4. bathroom privileges BRP
5. genitourinary GU
6. dyspnea on exertion DOE
7. coronary artery disease CAD
8. chief complaint CC
9. hypertension HTN
10. upper respiratory infection URI
11. within normal limits WNL

12. last menstrual period LMP
13. transient ischemic attack TIA
14. potassium K
15. treatment TX
16. congestive heart failure CHF
17. right lower quadrant RLQ
18. discontinue dc
19. date of birth DOB
20. electrocardiogram ECG, EKG
21. short of breath SOB
22. fetal heart rate FHR
23. health maintenance organization HMO
24. left lower lobe LLL
25. magnetic resonance imaging MRI
26. immediately stat
27. nothing by mouth NPO
28. physical therapy P.T.
29. range of motion Rom
30. urinalysis UA

MULTIPLE CHOICE

*Directions: Choose the **best** answer for each of the following questions.*

1. The patient's occupation and religious preference may be found on the
   1. physician's history and physical sheets.
   2. nursing admission assessment sheets.
   3. face sheet of the chart.
   4. admission and treatment consent form.

2. A specific advantage of source-oriented or narrative charting is that it
   1. is lengthy and thorough.
   2. provides subjective information about the patient.
   3. reflects the patient's conditions in chronological order.
   4. Is concise and often read by physicians.

3. A disadvantage of POMR documentation is that it
   1. provides for control of quality of care.
   2. reduces duplication of information and recording.
   3. speaks only to abnormalities in the patient's condition.
   4. fragments data due to much recording on flow sheets.

4. A FOCUS charting note contains
   1. description of the patient's present condition.
   2. data, action, and response.
   3. subjective information, objective information, assessment, and plan.
   4. statement of problem, action, and result.

5. Charting by exception's goal is to
   1. provide a comprehensive database.
   2. decrease lengthy narrative entries.
   3. utilize flow sheets only.
   4. make charting flow more smoothly.

6. The total amount of oral fluids consumed for the shift is recorded on the
   1. assessment database.
   2. intravenous fluid flow sheet.
   3. daily activity flow sheet.
   4. 24-hour intake and output flow sheet.

7. A notation of a physician's visit to the patient should be made by the nurse on the
   1. nurse's notes or activity flow sheet.
   2. consultation record.
   3. Kardex or computer care plan.
   4. physician's order sheet.

8. The type of IV catheter in use would be found charted on the
   1. physician's order sheet.
   2. daily activity flow sheet.
   3. medication administration record.
   4. intravenous flow sheet.

9. A legally acceptable way to correct a charting error is to
   1. use "white-out" to keep the chart neat.
   2. line through the word and write "error" above it.
   3. use ink to obliterate the word and write a word above it.
   4. tear out the page the error is on and begin charting for that shift again.

10. Which one of the following is NOT considered essential information to be included in documentation?
    1. number of friends who visited
    2. change in a sign or symptom
    3. changes in behavior
    4. physician's visit

11. The patient has redness of the left eye. "Left eye" is abbreviated as
    1. OD
    2. OS
    3. OU
    4. LE

12. One rule to follow when documenting is to
    1. use complete sentences.
    2. use only accepted abbreviations.
    3. include the patient's name.
    4. include your opinion.

13. If another nurse asks you to chart on a patient for him or her and gives you a list of the data, you should
    1. chart chronologically according to the list.
    2. refuse to chart what you have not done yourself.
    3. ask what else you can do to help as you cannot chart for the other nurse.
    4. chart on the activity flow sheets, but not in the nurse's notes.

14. A very important part of charting from the hospital's point of view is
    1. noting the physician's visits.
    2. noting the discharge time on the chart.
    3. documenting when visitors come.
    4. documenting equipment being used.

15. When documenting that a patient has refused a treatment, you should include
    1. consequences of refusing the treatment.
    2. why the treatment was refused.
    3. attempts to change the patient's mind.
    4. why the treatment is important to recovery.

CRITICAL THINKING ACTIVITIES

1. Compare the six different forms of charting and choose the one that seems to you to be the most logical and easy to use. ______________________

2. From the following scenario, list the assessment data, define the main problem in the form of a nursing diagnosis, and write an expected outcome.

   J.T., age 22, was involved in an automobile accident. She arrives via ambulance at the emergency room. She is able to answer questions and can follow commands, although she is strapped to a backboard to prevent spinal movement. Her pupils are equal and reactive to light. X-rays show a fracture of her right femur and she is unable to move her right leg without excruciating pain. There is a laceration on her right wrist. She complains of pain in the right wrist.

   Assessment data:

   Nursing diagnosis:

   Expected outcome:

MEETING CLINICAL OBJECTIVES

Directions: The following suggested activities will help you meet the stated clinical practice objectives for the chapter. Review your school's clinical objectives for the week and outline a plan of activities that will help you meet them. If unsure as to how to meet them, consult with your instructor at the beginning of the clinical day.

1. After obtaining permission, read nurse's notes that staff nurses have written and identify four characteristics of good documentation.
2. Review each of the flow sheet chart forms for the types of information to be recorded.
3. Write out nurse's notes daily on each assigned patient, trying to create a "picture" of the patient for someone else reading the notes. Edit your notes to make them more concise and objective.
4. Review the hospital charting/documentation manual for specific requirements of the assigned facility that may vary from what you learned in lecture or from textbooks.
5. Ask a staff nurse to show you how the computer is used in the facility to chart, update care plans, order supplies, discontinue charges, and so forth.

STEPS TOWARD BETTER COMMUNICATION

VOCABULARY BUILDING GLOSSARY

Term	Pronunciation	Definition
acronym	AC ro nym	a word formed from the first letters or parts of other words
adage	AD age	a saying
adhere to	ad HERE to	follow rules, pay attention to
ambiguous	am BIG u ous	not clear, not specific

audit	AU dit	an official examination of records
brevity	BREV i ty	not using a lot of words, shortness
compiled	com PILEd	to put together item by item
duration	du RA tion	the length of time
jot	JOT	make a quick written note
noteworthy	NOTE wor thy	important
offshoot	OFF shoot	a new development or direction
reimbursement	re im BURSE ment	to pay back someone for money that has been paid out
rule of thumb	RULE of thumb	a guideline
time frame	TIME frame	limits of a period of time

VOCABULARY EXERCISE

Directions: Substitute words from the glossary for the underlined words.

1. The saying was not clear.

   The adage was ambiguous.

2. The examination of records showed a need to pay back the patient's money.

   The audit showed a need to remburse the patient's money.

3. The guideline is that the length of time of the office visit should follow the rules.

   The rule of thumb is that the duration of the office visit should adheire the rules.

4. The student should make a quick note of the letters standing for words that she feels are important and put together a list.

   The student should jot down the acronyms that she feels are noteworthy and complites a list.

5. The limited time required the doctor use only a few words in talking about the new development in the problem.

   The time-frame required that the doctor use brevity in talking about the off-shoot in the problem.

PRONUNCIATION AND INTONATION SKILLS

A statement ends with a falling voice pitch or intonation, for example: She has completed the documentation.

A question may end with either a rising or a falling intonation of the voice.

Questions that can be answered "yes" or "no" end with a rising pitch: (N=nurse; S=student)

1. N: Did you complete the charting?

   S: Yes, I did.

2. N: Is the patient ready for surgery?

   S: Yes, he is.

3. N: Are there any donuts left in the coffee room?

   S: No, sorry. They are all gone!

Questions that ask for information with a question word ("who," "what," "when," "where," etc.) end with a falling pitch.

1. N: When did you give the meds?

   S: Fifteen minutes ago.

2. N: Who is working the second shift?

   S: M.A.

3. N: Why is the computer terminal still on?

   S: Oops, sorry. I forgot to turn it off.

Directions: Look at the following sentences and mark whether the pitch is rising (up) or falling (down). Practice asking and answering the questions with a partner.

1.	Where is the doctor?	up	down
2.	Have you finished taking the vital signs?	up	down
3.	Can I bring you some fresh water?	up	down
4.	What was K.J.'s temperature?	up	down
5.	Did you initial the error in the chart?	up	down
6.	Who ate all the donuts?	up	down

COMMUNICATION EXERCISE

Look at the method of charting you chose in Critical Thinking Activity #1 in the textbook chapter. Explain to a partner why you chose that method of charting. Listen to your partner explain his or her choice.

Review the chapter highlights, answer the study questions, and complete the critical thinking activities at the end of the chapter in the textbook.

NINE

Patient Teaching

TERMINOLOGY

Directions: Fill in the blank(s) with the correct term(s) from the terms list in the textbook chapter to complete the sentence.

1. Learning through lecture or discussion is termed auditory learning.
2. One teaching method used for visual learners is to show a videotape.
3. Performing procedures step by step in the laboratory promotes Kinesthetic learning.
4. A behavioral objections is a statement that represents the desired changes or additions to current behaviors and attitudes.
5. Obtaining current knowledge Base from the patient regarding what was taught assures that he or she understands.
6. Obtaining a return demonstration of the technique of changing a dressing is a good way to evaluate the success of your teaching on that subject.

SHORT ANSWER

Directions: Write a brief answer for each question.

1. When assessing learning needs of a patient, you would consider the following areas:
   Factors effecting learning — cognitive domain
   Cultural values & expectations OR — affective domain,
   Confidence & abilitities — psychomotor domain
2. When preparing a teaching plan for a 78-year-old patient, you should consider physical factors that might affect learning, such as:
   If patient wears glasses, needs a hearing aid, check for comprehension, use of large print
3. Situational factors that indicate it may not be a good time to begin teaching a patient are:
   If Patient has pain, fatigue, a sense of being overwhelmed by all this is happening & multiple people coming in & out of patient unit

4. Three types of resources for patient teaching and meeting patient learning needs are:
   a. book & Articles, Videotapes, pamplets, hands on equipment
   b. Hospital Social workers & patient representatives
   c. Nursing specialists

5. When teaching the elderly patient, it is important to be certain that:
   a. keep distractions & noice to a minimal
   b. provide good lighting
   c. printed materials should be lg. print
   d. Use short sentences & speak slowing
   Be sure glasses are on, hearing aid turned on
   check for comprehension

COMPLETION

Directions: Fill in the blank(s) with the correct word(s) to complete the sentence.

1. For teaching to be successful, it is necessary to work within the patient's values and cultural system.
2. To build confidence in the patient's ability to perform a task, break the task down into small steps.
3. Play techniques are very successful when teaching children.
4. When preparing a teaching plan that includes written materials, never assume that the patient is literate; find out.
5. The nursing diagnosis utilized for patients who have learning needs is "Knowledge Deficit" followed by the specifics such as "related to self-administration of insulin".
6. In order for the patient to master and retain new information, consistancy of teaching is important.
7. During a teaching session, it is wise to frequently ask if there are any questions.
8. When a patient is performing a return demonstration as a method of feedback, allow the patient to perform at his or her own speed.
9. Discharge teaching begins at the time of admission.
10. A teaching moment is when a patient is at an optimal level of readness to learn and apply a particular piece of information.
11. Learning to draw up a medication is an example of Kinesthetic learning.
12. When teaching the elderly, the pace is slowed to allow more time for processing the information.
13. Advanced age of the learner may interfere with dexterity or strength for performing certain tasks.
14. The reason for assessing what the patient knows about the topic to be taught is so that you can build upon the current Knowledge Base.
15. One aspect of preparing a patient for teaching is to show him or her the advantages of learning what he or she needs to know.
16. When several people are involved in the care and teaching of a patient, consistancy in teaching is important.

17. During a teaching session it is important to frequently ask for _feedback_.

18. Each ongoing teaching session should begin with a _review_ of what has been previously learned.

19. The best type of feedback for a psychomotor skill is a _return demonstration_

20. At discharge it is very helpful to send a _printed_ plan home with the patient.

MULTIPLE CHOICE

*Directions: Choose the **best** answer for each of the following questions.*

1. What type of learner is the person who learns best by practicing a skill, such as drawing up medication for injection?
 1. auditory
 2. visual
 3. kinesthetic ⟵
 4. motor

2. When considering a teaching plan, the knowledge base is what the patient
 1. needs to know about a subject.
 2. is taught about a subject.
 3. expresses a desire to learn.
 4. already knows about a subject. ⟵

3. Which one of the following would be considered a "situational" block to learning?
 1. pain ⟵
 2. blindness
 3. mental impairment
 4. illiteracy

4. Which one of the following would be the best feedback that the patient has mastered the material taught? The patient
 1. presents a written outline of the material.
 2. demonstrates the task that was taught. ⟵
 3. has questions regarding the specifics of performing the task.
 4. reads all of the written material the nurse presented.

5. An appropriate behavioral objective for a teaching plan to teach the patient to give his own insulin would be "The patient will" ✓
 1. explain the purpose of insulin.
 2. identify the signs of hypoglycemia.
 3. draw up the correct dose for each injection. ⟵
 4. identify the complications of diabetes.

6. An initial step in formulating a teaching plan is to ✓
 1. evaluate the patient's knowledge base.
 2. locate resources for teaching.
 3. write out the behavioral objectives. ⟵
 4. plan times when teaching can be accomplished.

7. Learning will be enhanced by
 1. a very specific teaching plan.
 2. a relaxed, quiet atmosphere. ⟵
 3. the sophistication of the teaching aids.
 4. use of one mode of learning.

8. A very important part of the teaching process is
 1. the type of materials used.
 2. the expertise of the teacher.
 3. documenting the teaching session.
 4. reinforcement of the material taught. ⟵

9. A patient's ability to learn would most likely be enhanced by his or her
 1. illness.
 2. anxiety.
 3. readiness. ⟵
 4. knowledge.

10. One of the best ways to increase motivation to learn is to
    1. make the environment comfortable.
    2. use a variety of learning tools.
    3. give timely feedback.
    4. explain the advantage of the learning.

11. A learning objective should contain
    1. performance criteria and conditions.
    2. encouragement and motivation.
    3. data and behaviors.
    4. learning activity and long-term need.

12. Affective learning is directed at a change in
    1. knowledge.
    2. skills.
    3. values.
    4. practices.

13. When several disciplines are involved in the care and teaching of a patient,
    1. collaboration on the plan is important.
    2. each discipline teaches one aspect of care.
    3. the nurse always oversees the teaching plan.
    4. the patient is not consulted.

14. Mr. T. is readmitted with a foot ulcer, a complication of her diabetes. She has received diabetic teaching in the past. When formulating her teaching plan, you should first
    1. tell her what she is doing wrong.
    2. assess her present knowledge base.
    3. determine her insulin requirements.
    4. write learning objectives.

15. A factor in the failure of Mr. T. to carry out the foot care teaching she had before might be
    1. a sedentary lifestyle.
    2. poor eyesight.
    3. family responsibilities.
    4. financial difficulties.

16. When Mr. T. gives you a return demonstration of the correct way to dry her feet, she does not dry between all her toes as you had instructed. The best comment would be
    1. "That's fine, Mr. T., you are making good progress."
    2. "You are reaching the bottom of the foot well, Mr. T., but you forgot to dry between your toes."
    3. "Oh oh, you forgot to dry between your toes."
    4. "Good, you've dried the top and bottom of the foot. What parts of the foot are still damp?"

17. Mr. T. is an auditory learner. Besides attending lecture, which of the following would be the best way for her to learn material?
    1. Read the chapters in the textbook.
    2. Listen again to the lectures on tape.
    3. Use flash cards to memorize facts.
    4. Practice the steps of the skills in the laboratory.

CRITICAL THINKING ACTIVITIES

1. List which modes of learning are best for you.
2. Considering your best mode of learning, what techniques might make learning nursing content easier for you?
3. Devise a general teaching plan outline for teaching patients about their medications.

MEETING CLINICAL OBJECTIVES

Directions: The following suggested activities will help you meet the stated clinical practice objectives for the chapter. Review your school's clinical objectives for the week and outline a plan of activities that will help you meet them. If unsure as to how to meet them, consult with your instructor at the beginning of the clinical day.

1. Consider the most frequent types of teaching needed on the unit to which you are assigned. Prepare teaching outlines for those topics.
2. Evaluate the learning needs of each patient to whom you are assigned.
3. Prepare a complete teaching plan and perform the teaching for a patient.
4. Practice teaching with a peer and obtain feedback.
5. Evaluate your teaching and revise the plan as needed.

STEPS TOWARD BETTER COMMUNICATION

VOCABULARY BUILDING GLOSSARY

Term	Pronunciation	Definition
admonishment	ad MON ish ment	scolding, criticizing, warning
cognition	cog NI tion	the process of thinking or perceiving
detach	de TACH	to remove, separate
deficit	DEF i cit	to lack, to be missing
dexterity	dex TER i ty	skill or ability, especially with the hands
domains	do MAINS	areas
frame of reference	FRAME of REF er ence	the knowledge and beliefs that affect one's understanding of new information
goes a long way	goes a LONG way	is very helpful
intact	in TACT	all in one piece, not broken
literate	LIT er ate	the ability to read and write
patient teaching	PA tient TEACH ing	teaching a patient
taut	TAUT	tight
teaching moments	TEACH ING MO ments	times that are best for teaching because of the situation, mood, and condition of the learner

COMPLETION

Directions: Fill in the blank(s) with the correct word(s) from the vocabulary building glossary to complete the sentence.

1. Teaching a patient how to self-catheterize requires some degree of __patient teaching__ on the part of the patient.
2. It is necessary to know whether the patient is __dexterous__ before using written materials as part of the teaching process.

3. The patient has a deficit in regard to knowledge about the side effects of his medication.

4. While administering the patient's medications after his afternoon rest, a good teaching moment appeared for teaching information about the side effects of the medication.

5. Learning usually takes longer when the subject matter is outside of the patient's cognition.

VOCABULARY EXERCISE

Look at these two words which have the same sound and spelling, but have two different meanings and are used differently. Can you explain the meanings and uses?

patient vs. patient

1. patient - person
2. patient - response to time frame situation

These next two words sound the same, but are spelled differently. What is their relationship to the words above?

patients vs. patience

3. patients - people
4. patience - response to situation

WORD ATTACK SKILLS

Directions: Look at the words below and think about how they relate to one another.

1. The root, CO +GNOSCERE, means to come to know.
   cognition (noun)—the process of thinking or perceiving
   cognitive (adj)—involving thought and knowledge; knowing
   cognizant (adj)—having knowledge; aware
   recognize (verb)—to see again and know or remember
   recognition (noun)—remembering someone or something when you see or hear it

   Example: The patient was not cognizant of his surroundings, but he recognized his family.

2. detach/attach (soft *ch* as in chair) mean to unfasten or separate/to fasten to.

   Example: She detached the call light from the bed rail and attached it to the pillowcase.

COMMUNICATION EXERCISE

1. Read the dialogue with a partner, giving feed back about pronunciation and comprehensibility (how easy it is to understand).

Nurse:	"Mr. O., I need to teach you how to cleanse your wound."
Mr. O.:	"I need to do that myself?"
Nurse:	"Yes, unless you can convince your granddaughter to come over and do it for you."
Mr. O.:	"She's awfully busy with school and work."

Nurse: "O.K. then. First you wash your hands and then put on the gloves. Next, you remove the old dressing and put it into a sealable plastic bag. Then, use some of this saline solution on a gauze pad to cleanse around the wound. You need to cleanse from the inside of the wound outward first on one side and then with another moistened gauze pad on the other side."

Mr. O.: "Do I have to cleanse down in the wound?"

Nurse: "No, that might disrupt the healing tissue. Then apply the new dressing and tape it in place."

Mr. O.: "Can I do the cleaning tomorrow before I go home so that you can watch to see if I do it correctly?"

Nurse: "Certainly. That is a good idea."

2. With a partner, write a short dialogue teaching a patient how to empty a Foley catheter leg drainage bag. Correct and practice your dialogue, then join another pair and teach them, using your dialogue.
3. Tell how you could use each of the three ways of teaching to teach a patient to develop a weight reduction diet.

CULTURAL POINTS

1. What teaching methods were used in your elementary and high school? Were they different than the methods used in schools today? Share your experience in a group with people of different ages and from different countries. How do your experiences differ?
2. Has your learning style changed through the years? Do you learn in the same way you did as a child, or have you learned a different way?
3. Are you aware of any traditional medicines or healing techniques that were/are used in your culture or your family? Any "folk" medicines or traditions your grandparents used? Share these in small groups, and talk about why they may have worked.

Review the chapter highlights, answer the study questions, and complete the critical thinking activities at the end of the chapter in the textbook.

TEN

Growth and Development: Infancy through Adolescence

TERMINOLOGY

A. MATCHING

Directions: Match the terms in column I with the definitions in column II.

Column I		Column II
1. ______ bonding	a.	knowledge and thinking processes
2. ______ cephalocaudal	b.	union of ovum and sperm
3. ______ cognitive	c.	male or female
4. ______ conception	d.	brother or sister
5. ______ egocentrism	e.	fertilized egg
6. ______ gender	f.	period of three months
7 ______ neonate	g.	able to survive outside the womb
8. ______ peers	h.	newborn
9. ______ puberty	i.	instinctive protective action
10. ______ reflex	j.	sense of attachment between two people
11. ______ sibling	k.	feeling that I am the center of the world
12. ______ trimester	l.	others of similar age and background
13. ______ vernix	m.	sexual maturation
14. ______ viable	n.	cheesy, waxy substance that protects fetal skin
15. ______ zygote	o.	proceeding from head to tail

B. COMPLETION

Directions: Fill in the blank(s) with the correct word(s) from the terms list in the chapter in the textbook to complete the sentence.

1. Theory about human development and behavior is based primarily on ____________________.
2. Ordinal position, the ____________________ in which siblings are born into a family, is thought to be a factor in growth and development by some people.
3. The ____________________ reflex is elicited by making a loud noise near the baby.
4. Children learn ____________________ during Erikson's stage of Initiative.

5. The development of __________________ is learning about what is right and wrong.
6. __________________ is a combination of verbal ability, reasoning, memory, imagination, and judgment.
7. During the middle years of childhood, children begin developing __________________ competence.
8. By the end of adolescence, __________________ should be fairly well established and this includes a moral code.
9. The chromosomes contained in the __________________ inherited from one's parents carry the blueprints of development for the child.
10. A __________________ is a method of discipline where the child spends quiet time alone without toys.

REVIEW OF STRUCTURE AND FUNCTION

Directions: Write a brief answer for each question.

1. In the germinal stage of prenatal development, how soon does cell division occur?
____
2. When does the blastocyst attach to the uterine wall and how does this occur? ____________
____
3. When does the embryonic stage begin?
____
4. At what point does the heart begin beating?
____
5. At what point in time are 95% of the body's parts already formed?
____
6. What is the approximate size of the fetus by the fifth month?
____
7. What causes multiple births? __________________________________
____
8. At what average age does puberty for a female occur?
____
9. What is the average age of puberty in the male?
____

IDENTIFICATION

Directions: For the following developmental milestones, identify the age at which they generally occur.

a. 0-1 b. 2-3 c. 4-5 d. 6-9 e. 10-12 f. 13-18

1. ______ full set of deciduous teeth
2. ______ toilet trained (bladder)
3. ______ knows 8,000–14,000 words

4. ______ develops some autonomy
5. ______ sexual preference is developed
6. ______ sexual maturation has occurred
7. ______ gender roles have been learned
8. ______ seeks friendships and experiences outside the home
9. ______ may show signs of prepuberty
10. ______ begins to want to accomplish things
11. ______ denial of privileges becomes a more effective discipline
12. ______ begins Piaget's stage of Formal Operations
13. ______ grows 10–12 inches in 12 months
14. ______ develops object permanence
15. ______ begins to engage in pretend play

SHORT ANSWER

Directions: Write a brief answer for each question.

1. Erik Erikson's theory of development defined eight psychosocial stages that lead to a healthy ego. Each stage is identified by:
____
____

2. Jean Piaget developed a theory about how children learn based on the need to adapt to the environment. He stressed two principles, which are:
   a. ______________________________
   b. ______________________________

3. Lawrence Kohlberg developed a theory of moral development. Identify a behavior that belongs in each of the following three stages of moral development.
   a. Preconventional reasoning: ______________________________
   ____
   b. Conventional reasoning: ______________________________
   ____
   c. Postconventional reasoning: ______________________________
   ____

4. Basic principles of growth and development are:
   a. ______________________________
   b. ______________________________
   c. ______________________________
   d. ______________________________
   e. ______________________________

5. List one behavior that indicates positive accomplishment for each of the following stages of childhood according to Erikson:
   a. Trust vs. Mistrust: ______________________________
   b. Autonomy vs. Shame and Doubt: ______________________________
   ____

c. Initiative vs. Guilt: ____

d. Industry vs. Inferiority: ____

e. Identity vs. Role Confusion: ____

COMPLETION

Directions: Fill in the blank(s) with the correct word(s) to complete the sentence.

1. The rate of growth and development is ________________.
2. According to Kohlberg, moral values are not internalized until about age ________________.
3. According to Kohlberg, children begin using conventional reasoning at about age ________________.
4. Growth occurs in orderly and ________________ ways.
5. Development is multidimensional and involves ________________, ________________, and ________________ aspects.
6. Each child has ________________, half from the mother and half from the father.
7. A full pregnancy lasts ________________ weeks.
8. It is best if a woman is well ________________ before becoming pregnant.
9. It is considered healthiest for a woman to gain about ________________ pounds during pregnancy.
10. Prolonged stress in the pregnant woman interferes with adequate ________________ and ________________ to the fetus.
11. Infancy is the period from birth through ________________.
12. A typical newborn sleeps for ________________ hours a day.
13. Most babies can be given table food at ________________ of age.
14. Permanent eye color develops in the infant by ________________ months.
15. Brain growth is very rapid during the ________________ year.

MULTIPLE CHOICE

Directions: Choose the ***best*** *answer for each of the following questions.*

1. If physical growth is normal, a child will
   1. double the birth weight by 2 months of age.
   2. gain 10–12 inches in length by 6 months of age.
   3. triple the birth weight by one year of age.
   4. double head size by 6 months of age.

2. Normal motor development results in a child being able to
   1. draw before he can walk.
   2. coordinate small muscles before large ones.
   3. lift the chest before being able to lift the head.
   4. sit before being able to stand.

3. The cognitive skill of object permanence occurs at about ______ months.
   1. 8
   2. 6
   3. 12
   4. 3

4. Insecurity with strangers begins at about ______ months.
   1. 4
   2. 6
   3. 9
   4. 12

5. The primary environmental influence on physical growth is
   1. nurturing
   2. attention
   3. nutrition
   4. heredity

6. A positive function of day care for the child is that it
   1. promotes socialization skills.
   2. helps build immunity to childhood illness.
   3. prevents separation anxiety.
   4. builds self-esteem.

7. It is important that the 6–12 year old child receive
   1. strict discipline when misbehavior occurs.
   2. encouragement and praise for tasks accomplished.
   3. lots of guidance when performing a task.
   4. opportunities to make his or her own decisions.

8. A major reason that adolescents need more sex education is that
   1. communities are identifying a need for it.
   2. adolescents are maturing physically earlier.
   3. statistics indicate that 50% of girls and 66% of boys have had intercourse by age 18.
   4. adolescents are curious about their bodies and want to participate in life in grown-up ways.

9. Conflict between the young adolescent and parents is partly influenced by
   1. growth in intelligence as the child matures.
   2. major hormonal shifts that occur at this time.
   3. the many activities in which the adolescent participates.
   4. the need for strong attachment to the parents while spending more time with peers.

10. A sign of anorexia nervosa in an adolescent girl might be
    1. spending all her time in her room.
    2. eating little and exercising a lot.
    3. refusing to participate in family activities.
    4. cutting classes and getting poor grades.

11. According to Piaget, the child starts seeing him- or herself as separate from others at age
    1. 4–8 months.
    2. 8–12 months.
    3. 18–24 months.
    4. 2–4 years.

12. A child cannot be expected to logically manipulate abstract and unobservable concepts until about age
    1. 4.
    2. 6.
    3. 8.
    4. 11.

13. Bonding is important for the infant because it helps the person develop
    1. relationships with others throughout life.
    2. a good relationship with its parents.
    3. interest in other people.
    4. full growth and development.

14. A milestone in motor development for the toddler is
    1. climbing stairs without holding on.
    2. becoming toilet trained.
    3. throwing a ball accurately.
    4. increasing height by 3–5 inches.

TABLE ACTIVITY

Directions: Fill in the table with the changes that occur to males and females during puberty.

PHYSICAL CHANGES OF PUBERTY

Male	Female

CRITICAL THINKING ACTIVITIES

1. What ways can you think of to assist adolescents with the areas of concern listed in the chapter?
2. What do parents need to know about the growth and development of their new infant?

MEETING CLINICAL OBJECTIVES

Directions: The following suggested activities will help you meet the stated clinical practice objectives for the chapter. Review your school's clinical objectives for the week and outline a plan of activities that will help you meet them. If unsure as to how to meet them, consult with your instructor at the beginning of the clinical day.

1. Visit a preschool and observe the types of play occurring among the children.
2. Teach a newly pregnant female about the type of prenatal care that she needs.
3. Perform a Denver Developmental Screening on a child.
4. Assist parents to develop consistent methods of discipline for children of various ages.

STEPS TOWARD BETTER COMMUNICATION

VOCABULARY BUILDING GLOSSARY

Term	Pronunciation	Definition
A. Individual Terms		
cyanotic	cy a NOT ic	bluish color of the skin
deciduous	de CID u ous	related to shedding or falling off of the old (later replaced by the new); i.e., deciduous trees lose their leaves in the winter and children lose their teeth at certain ages
direly	DIRE ly	urgently
erupt	e RUPT	come out, break through, such as teeth erupting through the gums
resilient	re SIL i ent	able to recover its original shape, recover from difficulty
suffer	SUF fer	to undergo pain, loss, or disadvantage
B. Phrases		
baby fat	BA by FAT	the layer of fat under a healthy infant's skin, not the fat of overweight people
bounce back	BOUNCE back	come back to an original position or condition (like a ball bounces)
gender stereotypes	gen der STER e o types	certain actions or roles are automatically assumed for a gender/sex
growth spurt	growth SPURT	a period during which growth happens very rapidly

COMPLETION

Directions: Fill in the blank(s) with the correct word(s) from the vocabulary building glossary to complete the sentence.

1. The bluish tint to the skin indicates that the newborn is ____________________.
2. Babies often become fussy when a tooth begins to ____________________.
3. Although children can become very sick quite quickly, they are usually ____________________ and get well just as fast.
4. The ____________________ on an infant is partly what makes it so soft and cuddly.
5. The idea that only boys become heavy equipment operators is a ____________________.
6. Children frequently stay the same size for weeks at a time and then have a ____________________ where they increase height by a half an inch or more.

VOCABULARY EXERCISE

1. English often has many words that mean basically the same thing, and can be used interchangeably with only slight difference in meaning. It is often thought to be good literary style to use different words rather than repeat the same one. Below is one example of words with similar meanings found in this chapter:

   resilient/flexible/bounce back

   Can you give two words that mean the same thing as the words below:

   a. vital   b. helping

2. Give examples of abilities a person might have related to the following kinds of intelligence:

   Linguistic   Bodily kinesthetic

   Mathematical   Interpersonal

   Spatial   Intrapersonal

   Musical

COMMUNICATION EXERCISE

1. With a partner, write a dialogue of a nurse helping the parents of a 2–4 year old child develop a consistent method of discipline. Among your classmates or friends, find a mother of young children and ask if the dialogue is realistic or useful.
2. Write and practice a dialogue with a partner, showing a parent or health care worker talking with a child about his feelings when he has to go to the hospital for surgery.

CULTURAL POINTS

1. Compare the raising of children as suggested in the chapter and the way children are raised in your native country. What are the similarities? What are the differences? Discuss these in a small group. How do you learn to parent in your country? How do people learn here?
2. Physical punishment, for the most part, is no longer considered an acceptable method for disciplining children. Many people, in this country as well as other countries and cultures, were raised with physical punishment and may resort to it as parents in moments of stress. Can you recall stories of how your parents were disciplined or do you have memories of physical punishment yourself? What is your feeling about its effectiveness versus the new methods? How would you help a person adapt to the new cultural norms?
3. Some language theorists say that people learn a second language in much the same way they learned their first language as children. First, they listen and begin to understand but do not speak, then they respond to questions with brief answers, and learn to communicate to make their needs known. Later, they become more fluent as they have need and opportunity to interact with other speakers of the language they are learning. They learn and speak better in a supportive, nonthreatening environment than when they are nervous and afraid. How do you feel about this? Is this the way you experienced learning a language? Share your experience with a first language speaker. How do they feel about the languages they have learned?

Review the chapter highlights, answer the study questions, and complete the critical thinking activities at the end of the chapter in the textbook.

ELEVEN

Adulthood and the Family

TERMINOLOGY

A. MATCHING

Directions: Match the terms in column I with the definitions in column II.

	Column I		Column II
1. d	baby boomers	a.	Being fully developed
2. b	career	b.	Work which requires specific training
3. h	empty nest	c.	Trade, professional, or occupational
4. j	intimacy	d.	People born between 1946 and 1964
5. g	libido	e.	Decreased flexibility of the eye lens
6. a	maturity	f.	Loss of hearing
7. i	mentor	g.	The sex drive
8. f	presbycusis	h.	Children have left the home causing a sense of loss
9. e	presbyopia	i.	Teacher or coach
10. c	vocational	j.	Close, meaningful relationship

B. COMPLETION

Directions: Fill in the blank(s) with the correct word(s) from the terms list in the chapter in the textbook to complete the sentence.

1. According to Schaie, the young adult stage of cognitive development is the achievement stage.
2. The responsiblity stage, concerned with real-life problems, occurs in middle adulthood.
3. Some middle adults who have multiple responsibilities are in the executive substage.
4. In Erikson's stage of generativity, the middle adult guides the lives of younger people.
5. Stagnation occurs if the middle adult is engaged in inactivity and self-absorption.
6. Offspring who return to the parental home for a period of time are termed boomerang children.
7. Middle adults who find themselves with both dependent children and dependent parents needing care giving are in the sandwich generation.

SHORT ANSWER

Directions: Write a brief answer for each question.

1. The first stage of cognitive development according to Schaie is the Achievement stage. List three goals of young adults in this stage.
   a. continuing education
   b. careers and
   c. psychosocial Development

2. List three types of responsibilities middle adults encounter when they enter the responsibility stage according to Schaie.
   a. caring for parents
   b. Going back to school
   c. changing lifestyle to become healthier

3. Three functions of those middle adults who are in the executive substage according to Schaie are:
   a. delegate
   b. juggle roles
   c. manage complex situations

4. In Erikson's stage of Intimacy vs. Isolation, a young adult who adjusts positively might exhibit the following behaviors.
   a. volunteering
   b. mentor to younger adults
   c. close family ties

5. When a middle adult is in the stage of Generativity vs. Stagnation, behaviors indicating a positive adjustment might be:
   concerned for others + want to contribute - become mentors, self-confident and nurture younger people

6. List three functions of families.
   a. physical maintenance - providing essentials
   b. protection - create atomospere for health & safety
   c. Nurturance - providing love, care & guidance

7. List three possible outcomes for the people involved in divorce.
   a. affects parents + other relatives
   b. major cause of poverty
   c. grandparents lose opportunities to be with children

8. Risky behaviors of young adults that may affect health are:
   a. chemical abuse
   b. over-eating
   c. in-adequate sleep
   d. inactive lifestyle
   e. sexual promiscuity

9. The major health problems of middle adults include:
   heart disease, cancer, vascular disease, obesity, diabetes, alcohol abuse, accidents, hypertension, mental illness

TABLE ACTIVITY

PHYSICAL CHANGES

Directions: Fill in the table with the typical physical changes of young and middle adults.

PHYSICAL CHANGES OF YOUNG AND MIDDLE ADULTS

Young Adult	Middle Adult
skeletal develpement completed Dental maturity Physical Growth of Brain continues Best years for Reproduction Physically at their Best sexual Preferences are Identified	changes of aging (declines begin) natural Redistribution of Body wt. Presbyopia occurs (decreased Flexibility eye lens) (cataracts may develop) Presbycusis (loss of hearing) Gradual Compression of Spinal Column (disks shrink) Muscles lose tone + elasticity Blood Pressure Increases skin becomes less resilient + wrinkles appear Digestive muscles change + cause food intolerances Graying hair – loss of hair Hormone Production slows Menopause Begins

COMPLETION

Directions: Fill in the blank(s) with the correct word(s) to complete the sentence.

1. Stress-related illnesses begin to be common after age 30.
2. Personality development continues throughout the lifespan.
3. Approximately 11% percent of adults of all ages live alone.
4. By age 40, a woman is statistically at high risk during a pregnancy.
5. The average age for menopause is 51.
6. Creativity is believed to peak during middle adulthood.
7. Leisure activities can be healthy ways to reduce stress.
8. It is vital to the marriage that middle adults develop mutual interests and activities.
9. Throughout adulthood, close family ties are very important.
10. Physical changes related to aging begin in the middle years of life
11. A factor that has greatly affected relationships among extended family members is divorce.
12. Nearly 70 % of two-parent families have two wage earners.
13. Divorce ends approximately 50 % of marriages.
14. The increasing incidence of divorce is seen as a major cause of poverty among women.
15. Biannual mammograms are recommended for all women beginning at age 40.
16. A Pap test is recommended for women to screen for cervical cancer.

17. The earning power of women continues to be 75%-80% of what men earn in similar work.
18. Noisy work settings and loud music contribute to eventual hearing loss.
19. mentor with others is the focus of psychosocial development in middle adults.
20. Middle adults who have centered their lives around their children may experience the empty nest syndrome when the children leave home.

MULTIPLE CHOICE

*Directions: Choose the **best** answer for each of the following questions.*

1. A 22-year-old female who has a back injury is assigned to you. You recall that a major developmental task for this age is
   1. establishing trust relationships.
   2. establishing close personal relationships.
   3. guiding other young people.
   4. balancing work with a multitude of other roles.
2. A major factor that will impact the health of young adults when they become older adults is
   1. length of the work week.
   2. compliance with recommended physical exams.
   3. lack of attention to good nutrition.
   4. degree of affluence that they will attain.

Situation: M.J. is 26 years old. She is married, has an executive position and works 50–60 hours a week. She gets little exercise and does not eat many balanced meals, often eating fast food between meetings. She complains of fatigue and insomnia.

3. M.J. has come into the clinic for a Pap smear. At this time you would reinforce teaching regarding
   1. the best years for child-bearing.
   2. the need to do monthly breast self-examination.
   3. prevention of sexually transmitted diseases.
   4. the necessity for practicing birth control.
4. You suspect her fatigue is partly caused by stress, and to combat it you recommend
   1. a daily walk.
   2. increased protein.
   3. changing jobs.
   4. A midday nap.
5. If M.J. continues her pattern of poor nutrition and eating lots of fast food, she will be at risk for
   1. obesity.
   2. chronic illness.
   3. loss of energy.
   4. malnutrition.
6. At this stage of her life, it is important that M.J. spend time maintaining
   1. activities that ensure a promotion at work.
   2. her intimate relationship with her husband.
   3. an efficient and tidy household.
   4. her heavy schedule of overtime at work.

Situation: L.Z. is 54. He has a wife and two children. He has been employed in his present job for 15 years.

7. An activity that would indicate that L.Z. is engaged in the stage of generativity is
   1. membership in the local golf club.
   2. time spent quietly working on his stamp collection.
   3. participation as a youth counselor at his church.
   4. taking his wife out to dinner at least once a week.

8. L.Z. should have his eyes examined every 2–3 years at this age because
   1. decreasing hormone levels affect vision.
   2. nutritional problems may cause vision changes.
   3. lack of exercise may affect vision.
   4. presbyopia may affect near vision.

9. As a healthy individual, L.Z. at this age can count on
   1. intellect remaining stable.
   2. a stable level of strength and endurance.
   3. an increased libido.
   4. a decline in responsibilities.

10. A physical change that L.Z. might have is
    1. steadily decreasing body fat.
    2. graying of the hair on the head.
    3. increasing muscle mass.
    4. a need for increasing amounts of sleep.

11. A blended family consists of
    1. a parent and child and a new parent.
    2. a mom, dad, and children.
    3. a single parent, a child, and a step-child.
    4. mom and her children, dad and his children.

12. A risk factor for divorce among couples is
    1. one or both partners did not finish high school.
    2. only one partner is employed.
    3. one partner's parents are deceased.
    4. one partner is over age 30.

13. A behavior indicating maturity is
    1. ability to earn a living.
    2. being respectful of elders.
    3. being able to tolerate frustration.
    4. continuing to pursue education.

CRITICAL THINKING ACTIVITIES

1. Determine which of your activities show that you are in a positive state of development according to Erikson.
2. Think about what health risks you face at this stage of your life. What can you alter in your lifestyle to decrease those risks?

MEETING CLINICAL OBJECTIVES

Directions: The following suggested activities will help you meet the stated clinical practice objectives for the chapter. Review your school's clinical objectives for the week and outline a plan of activities that will help you meet them. If unsure as to how to meet them, consult with your instructor at the beginning of the clinical day.

1. Assess an assigned patient's developmental stage.
2. Assess assigned patients for signs of the problems for which they are at the highest risk for within their age group.
3. Develop a teaching plan for the young adult to promote a healthy lifestyle that may help avoid health problems later in life.
4. Teach the middle adult about the preventive health care and diagnostic testing needed at this stage of life.

STEPS TOWARD BETTER COMMUNICATION

VOCABULARY BUILDING GLOSSARY

Term	Pronunciation	Definition
A. Individual Terms		
boomerang	BOOM e RANG	a curved stick that returns to the person who throws it (the children return home to live with their parents after living away for a while)
confidante	CON fi DANTE	a person with whom you share close personal feelings and information
down-sizing	DOWN siz ing	when companies decrease their size and expenses by letting employees go
family-friendly	FAM i ly FRIEND ly	a situation that is positive or encouraging for the well-being of a family
hot flashes	HOT flashes	a sudden sensation of extreme warmth, often accompanied by perspiration and reddening of the face caused by the hormonal changes of menopause, not external temperatures
juggle	JUG gle	keep many things happening at the same time
menopause	MEN o pause	the time when a woman ceases to have monthly menstrual periods
parenting	PAR en ting	the qualities and skills used in raising children
peak (verb)	PEAK	to be at a high point
skeptical	SKEP ti cal	not sure something is true or right, doubtful
susceptible	sus CEP ti ble	easily affected or influenced by
urbanization	ur ban i ZA tion	becoming more like a city than the country
volunteering	vol un TEER ing	helping others on a voluntary basis, not for pay
B. Phrases		
biological clock	bi o LOG i cal CLOCK	the natural growth and aging pattern of the human body, especially used about the period during which a woman can get pregnant
family ties	FAM i ly TIES	family relationships
life is all downhill	life is All DOWNhill	the best or highest part of life has been reached, and the rest of life will be worse, or going down
opposites attract	OPP o sites at TRACT	a saying that means a person is attracted to someone with opposite characteristics or qualities: a quiet person is attracted to an outgoing person, blondes to dark-haired people, etc.

COMPLETION

Directions: Fill in the blank(s) with the correct word(s) from the vocabulary building glossary to complete the sentence.

1. Young adult females often have a confidante with whom they can share problems and concerns.
2. P.T. lost his job due to down-sizing of his company.
3. Women often have a difficult time learning to juggle the responsibilities of both career and child-raising.
4. Many middle-aged couples have the problem of boomerang children who return home after being gone for a few years.
5. Unfortunately for middle-aged women, menopause often occurs at the same time that there are teenagers at home.
6. Once children leave the home, adults have more time for volunteering in the community.
7. The couple did not want the transfer the company was offering because they have family ties in the area and do not wish to be far away from all their relatives.

VOCABULARY EXERCISE

Directions: List some opposite types that might attract each other.

Example: urban vs. rural

1. quiet loud
2. blonde Brunette
3. athletic reader
4. tall short
5. large small

PRONUNCIATION AND STRESS

In the Vocabulary Building Glossary, we have indicated where the stress or accent falls in a word as it is normally used. For understanding, using the correct stress pattern is more important than using the correct sounds. There are a few basic rules for placing stress in words in English:

1. Not counting verbs, 90% of two-syllable words are stressed on the first syllable.

   healthy lifestyle caring people spinal column

2. In words with three or more syllables, one syllable gets the main stress (indicated by capital letters in the glossary), and sometimes there is a secondary stress.
3. There also are certain pronunciation patterns that can be found. In words with certain endings, like those below, the stress is on the syllable that comes before the ending.

Directions: Underline the stressed syllable, then practice the pronunciation aloud. Add other words to the list as you find them, and notice any that are different from the pattern.

-tion/-sion	-ic/-ical	-omy	-ogy	-ity
urbanization	pelvic	economy	biology	maturity
generation	chronic	autonomy	sociology	infidelity
question	biological		gerontology	validity
maturation	skeptical			flexibility
tension	physical			obesity
stagnation	cervical			promiscuity
				generativity
				personality

-ery	-edy	-istry
delivery	remedy	dentistry
grocery	tragedy	chemistry
nursery	comedy	
surgery		

COMMUNICATION EXERCISE

1. Read the following conversation. Discuss it with your classmates or a friend. Practice reading it aloud with a partner. How do you think Ms. L. will feel? What do you think she will do? Was this a good way to handle the problem?

Nurse: "Thank you for coming in today, Ms. L. I want to talk to you about your son."

Ms. L.: "Has he gotten into trouble again?"

Nurse: "No, but the kindergarten teacher brought him into the office because he has bruises on his upper arms. Do you know how he might have gotten them?"

Ms. L.: "No, not unless he got in a fight with the boys."

Nurse: "These look like an adult held him very tightly. Do you know when that could have happened?"

Ms. L.: "Well, two days ago when he wouldn't sit down and be quiet, I grabbed him and gave him a good shaking. But I didn't hurt him. That boy just won't listen!"

Nurse: "I know you think you didn't hurt him, but he is bruised. Did you know that severe shaking can cause brain damage and even death in young children?"

Ms. L.: "No! But I am sure I didn't hurt him that much."

Nurse: "It doesn't take very much when they are small. And we are required to report any suspected physical abuse—like repeated shaking, slapping, and hitting—to the authorities."

Ms. L.: "But how am I supposed to get him to listen? That is the way our parents treated us, and it didn't hurt us any!"

Nurse: "We know more now about the damage it can cause, and at any rate, there are laws about it now. Let me give you this pamphlet on discipline and make an appointment for you and your husband to come back so we can talk about other ways that you can use to discipline your son."

Ms. L.: "Well, I guess I had better do something. I don't want to hurt my son and I don't want to get in trouble with the law."

2. Discuss with a group whether you think opposites attract. Can you think of some examples? Why do you think it might be true?

CULTURAL POINTS

1. How do people in your native country learn about parenting? Are classes available or do they learn from their families? How have you learned? How do you feel about a different way of learning? What methods of discipline are common? Do you think they are effective? Would they be acceptable in the U.S.?

2. Do the three stages of adulthood follow the same pattern in your native country? In a group, talk about how they are the same or different.

Review the chapter highlights, answer the study questions, and complete the critical thinking activities at the end of the chapter in the textbook.

CULTURAL POINTS

TWELVE

Promoting Healthy Adaptation to Aging

TERMINOLOGY

A. MATCHING

Directions: Match the terms in column I with the definitions in column II.

Column I		Column II	
1. __f__	ageism	a.	Length of life
2. __c__	centenarians	b.	Statistics about populations
3. __d__	dementia	c.	People over 100 years old
4. __b__	demographics	d.	Degeneration of brain tissue
5. __h__	gerontologist	e.	Having good judgment based on accumulated knowledge
6. __a__	longevity	f.	Discrimination because of age
7. __g__	reminiscence	g.	Reviewing one's life
8. __e__	wisdom	h.	Specialists in the study of aging people

B. COMPLETION

Directions: Fill in the blank(s) with the correct term(s) from the terms list in the chapter in the textbook to complete the sentence.

1. __Benign senescence__, the normal changes of aging, begin in early adulthood.
2. Ways to look at the physical aging process are based on __biological__ theories.
3. Erikson's stage of development for older adults is called __ego integrity (state of being complete)__ vs. Despair.
4. A nurse must legally report __elder abuse__ to a law enforcement agency.
5. The __lifespan__ for human beings is 115–120 years.
6. The disengagement theory, a __psychosocial__ theory, states that it is normal for older people and society to withdraw from each other.

SHORT ANSWER

Directions: Write a brief answer for each question.

1. Identify five biologic theories on the aging process.
   a. biologic clock–body cells are programmed for a specific length of time + die
   b. free-Radical Theory–cells are damaged by toxins in environment, disease
   c. wear + tear theory–body cells + organs eventually wear out, like machinery
   d. immune system failure theory–system loses ability to protect from disease
   e. auto immune theory–body no longer recognizes self–begins to attack + break down

2. Give a probable response of an aging adult considering the following psychosocial theories of aging:
   a. Disengagement theory I don't like being ok
   normal to withdraw–no longer is credited for this idea
   b. Activity theory I Love playing cards at the rec Hall
   Remain interested + active will cont. to enjoy life + live longer
   c. Continuity theory I needed to slow down a bit, cont. to live +
   develop as unique person–will cope with aging

3. Four factors that contribute to longevity are:
   a. Good hygene–eliminates many illnesses
   b. Education–practice preventive health
   c. Life-style–healthy diet + regular excercise
   d. person's happy Personality
   Gender–women live long

4. Indicate one physical change that occurs with aging for each body system.
   a. Cardiovascular: increased heart size, thickened heart valves, less elasticity of Blood vessels
   b. Respiratory: weakened respiratory muscles, thick alveolar walls, decrease in cilia + vital capacity
   c. Musculoskeletal: thin intervertebral disks, decreased Bone Calcium, small muscle mass
   d. Integumentary: thinner, dryer skin, Loss of subcutaneous fat, Slow growth rate of hair + nails
   e. Urological: decreased bladder capacity, sphincter control, loss of nephrons
   f. Neurological: vision cataract developement, Hearing loss, Balance, increase wax production, Reflexes
   g. Endocrine: slow production of hormones, decrease metabolic rate, delayed insulin response
   h. Gastrointestinal: decrease saliva + dig. enzymes, slow peristalsis, Reduced absorption of nutrients
   i. Reproductive: decrease hormone production, Atrophy of ovaries, uterus, vagina, slowed sexual re

5. Describe the essence of Shaie's theory for cognitive development in the older adult.
   reintegrative stage–older adults are more selective about how they will spend their time.

6. Give two examples of behaviors that would indicate a person is in the stage of Ego Integrity.
   a. If satisfied with a good life–have ego integrity
   b. If unhappy about their life–will despair

7. Give three examples of activities that might help older adults maintain cognitive health.
   a. crossword puzzles
   b. books–reading + writing
   c. hobby–computer

8. Identify five signs that an older person needs assistance.
   a. soil clothing–irregular dressing
   b. Significant wt. loss
   c. Frequent Falls
   d. Social isolation
   e. Confusion about medications
   Unpaid Bills, suspicion of others, unkempt appearance

COMPLETION

Directions: Fill in the blank(s) with the correct word(s) to complete the sentence.

1. The average life span according to the U.S. Census Bureau is __79__ years.
2. Two lifestyle factors—a healthy __diet__ and regular __excercise__—are crucial to longevity.
3. A person's __personallty__ seems to affect the length of life as well as the quality.
4. Heredity seems to account for only __30%__ percent of longevity.
5. Nearly 75% of the population over age __75__ has some hearing loss.
6. __Arthritis__ is the most common chronic health problem in those over age 75.
7. About 10% of older adults are clinically __depressed__.
8. Others often think that older adults cannot continue to learn simply because they __think__ more slowly; they can and do continue to learn.
9. More severe memory losses and dementias of aging are often the result of __circulatory__ changes.
10. Having a __positive__ attitude is very important to successful aging.
11. Active involvement in the community through __volonteer__ work is a good way for an older adult to stay active and involved.
12. Older adults need to feel __needed__ as this contributes to their self-concept and emotional health.

MULTIPLE CHOICE

*Directions: Choose the **best** answer to each of the following questions.*

Situation: C.S. is 78 years old. She is a widow and lives alone. She has hypertension which is controlled and some rheumatoid arthritis that is worsening.

1. The arthritis in C.S.'s knees could possibly be explained by which of the following biologic theories of aging?
   1. Biological clock theory
   2. Free-radical theory
   3. Immune system failure theory
   4. Autoimmune theory

2. The continuity theory explains why C.S.
   1. copes as she has coped before.
   2. is more withdrawn than in younger years.
   3. wants to stay as active as possible.
   4. makes no effort to contribute to the community.

3. One reason C.S. might feel cold in rooms where younger people feel warmer is that
   1. her thyroid function has declined.
   2. she is not as active as she used to be.
   3. she has less subcutaneous fat at this age.
   4. the skin thins with advanced age.

4. C.S.'s appetite has waned. Her appetite might be improved by
   1. sharing meals with others.
   2. using a microwave oven to heat meals.
   3. eating a well-balanced diet.
   4. increasing the amount of fresh vegetables at meals.

5. When planning a teaching session with C.S., be certain
   1. she has had her afternoon nap.
   2. written materials are available.
   3. she has her glasses on.
   4. she has finished her meal.

6. C.S. is having trouble with recent memory. One technique that can assist her with remembering things is to
   1. repeat what she needs to remember out loud.
   2. concentrate on what needs to be remembered for 10 seconds.
   3. tell someone else to remind her of what she needs to remember.
   4. make written lists or mark appointments on a calendar.

7. One factor that may contribute to ego integrity for C.S. is
   1. setting goals for the future.
   2. being proud of the children she raised.
   3. regretting that she did not go to college.
   4. wishing that she had had a career.

8. C.S. has a better chance of adjusting to continued aging in positive ways if she
   1. remains actively involved with others.
   2. curtails her activities to prevent fatigue.
   3. depends on her daughter to do her errands.
   4. has a living will in place with her doctor.

9. It would be wise for C.S.'s daughter to speak with her regarding
   1. how she wishes to distribute her estate when she dies.
   2. granting her power of attorney before she becomes really ill.
   3. how various crises that may occur should be handled.
   4. having someone come and live with her now.

10. C.S.'s daughter would know that her mother needs more assistance if
    1. the dishes are not done before noon.
    2. the clothes she is wearing are often soiled.
    3. she starts spending all her time at the senior center.
    4. she repeats stories about the trips she has made.

CRITICAL THINKING ACTIVITIES

1. Create an educational program to assist older adults to maintain physical and mental health. Points to cover are:
2. Identify problems that will occur if an older adult mentally deteriorates.

MEETING CLINICAL OBJECTIVES

Directions: The following suggested activities will help you meet the stated clinical practice objectives for the chapter. Review your school's clinical objectives for the week and outline a plan of activities that will help you meet them. If unsure as to how to meet them, consult with your instructor at the beginning of the clinical day.

1. Assess an older adult for physical signs of aging.
2. Take a psychosocial history on an older adult and identify areas that contribute to ego integrity.
3. Assess an older adult who has a chronic disease and determine how this, along with the changes attributed to aging, affects the quality of life.
4. Identify problems related to psychosocial health in an elderly patient with a chronic health problem.

5. Using possible community resources, try to help an older adult improve the quality of his or her life.
6. Design a general educational program to assist older adults maintain physical and cognitive health.

STEPS TOWARD BETTER COMMUNICATION

VOCABULARY BUILDING GLOSSARY

Term	Pronunciation	Definition
benign	be NIGN	harmless, gentle
elder hostel	ELD er HOS tel	relatively low-cost programs where elders can travel or live in dormitories for a short period of time, and take classes and attend lectures or programs
irrelevant	ir REL e vant	not important, not connected with what is happening
lifestyle	LIFE style	the manner and habits of a person's life
myth	MYTH	a story told by many people as true, but without proof
nest egg	NEST egg	some money put aside for future use, such as retirement

COMPLETION

Directions: Fill in the blank(s) with the correct word(s) from the vocabulary building glossary.

1. The fact that there was a senior center in town was Irrelevent to C.S., as she had no way to get there.
2. It is hoped that each elderly person will not outlive his or her nest egg and have to rely on community and government services to survive.
3. It is a myth that elderly people have no power in this country.
4. One must put aside considerable money throughout life in order to maintain the same lifestyle after retirement.

VOCABULARY EXERCISE

MYTH VERSUS THEORY VERSUS FACT

A fact is something that has been proven to be true. Neither myths nor theories are proven facts; but a theory is based on facts, while a myth is based on tradition or on beliefs that may not be true.

Directions: Indicate whether the following statements are Myth (M), Theory (T), or Fact (F).

1. Gerontologists say heredity plays a part in determining longevity. F, T
2. Old people cannot learn new things. M
3. Heart and lungs are usually less efficient in the older adult. F

PRONUNCIATION AND STRESS

In the Vocabulary Building Glossary, we indicated where the stress or accent falls in a word as it is normally used. Using the correct stress pattern is often more important for people's understanding than using the correct sounds. Equally important for clear understanding of meaning is where the stress falls in a sentence or a phrase.

In English, the content words are usually given extra emphasis. Content words are words which have the most information. Even if you only heard those words you would have some idea of what was being said. You can emphasize a word by giving extra length to the stressed syllables.

She ATE all her MEAL.

Stress can change the meaning in the following phrases:

YOU did excellent work. (But your friend did not.)
You DID excellent work. (But this week, your work is not so good.)
You did EXCELLENT work. (It was very, very good.)
You did excellent WORK. (But your attitude was not very good.)

COMMUNICATION EXERCISE

Directions: Put a line in the sentence under the words that receive stress, then practice reading it aloud. With a partner read the following dialogue:

Mr. H. has hypertension, high cholesterol, and diabetes mellitus and his doctor has prescribed medications. The nurse is doing a regular home visit with him.

Nurse: "Good morning, Mr. H. How are you feeling?"
Mr. H.: "Pretty good for an old guy my age."
Nurse: "Now, what medications are you taking?"
Mr. H.: "Oh, I don't know. There are some pink ones and some red ones. There were some big horse pills too, but I stopped taking them."
Nurse: "Why? Did the doctor tell you to stop?"
Mr. H.: "No, but they weren't doing me any good and they stuck in my throat."
Nurse: "How do you know they weren't doing you any good?"
Mr. H.: "Well, I don't feel any different when I take them."
Nurse: "Mr. H., some medications don't make any difference in how you feel, but they are doing their job in your body. Your cholesterol and hypertension pills help keep the blood vessels open to your heart and brain so you won't have a stroke or heart attack. You don't want your wife to have to take care of you if you can't talk or feed yourself, do you?"
Mr. H.: "Oh gosh, no! Is that what will happen?"
Nurse: "Well, the medication helps prevent those types of complications. If you have some side effects or other problems taking those pills, talk to the doctor and maybe he can change the prescription. But you should continue taking them until you talk to the doctor."
Mr. H.: "Well, OK, but I sure don't like those horse pills!"
Nurse: "You know the old saying, healthy as a horse. Maybe that's how they stay healthy! Seriously, let's see if the pills can be cut in half."

Review the chapter highlights, answer the study questions, and complete the critical thinking activities at the end of the chapter in the textbook.

THIRTEEN

Cultural and Spiritual Aspects of Patient Care

TERMINOLOGY

A. MATCHING

Directions: Match the terms in column I with the definitions in column II.

Column I

1. e agnostic
2. d atheist
3. b belief
4. g bias
5. J egalitarian
6. K ethnocentricity
7. C faith
8. L generalization
9. O kosher
10. h matriarchal
11. I patriarchal
12. f race
13. a ritual
14. m values
15. n transcultural

Column II

a. Ceremonial acts or practices
b. Conviction or opinion considered to be true
c. Belief which cannot be proven
d. Person who does not believe in the existence of God
e. Person who doubts the existence of God
f. Biologic way of categorizing people
g. Positive or negative attitude or opinion that inhibits impartial judgment
h. Female-dominated
i. Male-dominated
j. Equal authority between male and female
k. Tendency of humans to think that their way of thinking, believing, and doing things is the only way
l. Identifies common trends, patterns, and beliefs of a group
m. Ideas and perceptions seen as good and useful
n. Recognizing cultural diversity
o. Way of ritually slaughtering, preparing, and packaging food

B. COMPLETION

Directions: Fill in the blank(s) with the correct term(s) from the terms list in the chapter in the textbook to complete the sentence.

1. Respecting accepted patterns of communication and refraining from speaking in ways that are disrespectful of a person's cultural beliefs displays cultural __sensitivity__.
2. Nurses must not __generalize__ a patient by applying an overall opinion of a cultural group to that individual person.
3. Different __dialet__ of a language reflect regional variations with different pronunciation, grammar, or word meanings.
4. The shared values, beliefs, and practices shared by a majority of a group of people is termed their __culture__.
5. ✓ A group's __beliefs__ is the way in which they explain life events and view life's mysteries.
6. An element of religion, __spiritualty__, concerns the spirit, or soul.
7. __Religion__ is a formalized system of belief and worship.
8. __Ethnic__ groups are differentiated by geographic, religious, social, or language differences.
9. Many Asians/Pacific Islanders believe that health is dependent on the flow of __qui__, the universal life force.
10. Many Asians also believe that the forces of __yin__ and __yang__ must be in balance in order to be in good health.
11. Some Hispanic Americans may seek the services of a __curandero__ when ill.
12. Many Native Americans will wish to consult a __shaman__ when ill.
13. In the Jewish religion, __circumcision__, removal of the penile foreskin, is performed on the 8th day of life.
14. The distance from each other at which people are comfortable when conversing is called __person__ space.

COMPARISONS

Directions: List three beliefs or values affecting health care for each cultural group.

Cultural Group	Beliefs or Values
Hispanic American	value family over individual, patriarchal, Health is a gift from God often seek help with family member 1st – then curandero (Folk Healer) may be superstitious (ex. staring at new baby OR commenting on beauty brings mal de ojo, the evil eye – Equilibrium achieved by prayer, rituals, rel. objects use of herbs + spices, treating others with respect
Asian American	Value self-control, age authority and harmony (Avoidance of conflict) maintain holistic view of health + illness – nature is dominant force. Dependent on flow of chi (life force, energy) Yin + Yang, Believe a misdeed leads to illness or accidents due to misdeed in previous life, Reluctant to express emotion to others, Consider it disrespectful to disagree with Authority, Buddhism, Taoism, Hinduism + Christianity are prominent faiths
Native American	Respect for the aged, work cooperatively with avoidance to individual gain Believe in keeping natural harmony with humans + nature. Each person has individual physical + spiritual dimension, Believe illness caused by disharmony with environment, individual or spirit world. Periods of silence and avoidance of eye contact show respect. Health care practices linked to spirituality + harmony with universe. Shaman (medicine man) herbal medicines, rituals, fasting, massage are treatments to illness

Cultural Group	Beliefs or Values
African American	health + illness intertwined with religion + good + bad forces, familys often close, Folk or home remedies, Faith healers used as well as Professional Heath care. Christianity and Islam are promimant faiths, Family structure Matriarchal. Believe all illness is preventable if they are attentive with God relationship, nature + other Persons,
European American	value youth, attractiveness, cleanliness, order, punctuality, education, individualism + hard work, Future oriented. Value self-care, self improvement + use preventive health Practices. maintain scientific view of health - often use home remedies before seeking professional help, Extended family support disrupted by geographic distance, Elderly may need outside help, Christianity + Judaism prominent religious faith, Use of med. Technology to treat illness

SHORT ANSWER

Directions: Write a brief answer for each question.

1. List three ways in which poverty often impedes adequate health care in our country.
   a. Lack of funds
   b. Lack of transportation/lack access to attend health care
   c. Lack of treating T.B, chronic Disease

2. Identify one dietary/nutritional practice or belief that is pertinent to the nursing care of each of the following cultural/religious groups:
   a. Hispanic American
      Spicy foods, beans, bananas
   b. Muslim
      no pork, Alcoholic Beverages, All meat is Blessed. Many don't eat traditional black American foods such as: corn bread, collard greens
   c. Judaism
      food is ritually prepared during slaughter, processing and packaging - (labeled Kosher) Use separate utensils for milk + meat, fasting during Yom Kipper Holiday, not eating raised breads during Passover, Thankgiving before + after meals,
   d. Hinduism
      most are vegetarians don't eat meat because harming a living creature.

3. Identify ways in which you can achieve cultural competence.
   Read literature, respect differences amoung groups, Learn to effectively communicate, Don't make judgements about cultural behaviors + practices, talking with people

4. Cultural awareness involves: "Knowledge of Peoples history, expressions of foods + celebrations" expressions
   Being resourceful + creative, fitting nursing interventions into belief system of patient, interpretor, Amount of space given to person, how to address someone, is touch acceptable, who makes decisions in family, is eye contact considered polite or rude

5. Areas in which cultural difference is evident are:
   a. Communication
   b. view of time
   c. Organization of the family
   d. nutrician
   e. issues related to Death + Dying
   f. Health care beliefs

COMPLETION

Directions: Fill in the blank(s) with the correct word(s) to complete the sentence.

1. Both spirituality and culture have to do with attempting to understand one's place in the world and life's ____meaning____ or ____purpose____.
2. During illness or when facing death are times when religious and spiritual beliefs may be strengthened, questioned, or ____rejected____.
3. ✓ Religious beliefs and rituals are interwoven into a group's ____world view____.
4. For Christians, death is viewed as a ____transition____ to a life with God.
5. The religious book of Muslims is the ____Koran____.
6. Circumcision of the Jewish male infant is to be done on the ____8th____ day of life.
7. Many Hindus are ____vegetarians____ and this must be considered when planning the diet.
8. Buddhists believe that liberation from ____anxiety____ through following Buddha's teachings is important in promoting health and recovery.
9. Taoists believe that illness or disease is due to an imbalance in ____yin____ and ____yang____.
10. Within cultures, the homeless are considered a ____subculture____ with distinct problems of their own.
11. Dr. M.M. claims that ____human caring____ is what all people need most to grow, remain well, avoid illness, and survive or face death.
12. Care must be taken not to let ____ethnocentrism____ affect one's attitude toward a patient.
13. The Vietnamese patient may avoid eye contact when talking with someone they consider an ____authority figure____ figure or who is ____older____.
14. In European American culture ____18 inches____ is the usual space between people that is comfortable when they are talking together.
15. An orientation toward the future is a ____European-American____ dominant cultural trait in the United States, but not of the African American or the Hispanic American cultures.
16. The Hispanic American family is essentially ____patriarchal____ in structure, while the African American family is ____matriarchal____.
17. Foods considered "hot" or "cold" within some cultures are based on characteristics other than ____temperature____.
18. All cultures have an element of ____folk____ medicine that is handed down through families for treatment of common illnesses.
19. Keloid formation is more common among ____African Americans____.
20. Diabetes is more common among the ____Hispanic____ and ____Native Americans____ population due to a genetic susceptibility.

APPLICATION OF THE NURSING PROCESS

Directions: Write a brief answer for each question.

1. Without looking in the textbook, list four assessment questions regarding culture and spirituality you would ask your patient.
   a. Are there any foods your religion forbids?
   b. Tell me about your beliefs?
   c. Would you like to speak to any religious leader?
   d. Is there anything staff should know about your religious practices?

2. List three common nursing diagnoses related to cultural and spiritual problems.
   a. Impaired verbal communication
   b. Decisional Conflict
   c. Spiritual distress

3. Write an expected outcome for each nursing diagnosis related to spirituality and culture.
   a. Express needs & opinions through an interpreter
   b. Cope with cultural differences of agency Routines
   c. Identify & employ spiritual support

4. List three general ways in which you could individualize nursing actions for a patient's culture while meeting basic needs.
   a. Enlist Family members to assist w/ Patients care if desirable
   b. Show cortesy & respect for the patient as an individual = therapeutic caring relationship
   c. praying with Patient

5. Identify how you would evaluate care to determine if the expected outcomes were met.
   when mutual trust & understanding developed Between patient & nurse. Advocate Rts. of patients to fit with their cultural & spiritual backgrounds.

MULTIPLE CHOICE

*Directions: Choose the **best** answer for each of the following questions.*

1. Assuming that all African Americans like grits with their breakfast is an example of
   1. ethnocentrism.
   2. stereotyping.
   3. values.
   4. culture.

2. A religious group that does not believe in using the services of physicians in most instances is
   1. Muslims.
   2. Jews.
   3. Taoists.
   4. Christian Scientists.

3. The Jewish religious leader is called a(n)
   1. imam.
   2. priest.
   3. rabbi.
   4. minister.

4. Orthodox Jews should never be served which two items at the same meal?
   1. milk and meat
   2. meat and bread
   3. milk and bread
   4. fruit and meat

5. Many Hindus believe that
   1. Christ was a prophet.
   2. what happens to them is the will of God.
   3. eating meat is necessary to keep healthy.
   4. praying will bring a favorable response from God.

6. A group within a larger culture that holds different beliefs, values, and attitudes is called a
   1. subculture.
   2. diversity.
   3. sect.
   4. ethnic group.

7. A group that does not view punctuality at all times to be of high value is
   1. European Americans.
   2. Arab Americans.
   3. Hispanic Americans.
   4. Asian Americans.

8. A cultural group in which families are often matriarchal is
   1. Hispanic American.
   2. European American.
   3. Asian American.
   4. African American.

9. Diabetes is more common among
   1. European Americans.
   2. Arab Americans.
   3. Asian Americans.
   4. Hispanic Americans.

10. The one culture that does **not** view foods as 'hot' or 'cold' based on their effect in the body is
    1. European American.
    2. Arab American.
    3. Asian American.
    4. Hispanic American.

11. Culture is the
    1. language, food preferences, and habits of a group.
    2. values, beliefs, and practices of a people.
    3. rituals, language, and traditions of a people.
    4. ethnicity, religion, and values of a people.

12. Knowing who is the dominant person in the family is important because the dominant person
    1. determines the family value system regarding health practices.
    2. is the main health care provider for the family.
    3. tends to make health care decisions.
    4. is the family member designated to communicate to the nurse.

13. Lactase deficiency is prevalent among
    1. European Americans.
    2. Chinese.
    3. Jews.
    4. Hindus.

14. Sickle-cell trait is most prevalent among
    1. European Americans.
    2. Native Americans.
    3. Asian Americans.
    4. African Americans.

15. A family with equality between the man and the woman is considered
    1. egalitarian.
    2. patriarchal.
    3. matriarchal.
    4. ethnocentric.

CRITICAL THINKING ACTIVITIES

1. Compare your own cultural beliefs toward health care with those of a peer from a different culture.

   Your beliefs:

   Peer's beliefs:

2. Plan how you would help meet the spiritual needs of a Hindu, a Buddhist, and a Muslim.

   Hindu:

   Buddhist:

   Muslim:

MEETING CLINICAL OBJECTIVES

Directions: The following suggested activities will help you meet the stated clinical practice objectives for the chapter. Review your school's clinical objectives for the week and outline a plan of activities that will help you meet them. If unsure as to how to meet them, consult with your instructor at the beginning of the clinical day.

1. Ask to be assigned to patients from different cultural groups.
2. Ask to be assigned to a patient whose language you do not speak.
3. Locate the health facility chapel so that you can offer its solace to family members when appropriate.
4. Contact a religious leader for a patient to whom you are assigned.
5. Identify spiritual distress in assigned patients and plan interventions to relieve it.
6. Discuss how to protect patients' rights when they wish to refuse a medical treatment because of cultural or religious beliefs.

STEPS TOWARD BETTER COMMUNICATION

VOCABULARY BUILDING GLOSSARY

Term	Pronunciation	Definition
A. Individual Terms		
attire	at TIRE	what people wear; clothing
impede	im PEDE	to slow down; get in the way of
prevalent	PREV a lent	common, observed frequently
refrain from	re FRAIN from	to avoid, or not do, something
sustained	sus TAINed	continued, constant
B. Phrases		
a wealth of information	a WEALTH of in for MA tion	a very large amount of information or facts
keep an open mind	keep an OPEN mind	to listen for new information before making a decision about something or someone

COMPLETION

Directions: Fill in the blank(s) with term(s) from the Vocabulary Building Glossary to complete the sentence.

1. She tried to refrain from making a quick judgment about the person from his appearance.
2. Her attire was that of a Hindu woman.
3. African Americans are very prevelent in our hospital population.
4. The nurse made a sustained effort to perform a cultural assessment on every patient.

5. The old chart contained a wealth of information about the patient's medical history and psychosocial needs.

PRONUNCIATION OF DIFFICULT TERMS

Remember that even if all the sounds in a word are correctly pronounced, placing the stress incorrectly can cause misunderstanding.

Directions: Practice pronouncing the following words.

agnostic	ag NOS tic
atheist	A the ist
egalitarian	e GAL i TAR i an
ethnocentricity	ETH no cen TRI ci ty
matriarchal	MA tri ARCH al
patriarchal	PA tri ARCH al

WORD ATTACK SKILLS

Directions: Find five words in the chapter in each of the following categories and underline the stressed syllable.

1. Accent or stress on the first syllable:

____

____

2. Accent or stress on the second syllable:

____

____

3. Accent or stress on the third syllable:

____

____

4. Accent or stress on the fourth syllable:

____

____

COMMUNICATION EXERCISE

1. With a native speaker, read the words you found in the exercise above to make sure you have the correct stress.
2. Number Practice: Stress makes a great difference in understanding numbers. Two different stress patterns are possible with numbers, but native speakers usually choose the one that makes the meaning clear. THIRty and THIRteen are possible, but when you are trying to distinguish or contrast the two, the stress changes: THIRty, not thirTEEN, or twenty-THREE, not twenty-FOUR.
3. Complete the following chart with a partner. Look only at your chart. Ask your partner questions to help you fill in the blanks in your chart, and answer your partner's questions.

STUDENT A

Room Number	Birthdate	Time of Admission
790	?	10:31 am
?	3/16/70	?
231	?	7:17 pm
?	8/15/80	?

STUDENT B

Room Number	Birthdate	Time of Admission
?	7/13/50	?
314	?	12:15pm
?	11/30/19	?
240	?	5:14 pm

CULTURAL POINTS

While it is important to be sensitive and observe all the considerations and precautions that are mentioned in the textbook, it may be somewhat reassuring to realize that most of the patients you will encounter have been living in this culture for some time and will be used to the predominant way of interacting. However, it is still respectful and caring, especially in a time of illness, to treat them with as much sensitivity and understanding as possible.

Review the chapter highlights, answer the study questions, and complete the critical thinking activities at the end of the chapter in the textbook.

FOURTEEN

Loss, Grief, and the Dying Patient

TERMINOLOGY

A. MATCHING

Directions: Match the terms in column I with the definitions in column II.

Column I		Column II	
1. ______	autopsy	a.	Philosophy of care for the dying
2. ______	bereavement	b.	Study of death
3. ______	coroner	c.	Treatment provided solely for comfort
4. ______	hospice	d.	Person with legal authority to determine cause of death
5. ______	obituary	e.	Examination of body tissues to determine cause of death
6. ______	palliation	f.	A notice of death published in the newspapers
7. ______	postmortem	g.	State of having suffered a loss by death
8. ______	rigor mortis	h.	Cover with which body is wrapped after death
9. ______	shroud	i.	After death
10. ______	thanatology	j.	Stiffening of a dead body

B. COMPLETION

Directions: Fill in the blank(s) with the correct term(s) from the terms list in the chapter in the textbook to complete the sentence.

1. ________________ refers to no longer possessing or having an object, person, or situation.
2. The emotional feeling of pain and distress in response to a loss is termed ________________.
3. ________________ may occur before a loss actually happens.
4. Dysfunctional grieving would be that which falls outside ________________.
5. Hope can be described as a feeling that what is desired is ________________.
6. ________________ spell out the patient's wishes for health care at that time when the person may be unable to indicate his or her choice.

SHORT ANSWER

Directions: Write a brief answer for each question.

1. In the high-tech hospital environment where equipment and medications can sustain a patient's breathing and heartbeat, what is necessary for death to be declared?

   ____

2. Today, a hospice is ______________________________
   ______________________________.

3. Identify three common fears a patient is likely to experience when dying.
   a. ______________________________
   b. ______________________________
   c. ______________________________

4. What is euthanasia?

   ____
   ____

5. Describe the difference between active and passive euthanasia.

   ____
   ____
   ____
   ____

6. How does assisted suicide differ from active euthanasia?

   ____
   ____
   ____
   ____

7. What parts of the ANA Position Statements make it a violation for a nurse to participate in active euthanasia or assisted suicide?

   ____
   ____
   ____
   ____

8. Which portion of the Rights of the Dying Patient guide the nurse's behavior regarding the patient's right to have treatment to extend life withheld?

   ____

9. Give one nursing intervention for comfort care particular to the dying patient for each of the following problems.
   a. pain ______________________________
   b. nausea ______________________________
   c. dyspnea ______________________________
   d. anxiety ______________________________
   e. constipation ______________________________
   f. incontinence ______________________________
   g. thirst ______________________________
   h. anorexia ______________________________

10. Describe a health care proxy.

____

____

11. It is essential to monitor bowel patterns daily in terminally ill patients because they tend to develop constipation due to:
    a. ______________________________
    b. ______________________________
    c. ______________________________

12. The bad taste in the mouth that many terminal patients develop can be improved by

____

13. A medication that can ease the secretions in the terminal patient that cause noisy respirations and a "death rattle" is ______________________________.

14. Encouraging a life review allows a patient to put his or her life in perspective. When doing this it is more important to ______________ than to ______________.

15. List five specific signs or symptoms of grief.
    a. ______________________________
    b. ______________________________
    c. ______________________________
    d. ______________________________
    e. ______________________________

CORRELATION

Directions: Correlate the behavior in column I with Kubler-Ross's stages of dying in column II.

		Column I		Column II
1.	______	Stays in bed most of the time.		
2.	______	Tells God, "I'll quit smoking if I can just live until after my daughter's wedding."	a.	denial
			b.	bargaining
			c.	anger
3.	______	"My family will be fine after I'm gone."	d.	depression
			e.	acceptance
4.	______	"My stomach is just easily upset; I don't have cancer."		
5.	______	"Go away, I don't want company."		
6.	______	Thinks "If Mom will just be OK, I'll do my homework every day."		
7.	______	"I'm going to sue that doctor for telling him that."		
8.	______	"She'll soon be at peace."		
9.	______	"She's not that sick!"		
10.	______	"I feel so hopeless about Mom's condition."		

APPLICATION OF THE NURSING PROCESS

Directions: Write a brief answer for each question.

1. Four other areas to specifically assess in addition to gathering a history and performing a physical assessment for a terminally ill patient would be:
   a. ______________________
   b. ______________________
   c. ______________________
   d. ______________________
2. List three nursing diagnoses you feel would be common at some point to most dying patients.
   a. ______________________
   b. ______________________
   c. ______________________
3. During the planning process, a first priority is to ______________________.
4. Write a realistic expected outcome for each of the nursing diagnoses listed above.
   a. ______________________
   b. ______________________
   c. ______________________
5. Interventions regarding pain control for the terminally ill often require adding prn medication for ______________ ______________.
6. A ______________ and ______________ program can be used to alleviate problems of constipation.
7. A point to remember when considering nutritional intake for the terminal patient is that decreased intake is ______________ for the patient than having ______________________.
8. Evaluation of success of the nursing care plan is based on ______________________.

MULTIPLE CHOICE

*Directions: Choose the **best** answer for each of the following questions.*

1. A major focus for the nurse in caring for the terminally ill patient should be
   1. assisting the patient to interact with family members.
   2. advocating medications and treatments that can prolong life.
   3. providing comfort measures that promote well-being.
   4. assuring the patient that things will get better.
2. Advanced directives usually do NOT
   1. direct disposition of the patient's belongings.
   2. state what measures the patient wishes to be used to prolong life.
   3. direct which organs may be donated after death.
   4. express whether resuscitation should be attempted.
3. When a patient who is dying continues to make concrete plans for next summer's vacation, it indicates he is in the stage of
   1. denial.
   2. acceptance.
   3. bargaining.
   4. depression.

4. A family member who is argumentative and rude to the dying patient may be going through the stage of
   1. denial.
   2. anger.
   3. bargaining.
   4. depression.

5. The nurse sometimes can tell when the terminal patient nears death because there is
   1. elevation of the blood pressure.
   2. a period of quiet acceptance.
   3. mottling of the dependent extremities.
   4. cyanosis around the mouth.

6. As death approaches in the terminally ill patient, there is often a change in
   1. facial color.
   2. patient behavior.
   3. skin odor.
   4. respiratory pattern.

7. Hospice care focuses on
   1. prolonging life as long as possible.
   2. working through the stages of grief.
   3. providing support and comfort measures.
   4. ending illness and hastening death.

8. Nurses may have a difficult time dealing with patient deaths if they
   1. did not foresee that the illness was terminal.
   2. have no friends among the unit staff.
   3. have not come to terms with their own mortality.
   4. cared for the patient for several days.

9. During assessment of the dying patient, it is good to ask
   1. "How did this illness come about?"
   2. "What are your concerns?"
   3. "Isn't your family coming to see you?"
   4. "How long do you think you will live?"

10. A continuing problem in caring for the dying patient is that
    1. families want the patient to die in the hospital.
    2. physicians expect nurses to tell them what the patient needs.
    3. narcotic regulations prevent adequate treatment of pain for the terminal patient.
    4. more than half of terminally ill patients die with uncontrolled pain.

CRITICAL THINKING ACTIVITIES

1. Your patient who suffered head trauma in an accident is on life support and expected to die at any time. Write out what you would say to the family regarding organ or tissue donation.
2. L.S., age 46, is dying of metastatic breast cancer. She becomes weaker every day and suffers from pain, constipation, incontinence, dyspnea, and anxiety. How can you support or instill hope in this patient and her family?

MEETING CLINICAL OBJECTIVES

Directions: The following suggested activities will help you meet the stated clinical practice objectives for the chapter. Review your school's clinical objectives for the week and outline a plan of activities that will help you meet them. If unsure as to how to meet them, consult with your instructor at the beginning of the clinical day.

1. Imagine you have just been diagnosed with a terminal illness. Think about what you would want to do with your remaining days. How would you go about getting your "affairs in order?"
2. Devise a will and plan your own funeral.

3. Accompany a nurse who is going to give postmortem care.
4. Role play with a peer measures to support a grieving family member.
5. Explain to a patient how to complete an advance directive and what the terms *health care proxy* and *DNR* mean in lay language.
6. Devise a plan of care for a dying patient that includes comfort measures for the problems of pain, nausea, dyspnea, anxiety, constipation, incontinence, thirst, and anorexia.

STEPS TOWARD BETTER COMMUNICATION

VOCABULARY BUILDING GLOSSARY

Term	Pronunciation	Definition
A. Individual Terms		
anticipatory	an tic i pa tor y	looking ahead at what might happen
cliches	cli CHES	sayings so common, or untrue, that they lose any meaning
closure	CLO sure	a condition where things are completed; a conclusion
collaboratively	col LAB or a tive ly	working together, sharing ideas and plans
commonalities	COM mon AL i ties	elements that are the same among a set of things
culmination	cul mi NA tion	final and total result
eradicate	e RAD i cate	to remove, to get rid of
enhance	en HANCE	to improve; add to
fluctuating	FLUC tu A ting	moving up and down; changing
grapple	GRAP ple	struggle; try hard to solve a problem
impending	im PEND ing	coming soon
inevitability	in EV i ta BIL i ty	happening no matter what action is taken
obituary	o BIT u ar y	an article in the paper announcing the death and describing the life of a person
proactive	PRO act ive	actively doing something for another person, not just standing by
prompted	PROMP ted	caused
proxy	PROX y	acting for another person
respite	RES pite	relief; rest
shielded	SHIELD ed	protected
validating	VAL i da ting	giving worth or value to something
B. Phrases		
anticipating the likelihood	an TIC i PAT ing the LIKE li hood	expecting that something will happen
first and foremost	FIRST and FOREmost	put the most important thing first
have a chilling effect	have a CHILL ing e FFECT	make something difficult, dangerous, or frightening

COMPLETION

Directions: Fill in the blank(s) with the correct term(s) from the Vocabulary Building Glossary to complete the sentence.

1. When the daughter heard about her father's metastatic cancer, she went into a state of __________________ grief.
2. The nurse worked __________________ with the respiratory therapist, the dietitian, and the occupational therapist to make the patient's remaining days as comfortable as possible.
3. Attending to the patient's problems with bowel function can __________________ his or her comfort level and quality of life during a terminal illness.
4. Active listening on the part of the nurse can assist a patient to __________________ with the issues facing him or her at the end of life.
5. The nurse needs to be __________________ in working with the physician to alleviate the patient's pain.
6. The daughter was designated the patient's __________________ regarding end-of-life care and desires.
7. Mr. O.'s wife badly needed a __________________ from the almost 24-hour-a-day care she was providing during his terminal illness.
8. Reviewing with Mr. O., his life accomplishments and major milestones was __________________ for him.

VOCABULARY EXERCISE

Directions: Read the short paragraph about cloning which uses the phrases in the Vocabulary Building Glossary. Then, write a similar paragraph about euthanasia, using the same phrases.

"Scientists are anticipating the likelihood of the cloning of the human embryo. Even if ethical and moral considerations are first and foremost, the idea has a chilling effect on most people."

WORD ATTACK SKILLS

Directions: Find the words in the Vocabulary Building Glossary that have more than four syllables and write them below, underlining the stressed syllable. Next, write the root word you find in the glossary word. What is its meaning?

Glossary Word	Root Word	Meaning

COMMUNICATION EXERCISE

ROLE PLAY

1. Look at your answer to Critical Thinking Activity #1 in the textbook chapter where you wrote out what you would say to a family regarding organ or tissue donation. Role play that dialogue with a partner until you feel comfortable with the words and the emotions.

2. Look at your answers for Critical Thinking Activity #2 in the chapter in the textbook. Write two short dialogues, one with the patient and one with her family, of what you might say for support and comfort. Role play the dialogues with a partner.

CULTURAL POINTS

1. Customs around death vary from culture to culture and are very important to families, as they mark an important passage in life. Most cultures and religions have rules and rites dealing with death and the disposal of the body. In the United States, people are often very removed from death, as it usually occurs in hospitals, and health and funeral professionals handle the body. Some people do not even wish to view the body of a friend or loved one. In other cultures, such as Islam, the family is expected to wash the body and prepare it for burial according to custom and ritual. Be sure you know the family's wishes and needs if death is approaching.

2. Some euphemisms (a more agreeable expression used in place of an unpleasant one) used in English to refer to death are death, passed away, expired, deceased.

   He died/passed away/expired an hour ago.

   My mother is dead/deceased/departed/gone to be with God.

   She is at peace/at rest/in no more pain/with God.

3. Words of sympathy or condolence you might use to the family and friends are:

   "I am sorry." "I am sorry for your loss." "You have my sympathy." "I'm so sorry this has happened to your family." "I'm so sorry things have ended like this." "I'm sorry that in spite of all efforts, we couldn't prevent his death." "I am sorry for your loss; is there someone I can call for you?"

Review the chapter highlights, answer the study questions, and complete the critical thinking activities at the end of the chapter in the textbook.

FIFTEEN

Infection, Protective Mechanisms, and Asepsis

TERMINOLOGY

A. MATCHING

Directions: Match the terms in column I with the definitions in column II.

Column I		Column II	
1. b	antibiotic	a.	Organism only visible with a microscope
2. h	antimicrobial	b.	Chemical substance that can kill microorganisms
3. i	antiseptic	c.	Process of destroying all microorganisms
4. f	asepsis	d.	Make unclean
5. d	contaminate	e.	Without pathologic organisms
6. G	debris	f.	Freedom from pathogenic microorganisms
7. j	disinfectant	g.	Dead tissue or foreign matter
8. a	microorganism	h.	Killing or suppressing growth of microorganisms
9. e	sterile	i.	Chemical compound used on skin or tissue to inhibit growth of microorganisms
10. c	sterilization	j.	Agent that destroys microorganisms

B. COMPLETION

Directions: Fill in the blank(s) with the correct word(s) from the terms list in the chapter in the textbook to complete the sentence.

1. aneorobic organisms can only grow when oxygen is absent.
2. A single-celled organism lacking a nucleus that reproduces about every 20 minutes is a bacteria.
3. viruses can only grow and replicate within a living cell.
4. protozoons are one-celled organisms that belong to the animal kingdom.
5. Rickettslas are rod-shaped microorganisms that are transmitted by the bites of insects that act as vectors.

6. Tiny primitive organisms of the plant kingdom that contain no chlorophyll and reproduce by means of spores are Fungi.
7. Roundworm and tapeworm are parasitic and are called Helminths.
8. Toxin is a poisonous protein produced by certain bacteria.
9. A nosocromial infection is one that is acquired in the hospital.
10. Microorganisms that are capable of causing disease are called Pathogens.
11. In order to determine which antibiotic will eradicate an infection, it is necessary to culture the bacteria.
12. One of the most effective ways to prevent the transfer of microorganisms from one person to another is to handwash.
13. Handwashing is performed before glouving and immediately after removing the gloves as they are not 100% protective.
14. Disposable sharp instruments such as syringes, scalpel blades, and suture needles are often called sharps.
15. Contaminated waste such as soiled dressings are disposed of in sealed plastic bags marked biohazard or Hazardous waste.

SHORT ANSWER

Directions: Write a brief answer for each question.

1. Characteristics that affect the virulence of microorganisms are the abilities to:
   a. adhere to mucosal surfaces or skin
   b. penetrate mucos membranes
   c. multiply once in the body
   d. secrete harmful enzymes or toxins
   e. resist phagotytosis (destruction of WBC)
2. Give one example for each of the links of the chain of infection.
   a. Causative agent bacteria, viruses, protzoa, rickettsia, fungi, helminths
   b. Reservoir infected wounds, human or animal waste, animals, insects (contaminated Food water)
   c. Portal of exit coughing, sneezing, feces skin, mucous membranes
   d. Mode of transmission contaminated items from another person, coughing, sneezing (droplet, vectors)
   e. Portal of entry contaminated Food, water, broken skin, mouth, nose, trachea,
   f. Susceptible host weak state of health, broken skin, virtue of age,
3. Describe the difference between medical asepsis and surgical asepsis.
   medical asepsis referred to as "clean technique" but not all microorganisms are destroy. surgical Asepsis is a "sterile tecknique" all microorganisms are destroyed.
4. Personal protective equipment (PPE) items include:
   goggles, gloves, gown, mask, hat, shoe covering

5. The most effective means for destroying viruses and all other kinds of microorganisms is to: expose them to moist heat (250°) for 15-20 minutes,

6. Four factors that may place an elderly patient at higher risk of infection compared to the younger adult are:
   a. poor nutrician
   b. immobility leading to poor hygiene
   c. chronic illness
   d. physiological changes

7. The first line of defense against infection is: skin

8. The five defense mechanisms that destroy pathogens via the second line of defense are:
   a. mechanisms of fever
   b. leucocytosis - increase production of WBC
   c. phagocytosis - work to destroy pathogens
   d. inflammation
   e. action of interferon - stimulate immune system & interfere with viral invasion

9. Phagocytes consist of ____________ and ____________ and work to remove cellular debris, destroy bacteria and viruses, and remove metabolic waste products by ____________.

10. Briefly describe the inflammatory process.
Blood vessels dilate, bringing more blood to damaged area causing redness & warmth. Chemicals histamine & serotonin are released. It neutralizes & destroy harmful agents, limit spread to other tissues, prepares damaged tissues for repair

11. Natural acquired immunity occurs when: body produces antibodies against an invader

12. To develop passive acquired immunity, a person must be given an antitoxin or antiserum that contains antibodies.

13. Artificially acquired immunity is achieved through: injection of vaccines or immunizing substances that contain dead or inactive microorganisms or their toxins
vaccine prompts body to produce antibodies

14. Considering standard precautions, a gown is to be worn when there's a chance of being splashed with blood or body fluid.

15. A mask is worn when there is a chance of contact with airborne pathogen or splashed body fluids.

16. Protective eyewear is worn whenever there is a possibility of fluid entering the eye or coming in contact of mucosa or surface of the eye.

17. To clean visibly soiled instruments or other items that are washable, gloves are always used and the following steps are taken:
    a. rinse object with cold water + remove organic material
    b. wash object in hot soapy water
    c. Use stiff-bristled brush or Abrasive to clean grooves + narrow spaces
    d. Rinse object well with moderately hot water
    e. Dry the object

MULTIPLE CHOICE

*Directions: Choose the **best** answer for each of the following questions.*

1. In the home care setting, contaminated dressings should be handled by ________________ before disposal.
    1. boiling them for ten minutes
    2. treating them with a 1:10 chlorine solution
    3. securing them in plastic zip-closure bags
    4. washing in hot soapy water

2. The hospital patient considered at high risk for nosocomial infection is the one who has
    1. been there more than three days.
    2. pneumonia.
    3. an indwelling catheter.
    4. just delivered a baby.

3. Considering the chain of infection and the way pathogens are spread, contaminated water is considered a
    1. reservoir.
    2. portal of exit.
    3. susceptible host.
    4. causative agent.

4. Many gram-negative bacteria are more dangerous than gram-positive bacteria because they
    1. multiply more rapidly.
    2. produce a dangerous endotoxin.
    3. cause severe diarrhea.
    4. are more virulent.

5. The liver participates in protection of the body against infection by
    1. phagocytic action in the liver tissue.
    2. action of bile inactivating bacteria.
    3. flushing bacteria from the blood.
    4. destroying bacteria via the Kupffer cells.

6. Another body defense occurs in the gastrointestinal system as the
    1. hydrochloric acid in the stomach destroys pathogens.
    2. bile in the stool kills bacteria.
    3. digestive enzymes in the small intestine kill bacteria.
    4. peristaltic action of the intestines eliminates pathogens.

7. Fever helps fight infection because heat
    1. kills most pathogens.
    2. slows the growth of pathogens.
    3. causes diaphoresis and flushing out of bacteria.
    4. causes more water consumption and urine production.

8. The redness and warmth in an inflamed area is due to
    1. dilation of blood vessels and increased blood flow.
    2. increased temperature in the affected tissues.
    3. phagocytosis and chemical action against pathogens.
    4. formation of debris, causing tissue swelling.

9. Normally, the immune system does not attack the self because
    1. only microorganisms cause antibody production.
    2. macrophages never attack one's own cells.
    3. cellular antigens help in distinguishing self from nonself.
    4. only foreign proteins cause antibody reaction.

10. Effective disinfection of surfaces contaminated with blood and possible HIV is accomplished by
    1. scrubbing with soap and hot water for three minutes.
    2. soaking with 70% alcohol solution for ten minutes.
    3. washing with iodine solution and then swabbing with alcohol.
    4. cleansing with a solution of 1:10 chlorine bleach and water.

11. Performing a culture and sensitivity test when a patient has a wound infection is important because
    1. antibiotics will kill the bacteria.
    2. different organisms are killed by specific antibiotics.
    3. some wound infections should not be treated.
    4. cleansing alone will not cure the infection.

12. Diarrhea is often caused by
    1. *Rickettsia.*
    2. fungi.
    3. protozoa.
    4. helminths.

13. Vaginal *Candidiasis* is caused by
    1. bacteria.
    2. virus.
    3. protozoa.
    4. fungi.

14. Nurses pay great attention to skin care for patients because
    1. cleanliness reduces the chance of infection.
    2. patients do not want pressure ulcers.
    3. everyone should have a bath every day.
    4. the skin is the first line of defense against infection.

15. Giving a patient a serum immune globulin injection will provide
    1. passive acquired immunity.
    2. naturally acquired passive immunity.
    3. artificially acquired immunity.
    4. passive artificially acquired immunity.

16. Considering handwashing as a measure to prevent infection, an important guideline is that
    1. a five-minute scrub is always appropriate.
    2. handwashing time should be adjusted to the amount of contamination of the hands.
    3. hands should be washed in very warm water to help kill any bacteria.
    4. only special antimicrobial soap will sufficiently kill the bacteria on the hands.

17. Standard precautions were developed by the CDC to
    1. protect patients.
    2. protect health care workers.
    3. break the chain of infection.
    4. prevent hospital-acquired infection.

18. Handwashing after removing gloves is necessary because
    1. powder from the gloves remains on the hands.
    2. gloves are not 100% protective.
    3. contamination occurs when removing the gloves.
    4. otherwise the gloves irritate the hands.

19. Which one of the following could be a vector capable of transmitting pathogens?
    1. tick
    2. eating utensil
    3. human
    4. water

20. Before sterilizing instruments, you should
    1. rinse off all visible matter with cool water.
    2. soak them in cool water.
    3. soak them in alcohol.
    4. soak them in hot water.

CRITICAL THINKING ACTIVITIES

1. Give specific examples of the methods of medical asepsis and surgical asepsis used in the health care setting.
2. Explain to a family member how the body's protective mechanisms work to prevent infection.
3. Explain to a patient why the use of standard precautions is essential to both the health care worker's and the patient's protection.

MEETING CLINICAL OBJECTIVES

Directions: The following suggested activities will help you meet the stated clinical practice objectives for the chapter. Review your school's clinical objectives for the week and outline a plan of activities that will help you meet them. If unsure as to how to meet them, consult with your instructor at the beginning of the clinical day.

1. Interview the infection control officer regarding how infection is prevented and tracked in the clinical facility.
2. Observe ten health care workers giving patient care and washing their hands. How many are following accepted protocols?
3. Teach a home care patient with a wound infection how to prevent the spread of infection to family members.

STEPS TOWARD BETTER COMMUNICATION

VOCABULARY BUILDING GLOSSARY

Term	Pronunciation	Definition
A. Individual Terms		
aerosolization	A er o sol i ZA tion	particles become suspended in a gas (air)
caustic	CAUS tic	able to burn or dissolve
commode	com MODE	toilet
impede	im PEDE	to get in the way, obstruct
impermeable	im PER me a ble	nothing can go through it
oozing	OO zing	coming out slowly
prevalent	PREV a lent	common
render	REN der	make
replicate	REP li cate	produce exact copies of
scrupulously	SCRUP u lous ly	carefully, perfectly
stringent	STRIN gent	strict, severe
vectors	VEC tors	carriers
virulent	VIR u lent	very harmful and rapidly spreading
B. Phrases		
wall off	wall off	to isolate

COMPLETION

Directions: Fill in the blank(s) with the correct word(s) from the Vocabulary Building Glossary to complete the sentence.

1. Bacteria can be very Virulent and their spread must be prevented.
2. A blood spill must be scrupulously cleaned up to prevent the spread of blood-borne pathogens.
3. A dressing over a wound will wall-off the transfer of microorganisms.
4. When there is likely to be splashing of body fluids, health personnel must wear an impermeable gown.
5. Autoclaving instruments should Impede caustic them free of microorganisms.
6. Unfortunately, nosocomial infection is prevalent in the hospital setting.
7. Mosquitos are a vectors for several diseases including encephalitis and malaria.

WORD ATTACK SKILLS

Directions: Match the word part with its meaning.

1. a -cyte
2. c -osis
3. b leuk-

a. white
b. cell
c. abnormal condition

PRONUNCIATION OF DIFFICULT TERMS

Directions: With a partner, practice pronouncing the following words.

immunosuppressive	im mu no sup press ive
leukocytosis	leu ko cy to sis
macrophage	mac ro phage
mucous	mu cous
mucosal	mu co sal
nosocomial	nos o co mi al
phagocytosis	pha go cy to sis
secrete	se crete
Streptococcal	strep to coc cal

COMMUNICATION EXERCISE

Directions: With a partner, write a dialogue teaching a home care patient with a wound infection how to prevent the spread of infection to family members (Clinical Activity #3 above). Explain in simple terms how infection occurs (infectious agents enter the body), and steps to prevent its spread in the home (handwashing, treatment and disposal of contaminated material, cleaning of surfaces, etc.). Include questions the patient might ask. Practice the dialogue with your partner until you feel comfortable with it.

CULTURAL POINTS

1. In modern cities, the government departments of public health and sanitation take much of the responsibility for infection control and sanitation. Some of these are garbage and trash collection, monitoring and purification of the water system, requiring inoculation of children before entrance to school, restaurant inspection, requiring permits for food service, and maintaining sewage treatment plants. These are necessary in densely populated areas with a concentration of people that can include hosts and carriers of disease. In a rural area with few people and less interaction among them, so many precautions might not be necessary.
2. How is infection control handled in your home country?

Review the chapter highlights, answer the study questions, and complete the critical thinking activities at the end of the chapter in the textbook.

SIXTEEN

Infection Control in Hospital and Home

TERMINOLOGY

A. COMPLETION

Directions: Fill in the blank(s) with the correct term(s) from the terms list in the chapter in the textbook to complete the sentence.

1. The incubation period is the time from invasion of the body by the microorganisms to the onset of symptoms.
2. The prodromal is the time from the onset of nonspecific symptoms to the beginning of specific symptoms of an infection.
3. Elevated temperature and malaise may occur during the prodromal period.
4. A systemic sign of infection is leukocytosis where the white blood cells increase in number.
5. When symptoms begin to subside, the convalescent period begins.
6. When a patient has a highly contagious infection, placing the patient in isolation helps prevent the spread of the infection.
7. Transmission Precaution are the guidelines established by the CDC to prevent the transmission of infection by one of two methods.
8. Standard precautions are an outgrowth of measures to prevent the spread of the HIV.
9. Standard Precautions require the use of a gown when entering the room if there is a possibility of contact with infected surfaces or items.
10. The transfer of microorganisms by transmission from the patient's wound to the nurse's hands can occur if the nurse does not wear gloves when cleansing a wound.

SHORT ANSWER

Directions: Write a brief answer for each question.

1. The four stages of an infectious process are:
   a. incubation period
   b. Prodomal period
   c. illness period
   d. convalescent period

2. Five ways to decrease the incidence of nosocomial infection are:
   a. proper handwashing before & after care of patient
   b. Clean incontinent patients promptly
   c. Keep urinary catheter drainage bags below level of bladder-All times
   d. Clean residual urine off catheter bag drainage tube after emptying
   e. Assist all patients on Bed rest to turn, deep breathe & cough every 2 hrs

3. The main reason transmission-based precautions have taken the place of previous isolation procedures is:
   because they did not apply to saliva, sputum, nasal secretions sweat, tears, feces, urine, or vomit unless visably contaminated with blood.

4. The difference in procedures between air-borne precautions and droplet precautions is:
   Airbourne - must wear hair covering plus other PPE and a special particulate filter mask must be worn & sterile glove
   drop-let - wear all PPE,

5. Three examples of nursing measures to meet the psychosocial needs of patients in an isolation room are:
   a. Listen to patients feelings
   b. educate & teach about the infection
   c. make positive comments & try to engage in conversation

6. In what ways do infection control procedures in the home differ from those in the hospital?
   none - must be taught - everythings must be kept clean, dust free & ventilation is important.

7. Special requirements for air-borne precautions when the patient has tuberculosis and needs to leave the isolation room for diagnostic tests are:
   people need to be notified, mask must be worn by patient

8. When a patient is immunocompromised, protective (neutropenic) isolation is required and everyone entering the room must
   wear PPE's - gloves, gown, hat, shoes, mask

9. The three main modes of occupational exposure to blood-borne pathogens through skin, eye, mucous membrane, or parenteral route are:
   a. puncture wounds from contaminated needles or other sharps
   b. skin contact allowing infectious fluids to enter thru broken skin
   c. mucous membrane contact to infectious fluids (eyes, mouth, nose)

10. The four rules of surgical asepsis are:
 a. Know what's sterile
 b. Know what is not sterile
 c. Separate sterile from unsterile
 d. Remedy contamination immediately

11. For the following situations, indicate ways to prevent nosocomial infection.
 a. C.O. is recovering from a colon resection. He has a Foley catheter, IV line, and a wound dressing.
 Use surgical asepsis technique, keep bag below bladder, make sure outer cover of catheter is kept clean + free of urine, use standard precaustions wear gloves, keep area clean, make sure wound dressing used is sterile. Use antiseptic to clean wound. Check date of IV fluid. Wash hands before + after procedures, Teach patient standard precaustions

 b. L.M. is admitted with urinary retention and requires the insertion of an indwelling catheter.
 Use surgical asepsis - use gloves - clean off excess urine around catheter, use antiseptic to cleanse area before inserting. Check dates for sterilization purposes. Don't talk while doing procedure, wash hands before + after, Teach patient standard precautions.

 c. R.C. had a hip replacement three days ago. He tends to dribble urine and needs assistance with turning.
 Make sure excess urine is cleaned around area. Change sheets and gown, use antiseptic when cleaning area + make sure you wash hands before and after procedure.

12. Considering the principles of aseptic technique, explain why the following are considered breaks in sterile technique.
 a. Turning your back to a sterile field:
 not with in visual limits - will not know if something dropped onto sterile field.
 b. Talking to the patient while performing a sterile dressing change:
 air-Bourne - droplets are a way of spreading nosocomial infection.
 c. Spilling sterile saline on the package wrapper that is used as your sterile field:
 package wrapped is contaminated - will contaminate sterile field
 d. Placing unopened packages of sterile 4 x 4 gauze on the sterile field for a sterile dressing change:
 packages are not sterile - should not introduce unsterile with sterile field.

MATCHING

Directions: Match the type of infection in column I with the required type of precautions in column II (may require more than one answer).

Column I			Column II
a 1.	c	pneumonia	a. Standard precautions
a 2.	d	diarrhea from *E. coli*	b. Air-borne precautions
a 3.	a	*Haemophilus influenzae* infection	c. Droplet precautions
a 4.	b	measles	d. Contact precautions
a 5.	c	herpes simplex virus	
a 6.	b	tuberculosis	
a 7.	d	impetigo	
a 8.	b	*Varicella* (chicken pox)	
a 9.	c	Streptococcal pharyngitis	
a 10.	c	viral influenza	

APPLICATION OF THE NURSING PROCESS

Directions: Write a brief answer reflecting application of the nursing process.

1. Assessment—Indicate four signs or symptoms in a patient that might indicate a need for transmission precautions.
   a. rash, swelling
   b. leucocytosis
   c. diahrea
   d. vomiting

2. Nursing diagnosis—The correct nursing diagnosis for a patient with an open wound regarding possible infection is:
   Risk of infection related to surgical wound, open wound or weakened condition

3. Besides writing expected outcomes for the patient, planning for the patient requiring transmission precautions includes:
   need for linens, are dressing supplies in room, Does patient need pain medication, need for ice & drinking water, PPE, are routine meds. due at this time

4. Implementation—The types of teaching required for the patient with an infection are:
   inform about the disease process, modes of transmission, precautions necessary to prevent spread of infection. Standard Precautions are explained

5. Disposable soiled equipment and supplies from the room of a patient under transmission precautions are handled by:
   central supply, laboratory, laundry, housekeeping

6. Evaluation—Evaluation of the patient who has had an infection includes:
   a. Surgical asepsis
   b. infection control

MULTIPLE CHOICE

*Directions: Choose the **best** answer for each of the following questions.*

1. For most nurses, one of the difficult things to remember to do regarding standard precautions is to always
   1. turn gloves inside out when removing them.
   2. instruct the patient when to use gloves.
   3. wash hands after removing gloves even when no contamination occurred.
   4. wash hands before gloving.
2. A sharps container should be replaced whenever it is
   1. completely full.
   2. 1/2 full.
   3. filled to an inch from the top.
   4. 2/3 full.
3. When changing the bed of an incontinent patient, you should wear both gloves and a gown because
   1. contamination of the uniform is likely.
   2. feces stains are hard to remove.
   3. the uniform will carry an odor after this task.
   4. urine will soak through the uniform to the skin.
4. When working with a patient who is under droplet precautions, you should
   1. talk to the patient over the intercom frequently.
   2. gather all needed equipment before entering the room.
   3. refrain from entering the room more than four times in a shift.
   4. avoid tiring the patient with a lot of conversation.
5. The goal of nursing actions is the same for surgical asepsis and for protective isolation; that is, to
   1. confine the organisms to the infected patient.
   2. protect the nurse from infection.
   3. protect other people from the microorganism.
   4. reduce the microorganisms in the vicinity of the patient.

Situation: You are assigned to the operating room to assist with a minor surgical procedure. The following questions refer to this situation.

6. When performing the surgical scrub, you use continually running water, an antiseptic agent, and scrub brush or pad and scrub the hands and arms for a distance of
   1. 4 inches above the elbow.
   2. an inch below the elbow.
   3. an inch above the elbow.
   4. 2 inches above the elbow.
7. When working with a sterile field, you should
   1. always face the sterile field.
   2. keep the field within 6 inches of the body.
   3. use only one hand within the field.
   4. open sterile packages toward your body.
8. When pouring a sterile liquid, you should
   1. pour it in short batches so as not to splash.
   2. pour with the label away from the palm of the hand.
   3. pour with the label toward the palm of the hand.
   4. place the cap open side down on a sterile surface.
9. If your hand touches the sink faucet while performing a surgical scrub, you must
   1. rescrub the area that touched the faucet.
   2. begin the entire scrub process over.
   3. rescrub the entire hand and arm.
   4. resoap the area and continue the scrub.
10. When opening a sterile package, you should
    1. open it toward your body.
    2. hold it down with one hand while opening it.
    3. open it away from your body.
    4. pull the package apart equally with each hand.

11. When working with a sterile field you know that
    1. the entire field is considered sterile.
    2. the area within 2" of the edge is not sterile.
    3. the area within 1" of the edge is not sterile.
    4. only the center 18" of the field is sterile.

12. You know that nosocomial infection often occurs because an opportunistic organism is more likely to cause infection when
    1. the patient's resistance is high.
    2. the patient's resistance is low.
    3. in the hospital environment.
    4. present in small numbers.

13. You wash your hands frequently because you realize that
    1. soap kills pathogens.
    2. patients expect it.
    3. it is required as part of standard precautions before gloving.
    4. it is the best method of preventing nosocomial infection.

14. The emphasis of protective (neutropenic) isolation is to
    1. protect the health care worker from infectious organisms.
    2. prevent the transfer of microorganisms outside of the patient's environment.
    3. protect the patient from microorganisms in the hospital environment.
    4. build up the patient's immunity to normal flora.

15. For which of the following procedures would sterile technique be *unnecessary*?
    1. surgical wound dressing change.
    2. insertion of a Foley catheter.
    3. insertion of a nasogastric tube into the stomach.
    4. changing a solution bag on an intravenous infusion.

CRITICAL THINKING ACTIVITIES

1. Decide how you would handle the situation if you were participating in a surgical procedure and you noticed the surgeon contaminate one glove.
2. Describe how to assess the psychosocial needs of a patient under transmission precautions and how you could plan to meet them.

MEETING CLINICAL OBJECTIVES

Directions: The following suggested activities will help you meet the stated clinical practice objectives for the chapter. Review your school's clinical objectives for the week and outline a plan of activities that will help you meet them. If unsure as to how to meet them, consult with your instructor at the beginning of the clinical day.

1. Ask to be assigned to patients under different types of transmission precautions.
2. Teach a home care patient and family how to dispose of used needles and syringes and how to sterilize implements used for dressing changes.
3. Practice the surgical scrub in the skill lab, or home-simulated situation, until you are comfortable with the procedure. Have a peer observe your technique.
4. Practice setting up a sterile field, opening sterile packages, and sterile gloving. Have a peer observe your technique.
5. Observe for breaks in asepsis when working with other nurses and decide how you would have avoided the break and how to remedy it.

STEPS TOWARD BETTER COMMUNICATION

VOCABULARY BUILDING GLOSSARY

Term	Pronunciation	Definition
affixed	af FIXed	fastened, attached, put on
curtail	cur TAIL	decrease, make less
enhance	en HANCE	improve
immunocompromised	IM mu no COM pro mised	poor immune response
impervious	im PER vi ous	nothing can go through it
intact	in TACT	whole, unbroken
integrity	in TEG ri ty	completeness, strength
muster	MUS ter	to collect, summon
onset	ON set	beginning
premise	PREM ise	a basis for reasoning, assumption
prudent	PRU dent	showing carefulness
residual	re SID u al	left over, remaining
rectified	REC ti fied	corrected, changed
scalding	SCALD ing	extremely hot, almost boiling
sensory deprivation	SEN so ry DEP ri va tion	a situation with little stimulation for the senses, like a dark, quiet room with no visitors
surveillance	sur VEIL lance	continually watching, looking for
tiers	TIERS	levels

COMPLETION

Directions: Fill in the blank(s) with the correct word(s) from the Vocabulary Building Glossary to complete the sentence.

1. The patient who has undergone radiation treatment or chemotherapy for cancer is immunocompromised.
2. A sterile package is only sterile if the package's onset is unbroken.
3. The resdual urine on the spout of a catheter bag can form a breeding area for bacteria.
4. One form of disinfection in the home is to pour scalding water over dishes and utensils.
5. The patient who is in an isolation room may experience sensorydepriation because people only enter when they have to perform some function and there is little social interaction.
6. A good handwashing program will enhance infection control in any agency.

VOCABULARY EXERCISE

Directions: Underline the word from the Vocabulary Building Glossary and fill in the blank.

1. What is the premise for handwashing? curtail
2. What is affixed to the hospitalized patient's wrist? affixed
3. What is a sign of the onset of infection? premise
4. We need to muster enough integrity to safely transfer the totally dependent 250 lb. patient.
5. If we curtail the noise, the halls will be sensory deprivation.
6. If you line out and note your tiers over the error in your nurse's notes, the error will be rectified.
7. If the skin is not broken, is it intact or enhanced? intact
8. A prudent nurse would maintain surveillance over a patient. True or false? ______________
9. The disposable gown was impervious to __________________.
10. The tiers of nursing administration end with the ____________________.

PRONUNCIATION OF DIFFICULT TERMS

Directions: Practice pronouncing the following words with a partner.

adenovirus	ad en o vir us
antimicrobial	an ti mi CRO bi al
epidemiology	EP i de mi OL o gy
epiglottitis	ep i glot TI tis
hemorrhagic	hem or rhAG ic
immunodeficiency	IM mu no de FI cien cy
leukocytosis	leu ko cy TO sis
Neisseria meningitidis	NES ser i a me NIN gi tid is
pharyngeal	pha ryn ge al
serosanguineous	ser o SAN gui ne ous
staphylococcal	STAPH y lo COC cal
furunculosis	fur UN cu los sis
streptococcal pneumonia	strep to CO cal pneum mon ia

COMMUNICATION EXERCISE

Directions: With a partner, write one of these dialogues and practice it together.

1. Describe to the patient's wife or husband how to remove contaminated gloves.
2. Explain to your home care patient's spouse why and how to keep the patient's room clean.
3. Explain to an extended family who wants to gather around the bed of their grandfather who has active tuberculosis why they must gown and mask when visiting him.

CULTURAL POINTS

Many of the procedures used for infection control are commonly known and accepted by the general public, even if they are not always followed: handwashing after using the toilet and before handling food, covering the mouth and nose when sneezing and coughing, disposing of soiled tissues in the trash, isolating oneself from people when contagious, not spitting or cleaning the nose with fingers.

However, in some cultures it is common and accepted practice for the family and friends to gather around the sick person. They may prefer to be very close to each other when they talk, and may commonly share drinking vessels and dishes. They may not have facilities for handwashing, or have a way to keep themselves and their belongings washed, and may not consider it important. They may not put used toilet paper in the toilet because they have not had modern plumbing or have been trained that it will clog the pipes. Some people commonly spit on the ground, and reuse the same dirty handkerchiefs.

Where have you observed these behaviors? Can you think of others? Do you think it affects those people's health? How would you explain to them the need for a change in behavior during illness, without offending them or saying anything negative about their culture?

Review the chapter highlights, answer the study questions, and complete the critical thinking activities at the end of the chapter in the textbook.

SEVENTEEN

Lifting, Moving, and Positioning Patients

TERMINOLOGY

A. MATCHING

Directions: Match the anatomical terms in column I with the definitions in column II.

Column I		Column II	
1. f	bone	a.	Cords of fibrous connective tissue connecting muscle to bone that are necessary for movement
2. d	bursa	b.	Fibrous connective tissue that acts as a cushion
3. b	cartilage	c.	Supports and strengthens the bones of joints
4. e	joint	d.	Small, fluid-filled sacs that provide a cushion in movable joints
5. c	ligament	e.	Union of two or more bones in the body
6. a	tendon	f.	Dense and hard type of connective tissue

B. COMPLETION

Directions: Fill in the blank(s) with the correct term(s) from the terms list in the chapter in the textbook to complete the sentence.

1. When a patient is positioned in bed, the body should be kept in proper body allignment to prevent strain on joints and promote comfort.
2. A pivot movement, when moving a patient from bed to chair, will help prevent twisting of the body and possible injury to the nurse.
3. A pressure ulcer is one that forms from a local interference with circulation.
4. Unrelieved pressure on an area can cause death of tissue referred to as necrosis.
5. When a patient slides down while sitting in a chair, a shearing force can occur which may cause a pressure ulcer.
6. During musculoskeletal assessment, observe for muscle weakness, paralysis, and symmetry of the extremities.

7. When assessing ability to perform activities of daily living (ADLs), assess the patient's ability to ambulate and change position independently.

8. The style of walking, called gait, is assessed to see if it is even and unlabored.

9. The logrolling method is used to turn patients in bed who have spinal injuries.

10. Positioning the patient on the side of the bed with the legs and feet over the side is called having the patient dangle.

11. A device that makes ambulating or transferring a patient much safer for both the nurse and the patient is a wheelchair.

12. If the arm is not placed in correct alignment and exercised regularly, the complication of elbow contractures may occur.

13. The study of movement of body parts and positioning is called Kinesiology.

SHORT ANSWER

Directions: Write a brief answer for each question.

1. Give two reasons that correct body alignment and body mechanics are important:
   a. body functions best when it's in correct alignment
   b. To prevent Injuries

2. Changing the patient's position accomplishes four things:
   a. it provides comfort
   b. relieve pressure on bony prominences + other parts
   c. helps prevent contractures, deformaties + respiratory problems
   d. it improves circulation

3. Principles of body mechanics to be used when transferring or repositioning a patient are (*complete the sentences*):
   a. Keep your feet about a shoulder's width apart (For a wide Base)
   b. Use smooth coordinate movements.
   c. Keep your elbows and work close to your body.
   d. Work at the same level or height as the object to be moved.
   e. Pull and Pivot.
   f. Face in the direction of movement.

4. Give an example of use of each of the principles in question #3 above.
   a. lifting a pt. from Bed
   b. tranferring pt. for stretcher
   c. tranferring pt. From bed to stretcher
   d. making a bed
   e. guiding pt. to wheelchair
   f. when picking up something

5. The three main hazards of improper alignment and positioning are:
   a. Interference with circulation - may lead to Pressure Ulcers
   b. muscle cramps, & contractures (Joints that are frozen because of muscles pulling
   c. fluid collection in the lungs

6. Indicate ways to help maintain correct alignment and position for each of the following patients.

   a. A 26-year-old male with a head injury who is on bed rest. He is in the supine position and is comatose.
   place pillow under patients head, neck, and upper shoulders, check symmetry, observe any noticable curves.

   b. A 76-year-old female with congestive heart failure and shortness of breath. She is in high Fowler's position and is very weak.
   Place head & neck against small pillow, Support arms and hands with Pillows, Place small pillow or towel roll under thighs. Use heel pads or small pillow or rolled towel under ankles to protect heals.

7. Describe the steps you would take to transfer a patient from the wheelchair to the bed.
   Use your leg muscles, provide your feet about a shoulders with apart, Use smooth coordinate movements, keep close to body, & center of gravity Pull or Pivot. Gather wheelchair & lock. Place chair parrellel to side of Bed explain procedure, Lower Bed rail, place slippers on Pt. Assist Pt. to turn on side, Support pt. shoulders and thighs with each hand, help pt. sit up & dangle legs, Place Robe on, Recheck locked wheels, Place arms under Axillary & Scapula, on a ct. of 3 raise pt. & Pivot 90° Flex knees & lower pt.

8. Pulling is easier than pushing because It brings patient closer to nurses center of gravity. & requires less effort.

√ 9. How do you provide lateral stability when reaching?
   Keep your feet about a shoulder's width apart.

10. Describe ways to decrease the risk of a patient falling while ambulating.
   use gait belt, use of wheelchair, assess patients balance or dizziness, get 2 People to help.

11. When performing passive ROM exercises, all muscles over a joint are maximally stretched to achieve or maintain flexibility.

12. Each set of movements for ROM exercises should be performed a minimum of 2 times.

13. When performing passive ROM exercises, it is important to always support the limb above and below the joint.

14. Pick up your heaviest book or a similar object and hold it out at arm's length for at least 30 seconds. Now bring it close to your body for the same length of time. What difference did you notice in its apparent weight?
   It seems less heavier. Back pressure was eased.

MATCHING

Directions: Match the position in column I with its description in column II.

Column I

1. __c__ supine
2. __e__ side-lying
3. __a__ prone
4. __f__ Fowler's
5. __d__ semi-Fowler's
6. __b__ Sims'

Column II

a. Lying face down
b. On left side with left arm behind the body and the right knee and thigh up above the left lower leg
c. Resting on the back
d. On back with head of bed between 30–60 degrees
e. Weight on dependent shoulder and hip
f. On back with head of bed between 60–90 degrees

APPLICATION OF THE NURSING PROCESS

Directions: Write a brief answer for each question.

1. When assessing the patient's position in bed for correct alignment you would check: problems associated with mobility, pillow under head - the vertebral column is centered under head, in alignment & there aren't any observable curves. Mattress should support the body in this position
2. The main or most common nursing diagnosis for patients who have a problem with body movement is risk for injury
3. An expected outcome for the nursing diagnosis in question #2 above is: patient will experience no musculoskeletal injury
4. When implementing ROM exercises, you know that they should be performed actively or passively several times a day.
5. When a patient has been lying in bed and is to ambulate or sit in a chair, the patient should be properly instructed before arising from the bed. (Assessed)
6. When moving a patient in or out of a wheelchair it is extremely important to first lock of wheels.
7. Evaluation should include your own use of proper Body mechanics.
8. Write two evaluation statements that would indicate that the above expected outcome is being met.
   a. Patient's positioning was safe & done correctly
   b. Pressure areas did not develop on skin

MULTIPLE CHOICE

*Directions: Choose the **best** answer for each of the following questions.*

1. To ensure good stability of the base of support of the body, the feet should be positioned
   1. parallel and very close together.
   2. about 8" apart, one a little ahead of the other.
   3. about 6" apart with toes pointed slightly laterally.
   4. parallel and about shoulder-width apart.

2. Areas that should be checked for problems due to pressure when the patient has been in the supine position are
   1. hip and shoulder.
   2. scapula, sacrum, elbows, and the heels.
   3. shoulder, elbow, and ankle.
   4. hip, elbow, and ankle.

3. The position most commonly used for inserting a rectal suppository is the
   1. prone position.
   2. Sims' position.
   3. side-lying position.
   4. knee-chest position.

Situation: O.B., a 67-year-old male, suffered a stroke three days ago. He has left arm and leg weakness (hemiparesis) and aphasia. His speech is limited to "boler," "soup," and "no." He is conscious and quite depressed.

4. While performing passive ROM to his affected extremities, O.B. says, "Boler, boler, boler." You don't understand what he is trying to say. What would you do now?
   1. Report to the charge nurse that he is crying and might be having pain or discomfort.
   2. Go ahead and carry out the bath and exercises, since he must be confused.
   3. Ask the patient to nod his head for "yes" and shake his head for "no," then explain again and ask questions to see if he understands what you mean.
   4. Tell him not to cry and reassure him that everything will be all right.

5. O.B.'s tray arrives with his lunch. As you feed him, you hand him a piece of bread, which he holds in his unaffected hand. As he moves his hand to his mouth to eat, what movement does he use?
   1. flexion of the wrist
   2. external rotation of the shoulder
   3. internal rotation of the shoulder
   4. pronation of the wrist

6. When performing ROM exercises, you raise the left arm straight out from the side to shoulder height. This movement is called
   1. flexion.
   2. abduction.
   3. extension.
   4. adduction.

7. Before transferring O.B. from the bed to a wheelchair, the most important step is to
   1. position the chair so you can pivot him into it.
   2. engage the lock on the wheelchair.
   3. assist him with putting on his robe and slippers.
   4. raise the head of the bed to Fowler's position.

8. O.B. has made very good progress in physical therapy. An order has been written to ambulate him with assistance. Before you assist him to walk for the first time, you help him to dangle his legs. The reason(s) for this could be to
   1. strengthen his leg muscles before he stands.
   2. improve the circulation of the paralyzed leg and foot.
   3. prevent contractures of the paralyzed arm and leg.
   4. help him adjust to the change of position and recover from any dizziness.

9. You are going to walk O.B. in his room for the first time with the assistance of another nurse. Which of the following will you do?
   1. Use a gait belt and walk on his weaker side.
   2. Provide support by having one walk in front of the patient and the other behind him.
   3. Hold him at the waist, walk backwards in front of him with the other nurse at his side.
   4. each support one arm and match his steps.

10. Considering O.B.'s state of weakness, when planning to ambulate him it is important to
    1. ambulate after a meal when he is strongest.
    2. remember to plan the distance for a 'round trip.'
    3. ambulate him as far as he can possibly go.
    4. have someone follow with a wheelchair in case of weakness.

CRITICAL THINKING ACTIVITIES

1. If your patient is in leg traction, what can you do to try to prevent pressure ulcers that often occur when a patient is in a supine position?
2. An unconscious patient does not move voluntarily at all. If you place him in Sims' position, which areas would need to be closely watched for signs of undue pressure?
3. Which positioning devices would be useful for the patient who is unconscious?

MEETING CLINICAL OBJECTIVES

Directions: The following suggested activities will help you meet the stated clinical practice objectives for the chapter. Review your school's clinical objectives for the week and outline a plan of activities that will help you meet them. If unsure as to how to meet them, consult with your instructor at the beginning of the clinical day.

1. Practice principles of body alignment and movement when performing daily tasks such as carrying groceries, reaching for things on high shelves, vacuuming, picking up a child, carrying your school books, and so forth.
2. With a peer or family member, practice placing the body in the various positions used for positioning the bed patient.
3. Work with another nurse on the unit to which you are assigned and learn how pillows and other aids are used to position patients.

STEPS TOWARD BETTER COMMUNICATION

VOCABULARY BUILDING GLOSSARY

Term	Pronunciation	Definition
alleviates	al LE vi ates	reduces
dispersed	dis PERSed	spread out over an area
hyperflex	HY per FLEX	bend too much
inertia	in ER tia	lack of movement or change

predisposes	pre dis POS es	makes vulnerable, more likely to happen
striated	STRI a ted	having long streaks, composed of long bands
sway	SWAY	move back and forth

VOCABULARY EXERCISE

Directions: Using terms from the Vocabulary Building Glossary, fill in the sentences in the following paragraph.

The ____Striated____ muscle works to move the extremities. ____mertia____ for long periods tends to make the muscles atrophy. When muscles are not exercised and joints are not moved, the joints are ____predisposed____ to contractures. Exercising the joints also ____alleviates____ the pain that can occur with inactivity. Proper positioning insures that the weight of the body is ____disperse____ over a broad area. When performing ROM exercises, it is best not to ____hyperflex____ a joint, as that may cause injury. When transferring a patient from the bed to a chair, a wide base of support is used so that you do not ____Sway____ while moving the patient.

WORD ATTACK SKILLS

ABDUCTION VERSUS ADDUCTION

1. "Ab" means away from, so *ab*duction would mean movement away from the body. Think of a hand open with the fingers spread away from each other.
2. "Ad" means toward, so *ad*duction would mean movement toward the body. Think of a hand that is open but with the fingers touching each other.
3. *Flex* means to bend.
4. A flexion position would mean a bent neck, elbow, knee, etc. Think of a hand with the fist closed.
5. *Extend* means to stretch out. Therefore, an extension position would be one where joints (the elbow, knee, neck, or wrist and finger) are not bent. Think of a hand held open and straight.

PRONUNCIATION OF DIFFICULT TERMS

Directions: Practice pronouncing the following words.

alignment ligament

When the consonant combination "gn" falls in the same syllable, the "g" is silent. Examples: sign (SIgN), malign (ma LIgN), gnaw (gNAW)

When the two consonants fall in different syllables, they are both pronounced. Examples: ignore (ig NORE), ignite (ig NITE), designation (des ig NA tion), dignitary (DIG ni tary)

Mark the syllables in these words and pronounce them:

prognosis design aligned magnificent

COMMUNICATION EXERCISE

Write a short dialogue explaining to O.B. (Questions 4-10 in the multiple choice section) what you are doing as you prepare to ambulate him/move him to a wheelchair. O.B. has very limited speech.

Review the chapter highlights, answer the study questions, and complete the critical thinking activities at the end of the chapter in the textbook.

EIGHTEEN

Assisting with Hygiene and Personal Care, Skin Care, and the Prevention of Pressure Ulcers

TERMINOLOGY

A. MATCHING

Directions: Match the terms in column I with the definitions in column II.

Column I			Column II
1. g blanch		a.	System of skin hair, nails, sweat and sebaceous glands
2. a integumentary		b.	Outer, thicker layer of skin
3. i maceration		c.	Substance secreted by sebaceous glands
4. d cerumen		d.	Substance secreted by ceruminous glands in the ear
5. j dermis		e.	Practice of cleanliness
6. b epidermis		f.	Foul-smelling breath
7. f halitosis		g.	Turn white or become pale
8. e hygiene		h.	Hardening of an area
9. h induration		i.	Softening of tissue
10. c sebum		j.	Inner, thinner layer of the skin

B. COMPLETION

Directions: Fill in the blank(s) with the correct term(s) from the list of terms in the chapter in the textbook to complete the sentence.

1. The redness that occurs at the beginning of a pressure ulcer is caused by local interference and vasodilation.
2. A patient that is experiencing diaphoresis is at risk of skin breakdown from the excess moisture.
3. Stage IV pressure ulcers often have dry, black, necrotic tissue called eschar within them.

4. If teeth are not brushed regularly, halitosis may form.
5. Skin color is determined by the amount of melanin secreted by the melanocytes in the epidermis.
6. Sebum is an oily substance secreted by the Sebaceous glands.
7. When assisting a patient out of a very warm bath, the patient should move slowly to avoid dizziness and fainting.
8. Constriction of the opening in the foreskin of the penis, ____________, sometimes occurs and prevents retraction of the foreskin back from the head of the penis.

REVIEW OF STRUCTURE AND FUNCTION

Directions: Note the structure that fits with the function listed.

1. melanin absorbs light and protects against ultraviolet rays.
2. skin (sweat glands) helps regulate temperature by dilating and constricting blood vessels.
3. sebaceous gland make skin waterproof.
4. Sebum lubricates the skin and hair.
5. Sweat Glands help maintain homeostasis of fluid and electrolytes.
6. mucous membranes protect against bacterial invasion, secrete mucus, and absorb fluid and electrolytes.
7. skin contains sensory organs for touch, pain, heat, cold, and pressure.
8. skin is the first line of defense in protecting the body from invading organisms.

SHORT ANSWER

Directions: Write a brief answer for each question.

1. List the five factors that affect hygiene practice:
   a. sociocultural background
   b. economic status
   c. knowledge level
   d. ability to preform self-care
   e. personal preference
2. List the five risk factors for pressure ulcers and give one rationale for each factor.
   a. Bed or chair confinement
      edema
   b. inability to move
      obesity
   c. loss of Bowel or Bladder control
      excessive diaphoresis
   d. Poor nutrition
      Dehydration
   e. Lowered mental awareness
      extreme age due to fragile skin

3. What are the other factors that may contribute to pressure ulcer formation?
Lowered mental awareness may be caused by meds, anesthesia or health problem

4. List five nursing interventions that you feel are most important in preventing pressure ulcers.
   a. Change patients position at least every 2 hrs.
   b. Keep heels of totally immobile patients off the bed
   c. observe color of skin carefully & frequently
   d. Restore circulation of deprived area by rubbing around reddened area
   e. wash & dry incontinent patients quickly
   f. Provide adequate nutrition & fluid intake

5. For each of the following positions, list pressure points to be checked when the patient's position is changed.
   a. Sitting in a wheelchair:
   Shoulder Blade, sacrum & coccyx, posterior knee, ischial tuberosity, foot
   b. Supine in semi-Fowler's position:
   rim of ear, elbow, occiput, Dorsal thoracic area, Sacrum & coccyx, heel
   c. Sims' position:
   side of head, shoulder, ischium, trochanter, malleolus anterior, knee, perineum

6. A thorough skin assessment should be done upon admission and every 24 hrs. thereafter.

7. A reddened area caused by pressure should subside within 30-45 mins. when the patient's position is changed.

8. Give three characteristics of each stage of pressure ulcer.
   a. Stage I:
   area of red, deep, pink or mottled skin that does not blanch discoloration, edema, warmth, induration - area feels hard
   b. Stage II:
   area surrounding damaged skin feels warm, partial-thickness skin loss of epidermis or dermis, Looks like abrasion, blister or shallow crater
   c. Stage III:
   Full thickness skin loss - looks like deep crater & may extend to fascia, Bacterial infection causes drainage of ulcer, may be damage to surrounding tissue
   d. Stage IV:
   extensive tissue necrosis or damage to muscle, bone, sinus tracts may be present, ulcer appears dry, black in color - appears wet & oozing, eschar present

9. Older adults have an increased risk of developing impaired skin integrity because:
of decreased subcutaneous fat, sebaceous gland activity and elasticity in their skin.

10. The four basic purposes for bathing are:
    a. accesses the condition of skin
    b. over-all physical appearance
    c. emotional & mental status
    d. learning needs

11. A partial bath done by a patient alone consists of washing the:
    face, hands, axillae, back & perineal area

12. Whirlpool baths are therapeutically used to:
    a. to cleanse
    b. stimulate peripheral circulation
    c. provide comfort

13. A sitz bath is used to promote healing by applying moist heat which increases circulation in the perineal area.

14. Sitz baths are used after vaginal or rectal surgery and after childbirth.

15. A back rub is essential for patients who are confined to bed.

16. Full mouth care for the unconscious patient should be provided at least once every 8 hours.

17. When not in the mouth, dentures should be cared for by placing them in labeled denture container

18. Nail care is important, but a physician's order is needed to cut the toenails of the diabetic patient or one with a disease of the lower extremities.

19. A contact lens should be cleansed by moistening and rubbing gently between the fingers while holding over a basin of water or stopped sink.

20. A hearing aid should never be cleaned by soaking it in water.

21. In the older adult, dry and itchy skin is caused by the decreased activity of the sebum or sebaceous glands.

APPLICATION OF THE NURSING PROCESS

Directions: Write a brief answer for each question.

1. Two primary areas to assess when considering hygiene needs and problems are:
    a. cognitive
    b. physical function

2. Most patients with a problem of mobility or who are on bed rest will have the following nursing diagnosis related to hygiene: risk for impaired skin integrity

3. Write an expected outcome for the above nursing diagnosis:
    patient will maintain intact skin while on bed rest

4. When implementing a bed bath for an elderly patient, you would alter your bath procedure by:
    on alternate days - use soap only on areas visibly soiled

5. Write an evaluation statement that would indicate that the expected outcome, "patient will maintain intact skin while on bed rest" is being met.

no evidence of redness, irritation or breaks in skin integrity
skin integrity is maintained

MULTIPLE CHOICE

*Directions: Choose the **best** answer for each of the following questions.*

Situation: P.S., age 76, is hospitalized with dehydration and pneumonia. She also has peripheral vascular (circulatory) disease of the lower extremities. She has been confused and in bed for several days before admission.

1. An especially important aspect of giving a bed bath to an elderly patient is to
   1. move very slowly to prevent agitating the patient.
   2. seek assistance in order to finish the bath quickly.
   3. keep the patient covered well to prevent chilling.
   4. use vigorous rubbing to remove soil from the skin.

2. When washing P.S.'s face you wash the eye area from the inner to the outer canthus with separate parts of the washcloth to
   1. promote circulation.
   2. prevent infection.
   3. avoid getting soap in the eye.
   4. prevent visual obstruction.

3. When washing P.S.'s arm, you use long, firm strokes, moving from the hand to the axilla to
   1. fully assess the skin on all sides of the arm.
   2. improve circulation in the extremity.
   3. prevent infection by cleansing from dirty to clean.
   4. provide range of motion exercise for the joint.

4. P.S. refuses perineal care. You know that this is probably because she
   1. can do it well by herself.
   2. has no vaginal secretions and does not need it.
   3. is embarrassed to have someone else perform it.
   4. prefers to do this only once a week.

5. When preparing to store P.S.'s dentures in a denture cup, you must be certain to
   1. label the cup with her name and room number.
   2. place denture solution in the cup.
   3. line the cup with a paper towel.
   4. send the dentures home with the family.

6. When turning P.S., you provide skin care by
   1. bathing the area that has been against the mattress.
   2. providing a back massage after turning.
   3. rubbing all areas that were against the mattress.
   4. checking all bony prominences that were dependent for reddening.

7. P.S. has a reddened, slightly abraded area on the inner aspect of her right knee. This would be considered a ________________ pressure ulcer.
   1. Stage I
   2. Stage II
   3. Stage III
   4. Stage IV

8. Because of this pressure area, it would be best to position P.S.
   1. on her back or right side.
   2. on her back or left side.
   3. supine in Semi-Fowler's only
   4. in Sims' position or supine.

9. A contributing factor for pressure ulcers for P.S. is
   1. respiratory infection.
   2. intravenous therapy.
   3. dehydration.
   4. weakness.

10. P.S.'s toenails are in need of trimming. You would
    1. ask the family to bring clippers from home.
    2. ask her daughter to perform this function for her.
    3. call her podiatrist to come and trim them.
    4. seek an order from the physician to cut her toenails.

CRITICAL THINKING ACTIVITIES

1. What should you do if your patient refuses to bathe?
2. Your male patient normally shaves with an electric razor. He was admitted as an emergency patient and does not have his razor with him. You would like to shave him. How would you plan to do this?

MEETING CLINICAL OBJECTIVES

Directions: The following suggested activities will help you meet the stated clinical practice objectives for the chapter. Review your school's clinical objectives for the week and outline a plan of activities that will help you meet them. If unsure as to how to meet them, consult with your instructor at the beginning of the clinical day.

1. Practice the bed bath procedure at home on a family member or friend until you are comfortable and efficient with the procedure.
2. Practice shaving the face of a male family member or friend to decrease initial anxiety and awkwardness when performing the procedure in the health care agency.
3. Accompany another nurse when she gives hygiene care to an unconscious patient. Pay particular attention to the technique of giving safe mouth care.
4. When observing hygiene care being given by other nurses, notice how the patient's privacy is protected or invaded. Discuss this issue in clinical conference.
5. Assist another nurse in giving a bed shampoo in order to become more familiar and comfortable with this task.
6. Provide personal care for a patient.
7. Attempt to stage a pressure ulcer and describe appropriate care.

STEPS TOWARD BETTER COMMUNICATION

VOCABULARY BUILDING GLOSSARY

Term	Pronunciation	Definition
acuity	a CU i ty	sharpness of perception
adipose	AD i pose	containing fat

debridement	de BRIDe ment (day breed maw) (French pronunciation)	removal of foreign, contaminated, or dead tissue from a wound
don	DON (verb)	to put on
exacerbation	ex a CER bA tion	increase in severity of symptoms
mottled	MOT tled	irregular patches of color
nick	NICK (verb)	very small cut, usually accidental
slough off	SLOUGH (pronounced "sluff") off	to shed, to drop off
stratified	STRA ti fied	in layers
subside	sub SIDE (verb)	to gradually go away, become less

COMPLETION

Directions: Fill in the blank(s) with the correct word(s) from the Vocabulary Building Glossary to complete the sentence.

1. Sometimes using soap on a patient's skin causes an exacerbation of a dry skin condition.
2. When shaving a patient with a safety razor, be careful not to nick the skin.
3. While bathing the patient, she noticed that the skin around the ankle was mottled.
4. It is essential to don gloves before cleansing the perineal area.
5. The patient who has sustained a deep burn often must undergo debridement of the burned area.

VOCABULARY EXERCISE

Directions: Match the following words in column I with their meanings in column II.

Column I		Column II	
1. e	blanched	a.	hardened
2. d	mottled	b.	blocked
3. b	occluded	c.	softened
4. c	macerated	d.	covered with patches of color
5. a	indurated	e.	lost color

WORD ATTACK SKILLS

Directions: Match the following words with their meanings.

1. If <u>dermis</u> is the inner layer of the skin, and <u>epidermis</u> is the outer, thicker layer of the skin, what does EPI mean? outer

2. What does DERM- mean? skin

3. If induration means hardening, and durable means sturdy or long-lasting, what does DUR- mean? hard + sturdy

PRONUNCIATION OF DIFFICULT TERMS

Directions: Practice pronouncing the following terms.

débridement	day breed MAW
decubitus	de CU bi tus
diaphoresis	di a pho RE sis
eschar	ES kar; ESC har
mottled	MOT ulled (this word is pronounced with a quick stop of breath between the two "t"s, and sounds almost like "modeled")
phimosis	phi mo sis
sebaceous	se BA ceous
syncope	SYN co pe

COMMUNICATION EXERCISE

What would be some things you could talk about as you give your patient a bath? Or should you talk?

CULTURAL POINTS

Americans today are very concerned about cleanliness and bathing often, usually every day, and about how they smell. Any natural body odor is usually considered bad. Perhaps this has been influenced by an over-application of the theory of health hygiene. On the other hand, as the public health environment has become "cleaner" we may have become lax about such things as handwashing.

What habits of hygiene are different here in the U.S. than they were in your country? Which ones make a difference for health, and which are only cosmetic—for looks or comfort?

Why would sociocultural or economic background affect hygiene? In what ways?

Is there a difference between personal hygiene and community hygiene? Can you think of ways in which hygiene makes a difference for the health of people in your native country?

Discuss these issues with your peers.

Review the chapter highlights, answer the study questions, and complete the critical thinking activities at the end of the chapter in the textbook.

NINETEEN

Patient Environment and Safety

TERMINOLOGY

A. COMPLETION

Directions: Fill in the blank(s) with the correct term(s) from the terms list in the chapter in the textbook to complete the sentence.

1. Room temperature, furniture arrangement, neatness of the area, and lighting are all part of the patient __environment__.
2. When a person is ill, __temperature__ of the room is even more important as fresh air is essential.
3. A very low __humidity__ dries respiratory passages and the skin.
4. A __poison__ is a substance that may cause functional or structural disturbances if it is ingested, inhaled, absorbed, injected, or developed within the body.
5. A biological agent or condition that can be harmful to a person's health, such as a contaminated needle, is called a __biohazard__.

SHORT ANSWER

Directions: Write a brief answer for each question.

1. The goal in caring for the patient environment is to provide __safety__ while making the patient as __comfortable__ as possible.
2. The patient's room temperature should be kept at __68°__ to __74°__.
3. Lighting should meet these three requirements:
   a. bright enough to see without glare — For tasks
   b. be soft + diffuse - avoid eye strain — to prevent injury
   c. prevent sharp shadows — sunny + cheerful
4. Two important measures that can assist in reducing odors that seem unpleasant to patients are to:
   a. Good ventilation
   b. cleanliness

5. Since the major source of noise is people, staff can assist in reducing the problem by:
avoid long conversations on intercom by going to patients room to talk, speak in lowered voices, talk in hallway

6. To maintain neatness in the patient unit, the area should be straightened whenever
making the bed, Old dishes + unused equipment should be removed

7. For safety, whenever a bed is not being moved, it is important to make certain that the
bed wheels are locked.

8. Principles of body mechanics used when making a bed are:
   a. Use good Body Alignment
   b. a wide base for support
   c. a proper working height when making bed
   d. Face toward direction of movement
   e. Bend at knees - not back

9. A measure to prevent falls for the ill patient is to prevent attempts to get out of bed unassisted by
Bed rails

10. List four measures to be used in the home environment that you consider to be most important in preventing patient falls.
   a. non-skid Bath mat
   b. use night lights
   c. encourage removal of extension cords
   d. install GRAB Bars for BR.

11. Extra vigilance to prevent burns is essential for these four types of patients:
   a. diabetics
   b. poor circulation
   c. paralized patient
   d. on drugs that alter mental awareness

12. Smoking is never allowed when oxygen is in use as
a spark could cause a fire

13. For fire safety, each staff member must know:
   a. location of fire extinguishers
   b. location of fire Alarms
   c. escape routes
   d. how to notify operator of a fire

14. The acronym RACE stands for:
R escue any patients in immediate danger by removing from area
A ctivate fire Alarm system
C ontain the fire by closing doors and any open windows
E xtinguish the flames with appropriate extinguisher

15. An important aspect of preventing poisoning in the home is to always keep poisonous substances in their origional labeled container.

16. Protective devices are to be used only as a last resort.

17. Measures that may help to decrease confusion in older adults when they enter a health care facility are: Frequently reorient them, have family bring familiar items from home

18. When applying a protective device, it is essential to be certain that the patient's movements or tugging will not impair blood circulation or nerve function.

19. To check the safe application of a protective device, see if you can insert your index & middle fingers between the patient and the device.

20. Ties for a protective device should be secured to immovable part of the bed frame, or under armrests of a chair.

21. A protective device that immobilizes a body part should be removed every 2 hours and excercises performed to immobilized joints and muscles.

MULTIPLE CHOICE

*Directions: Choose the **best** answer for each of the following questions.*

1. Safety precautions when serving meal trays include
   1. opening all containers on the tray.
   2. providing sufficient napkins.
   3. cutting up meat before serving.
   4. warning the patient about hot liquids.

2. One intervention by the nurse that helps prevent patient falls is to
   1. keep side rails up at all times.
   2. allow the patient to walk only with assistance.
   3. keep the pathway between the bed and bathroom clear.
   4. allow minimal patient belongings in the room.

3. When planning for patient safety, consider the patient's
   1. age.
   2. sex.
   3. educational level.
   4. occupation.

4. Infection control guidelines for patient safety require that infectious waste such as soiled dressings be treated as biohazards and be
   1. sterilized before disposal.
   2. placed in impermeable, sealed bags.
   3. burned as soon as possible.
   4. placed in the utility room trash.

5. In order to prevent falls by elderly patients, you should
   1. encourage the use of nonskid mats in tub or shower.
   2. insist on bright lighting at all times.
   3. keep side rails up when patient is in bed.
   4. encourage use of smooth-soled slippers.

6. When securing the ties on a protective device it is essential that
   1. the knot be easily undone in case of fire.
   2. the knot be difficult to undo.
   3. a double knot be used.
   4. only a square knot be used.

7. When utilizing a safety belt for a patient in a wheelchair, you must
   1. explain to the family exactly why it is being used.
   2. document the specific reason the belt is needed.
   3. fasten it to the chair loosely.
   4. obtain the patient's permission for use.

8. When utilizing a limb immobilizer there must be a written order and device must be removed & patient's position changed at least every 2 hrs.

protective device, you must
1. massage the area proximal to its attachment frequently.
2. flex the joint before applying the device.
3. check the circulation and sensation distal to the device frequently.
4. exercise all joints at least twice per shift.

9. When evaluating a patient's drugs for side effects that may increase the risk of falling, look at those that affect the
    1. central nervous system.
    2. integumentary system.
    3. gastrointestinal system.
    4. respiratory system.

10. A measure to promote patient safety after finishing a nursing procedure is to
    1. explain the reason for the procedure.
    2. elevate the head of the bed to semi-Fowler's position.
    3. replace the bed in the lowest position.
    4. tell the patient when you will return to the room.

11. A safety measure for the patient during ambulation is the use of
    1. a gait belt any time the patient is unsteady.
    2. two people at all times for ambulation.
    3. a rolling IV pole for stability.
    4. only rubber-soled shoes.

12. One measure to prevent nighttime wandering in the elderly is
    1. administer sleeping medication at bedtime.
    2. give a back rub and warm milk at bedtime.
    3. place the patient in a room with another patient.
    4. increase daytime stimulation to decrease napping.

13. The best choice for a protective device to assist a patient who cannot maintain an upright sitting posture in a wheelchair would be
    1. a security vest.
    2. a safety belt.
    3. a protective jacket.
    4. wrist immobilizing devices.

14. An important nursing action for the patient using wrist and ankle immobilizers is to
    1. attach the ties properly to the side rails.
    2. offer fluids at four-hour intervals.
    3. check on the patient every two hours while immobilized.
    4. document their removal and exercises performed every two hours.

15. The first action to be taken in the event of a fire is to
    1. activate the fire alarm.
    2. rescue the patient.
    3. contain the fire.
    4. extinguish the flames.

CRITICAL THINKING ACTIVITIES

1. Your patient is a 78-year-old male with pneumonia who is quite confused. He is prone to falls. He has just been admitted and keeps trying to get out of bed. What measures should you use to keep him in bed without using a protective device?
2. In reviewing Table 19-4, what would you need to do in your home to make it safer from fire?
3. Check your home for poison safety. What do you need to do to protect people in your home from poisoning?

MEETING CLINICAL OBJECTIVES

Directions: The following suggested activities will help you meet the stated clinical practice objectives for the chapter. Review your school's clinical objectives for the week and outline a plan of activities that will help you meet them. If unsure as to how to meet them, consult with your instructor at the beginning of the clinical day.

1. Practice hospital bed-making at home until you can quickly and smoothly make the bed.
2. Locate the fire extinguishers, fire alarms, and escape routes for the unit to which you are assigned for clinical experience.
3. Review the procedures for the handling of biohazards in your clinical facility.
4. If protective devices are available in the skill lab, work with a peer in applying and securing the devices. Take turns being the patient to experience how it feels to have such a device in place.
5. Practice securing the ties of a protective device to the bed properly.
6. When assigned to a patient who is wearing a protective device, think of an alternate solution to the underlying problem.

STEPS TOWARD BETTER COMMUNICATION

VOCABULARY BUILDING GLOSSARY

Term	Pronunciation	Definition
A. Individual Terms		
acronym	AC ro nym	a word made from the first letter of a related list of words (RACE)
altercations	al ter CA tions	arguments, disagreements
clutter	CLUT ter	lots of things around, messy
compromise	COM pro mise	to expose to danger by unwise action
diffused	dif FUSEd	spread around, scattered
frayed	FRAYed	worn at the edges, especially fabric with loose strings
glare	GLARE	a strong reflected light
hazard	HAZ ard	danger
miter	MI ter	joining two flat pieces together at an angle
noxious	NOX ious	harmful
predispose	pre di SPOSE	to make vulnerable, more likely to suffer from
prone	PRONE	likely to happen
slump	SLUMP	to slide or bend into a low position
solaria	so LAR i a	(plural of solarium) sun rooms
stifling	STI fling	preventing, or restricting from getting air
tact	TACT	to speak carefully about an uncomfortable subject so you will not offend
vigilance	VIG i lance	watching carefully over a period of time
warrant	WARR ant	to give sufficient reason or justification for some action

B. Phrases

holistic patient care	ho LIST ic patient care	caring for the whole or total patient—the physical, mental, social, and spiritual parts of life
last resort	LAST re sort	something to do when nothing else works
neat and tidy	NEAT and TI dy	things picked up and organized in their proper places
refrain from	re FRAIN from	to hold back; not do something

COMPLETION

Directions: Fill in the blank(s) with the correct term(s) from the Vocabulary Building Glossary to complete each sentence.

1. Soft, diffused light prevent shadows in the room which can interfere with vision and predispose a patient to a fall.
2. Leaving used equipment in the room trash can lead to noxious odors.
3. A Frayed cord for the electric bed presents a fire hazard.
4. When correcting an nursing assistant's action, it is best to use tact.
5. Nursing instructors like patient rooms to be neat & tidy without clutter lying about.
6. A patient who has a fever may find glare from light uncomfortable.
7. Leaving a spill on the floor will compromise the safety of those working in the area.
8. The patient who has one-sided weakness is prone to falls if allowed to ambulate unassisted initially.
9. One must be careful about intervening in altercation between angry family members.
10. It is necessary to stifling restricting a patient's movements unnecessarily.

VOCABULARY EXERCISE

English words may have many different meanings, as you have discovered. Sometimes these meanings are physical or tangible (meaning they can be touched or felt) and sometimes they are intangible (meaning they can not be touched—like an idea).

1. Below are Glossary words with two correct meanings. Some words have both tangible and intangible meanings. For those words, put the meanings in the correct place.

Word	Physical/Tangible	Emotional/Intangible
Example: frayed	*worn at the edges*	*irritated, annoyed*
glare	strong, reflected light	a look of anger, or hatred
miter	making a corner with 2pcs.	a tall Pointed Bishops hat
prone	likely to happen	lying face down
slump	to slide or bend	financial market
stifle	Restriction of air	Prevent someone from doing something

glare — (n) a strong reflected light/a look of anger or hatred, a harsh stare
(v) to look hard at someone with anger or hatred

miter — making a corner with two pieces at an angle
a tall pointed bishop's hat

prone — likely to happen
lying face down

slump — to slide or bend into a low position
to fall or sink down—financial market, sports record, etc.

stifle — preventing, or restricting from getting air
prevent someone from doing something

2. Opposites: Make sentences using these opposites from the Glossary.
   a. clutter/neat and tidy The clutter in the room became neat & tidy.
   b. glare/diffuse The glare from the light became diffused when adjusted.

COMMUNICATION EXERCISE

Directions: Write what you would say in each of these situations:

1. to a patient before raising the bed rails?
   This is for protecting you from falling out of bed
2. to visitors talking and laughing loudly in the hall?
   Please, lower your voices so our patients can get their proper rest
3. to a family whose elderly mother was put in restraints?
   we are using restraints temporarily for her safety because she keeps falling
4. to a patient when serving morning tea?
   Be careful - this is hot - wait till it cools abit.

GRAMMAR POINTS

The little word "as" has many important uses.

- Here it is used as a conjunction to hold two short clauses together. It means "because."
  "Floor or table fans are discouraged, as moving air currents spread microorganisms."
- Sometimes it is a preposition meaning "in the role of."
  "This medicine is used as a diuretic."
- Sometimes it is an adverb meaning "to the same amount."
  "Can you find something as effective as restraints?"
- "As" may mean "for example."
  "Immobility can cause such physical problems as muscle weakness, atrophy, contractures, constipation, and cognitive impairment."

Directions: What is the meaning of "as" in these sentences?

1. The physician's assistant can often act as a doctor.
   in the role of
2. Restraints should be checked often as they can impair circulation.
   to the same amount
3. Patient rooms are often as nicely furnished as hotel rooms.
   for example
4. Patients can be bothered by such loud noises as inconsiderate talking, noisy equipment, or blaring televisions.
   for example

CULTURAL POINTS

In the United States environmental security and safety are important not only for the patient's comfort and safety, but because there are so many laws requiring it. Hospitals, institutions, agencies, and even individuals run great risks of legal action if they do not provide for the safety and security of the patients and staff. It is for this reason that the administrators and inspectors are so careful to see that the rules are enforced.

Review the chapter highlights, answer the study questions, and complete the critical thinking activities at the end of the chapter in the textbook.

TWENTY

Measuring Vital Signs

TERMINOLOGY

A. MATCHING

Directions: Match the terms in column I with the definitions in column II.

Column I		Column II
1. f apnea		a. State of having a fever
2. b bradycardia		b. Pulse rate less than 60 bpm
3. h bradypnea		c. Pulse rate greater than 100 bpm
4. a febrile		d. Difference between the radial and apical pulse
5. i hypoxia		e. Irregular heart rate
6. e. arrhythmia		f. Absence of breathing
7. d pulse deficit		g. Rapid respiratory rate
8. j stridor		h. Slow, shallow breathing
9. c tachycardia		i. Decreased oxygen in the blood
10. G tachypnea		j. High-pitched crowing sound on inspiration

B. COMPLETION

Directions: Fill in the blank(s) with the correct word(s) from the terms list in the chapter in the textbook to complete the sentence.

1. The normal pattern of breathing is described as Eupnea.
2. The term used to describe difficult and labored breathing is dyspnea.
3. The diastolic pressure is written below the line for BP.
4. When a fever begins to come down, the patient is in a state of defervescence.
5. If a silence is heard between sounds when auscultating blood pressure, it is termed an pulse pressure.
6. The rate at which heat is produced when the body is at rest is the BMR (Basal metabolic Rate)
7. Heat production is a by-product of ~~temperature~~ metabolism
8. The Hypothalamus controls temperature by a feedback mechanism.

9. The pulse rate multiplied by the stroke volume equals the cardiac output / heart rate.

REVIEW OF STRUCTURE AND FUNCTION

Directions: Write a brief answer for each question.

1. Fever occurs when pathogens invade the body & body attempts to destroy them.
2. Factors that affect the BMR are hormones & muscle movement of exercise.
3. The mechanism of diaphoresis attempts to cool the body by evaporation when a high fever occurs.
4. The pulse is produced by cardiac contractions.
5. The pulse rate is normally dependent on the impulses emerging from the SA NODE in the heart. electrical impulse emerging from Rt. atrium
6. The character of the pulse is affected by the stroke volume.
7. Cardiac output is calculated by multiplying the stroke volume by the pulse rate.
8. Ventilation is the mechanical movement of air in and out of the lungs.
9. Diffusion of oxygen and carbon dioxide occurs across the aveolar membrane.
10. Structures directly involved in respiration are nose, pharynx, larynx, trachea, bronchi & lungs.
11. A substance necessary in the alveoli to keep them open is surfactant.
12. The respiratory center is located in the pon and medulla of the brain stem.
13. The respiratory centers are signaled to alter rate or depth of respiration by the carotid body receptors in the carotid arteries and by the aortic Body receptors adjacent to the aortic arch.
14. Systolic pressure is when there is the maximum pressure exerted on the artery during left ventricular contraction.
15. Diastolic pressure occurs when the heart is at rest between contractions.
16. Blood pressure increases as stroke volume increases.
17. Arterial blood pressure rises when there is an increase in vascular resistance.
18. If blood volume decreases, the blood pressure decreases.
19. When vascular wall elasticity decreases, the blood pressure will increase.
20. The lower-than-average temperature often found in the older adult may be a result of a decrease in metabolic rate.
21. The respiratory rate may be slightly rise in the older adult to compensate for a decrease in vital capacity and respiratory reserve.

SHORT ANSWER

Directions: Write a brief answer for each question.

1. Name at least four factors that influence body temperature.
   a. time of day - lower in morning, Afternoon - High Normal
   b. environmental temp.
   c. Age of patient
   d. disease conditions

2. What is the normal range for temperature in Fahrenheit and in Celsius?
   98.6 F. 37.0 C.

3. What is the normal pulse rate in the adult? 72 bpm

4. In addition to the rate, what characteristics of the pulse should you note and be able to describe? strength - rate, rythm, + volume (weak, regular, bounding, thready, feeble)

5. List the points on the body where the pulse can be palpated.
   radial, temporal, Carotid, Femoral, Apical, popliteal, Pedal Pulses

6. When counting the apical pulse, the stethoscope is placed at the 5th intercostal left and apex of heart and counted for 1 min.

7. What are four pulse findings that should be reported?
   a. tachycardia - pulse ≥ 100 bpm Fast
   b. bradycardia - pulse ≥ 60 bpm Slow
   c. Arrhythmia - irregular
   d. Normal

8. The normal range of respirations for a healthy adult is 12-20.

9. The respiratory center of the brain is more sensitive to changes in the Carbon dioxide levels.

10. The average blood pressure of a healthy young adult is 120/80.

11. Name at least five conditions/factors that are helpful in taking an accurate blood pressure reading.
    a. Have patient Lie down or sit for 5 min.
    b. Use correct cuff size
    c. check condition of equipment
    d. place cuff & stethoscope on bare skin of arm
    e. do not stop midway to inflate again

12. Low blood pressures are dangerous when they occur with symptoms of dizziness or cold clammy skin, increase in pulse Rate, blurred vision.

13. One problem that the elderly may have related to blood pressure is orthostatic or hypotension.

14. To determine if the patient has a pulse deficit you would:
    take radial pulse + apical pulse - radial subtracted by apical pulse. Take a pedal pulse or pulse - in radial

APPLICATION OF THE NURSING PROCESS

Directions: Write a brief answer for each question.

1. Jamie, age 14 months, has been ill with vomiting and diarrhea. He has been running an elevated temperature. His parents bring him to the clinic to see the nurse practitioner. Which type of thermometer would be best to use for Jamie and which route would you use to check his temperature? tympanic

2. How would you take a pulse on a crying 4-year-old child?
radial

3. If you check the radial pulse on your patient and find that it is irregular, what would you do next?
take apical

4. If your patient weighs 280 lbs., what type of equipment would you use to take the blood pressure?
large cuff size

5. What is the best way to measure respirations on a clinic patient who has on a shirt and sweater?
place hand on chest

6. List one appropriate nursing diagnosis for each of the following situations:
   a. Patient with a temperature of 102.2° F. (39.0° C.) who is acutely ill:
   febrile – pyrexia
   b. Patient with a respiratory rate of 28 who is quite short of breath: ✓
   dyspnea
   c. Adult patient with a heart rate of 128 who is dizzy:
   shock
   d. Adult patient whose blood pressure has been 168/98 on three readings on three different occasions:
   hypertension

7. Write one expected outcome for each of the above nursing diagnoses:
   a. febrile – brain damage – antibiotics
   b. dyspnea – death –
   c. shock – brain damage
   d. hypertension – heart attack

8. What evaluation data would you need to determine if each of the above expected outcomes was being met or was met?
   a. febrile (pyrexia) – normal temp reading
   b. dyspnea – oxygen level readings are normal
   c. shock – normal B/P reading
   d. hypertension – normal B/P reading

9. What would you do if your ill, hospitalized patient's temperature registers 95.2° F. (32.1° C.) on the thermometer? electric blanket, give hot fluids

10. What would you do if when taking your patient's blood pressure, you hear the first sounds, they disappear, and then you hear them again?
record B/P

MULTIPLE CHOICE

Directions: Choose the ***best*** *answer for each of the following questions.*

1. Respiration is controlled by the
   1. hypothalamus.
   2. pons and medulla.
   3. sinoatrial node.
   4. lungs.

2. Systolic blood pressure is the pressure
   1. exerted on the artery when the heart is at rest.
   2. equal to that in the arteries at any given time.
   3. in the arteries when intrathoracic pressure is greatest.
   4. exerted on the artery during left ventricular contraction.

3. If overhydration occurs, the blood pressure will
   1. increase.
   2. decrease.
   3. remain the same.
   4. become muffled.

4. Which one of the following is *true* regarding vital sign changes that occur with aging?
   1. Normal temperature is higher than that of the average adult.
   2. Pulse beats become more pronounced as arteries stiffen.
   3. Vital capacity increases as subcutaneous fat is lost.
   4. Respiratory rate my rise as a decrease in vital capacity occurs.

5. When measuring a patient's blood pressure in the arm, the center of the bladder in the cuff should be placed
   1. at the right outer edge of the arm.
   2. over the antecubital space.
   3. over thc brachial artery.
   4. at the inner edge of the arm.

6. When measuring respirations, the patient should NOT be
   1. sitting up in bed.
   2. talking to anyone.
   3. resting quietly.
   4. lying on the side.

7. An apical-radial pulse is taken to determine if there is
   1. an arrhythmia.
   2. skipped heart beats.
   3. an abnormal heart sound.
   4. a pulse deficit.

8. A type of Korotkoff sound that indicates the diastolic pressure in children and in some adults is
   1. tapping.
   2. knocking.
   3. muffling.
   4. silence.

9. When measuring blood pressure with a mercury manometer, it is important to
   1. read the manometer at eye level.
   2. support the arm above the level of the heart.
   3. take a reading from both arms.
   4. retake the pressure to verify the reading.

10. Biot's respirations occur in patients with increased intracranial pressure and are characterized by
    1. increasing rapidity of breathing followed by slowing of the rate.
    2. excessively slow, deep respirations followed by a period of apnea.
    3. increase-decrease of rate and depth of respiration.
    4. two or three shallow breaths followed by a period of apnea.

11. A heart rate within normal limits for a 6-month-old infant is
    1. 124 bpm.
    2. 65 bpm.
    3. 156 bpm.
    4. 76 bpm.

12. A normal respiratory rate in the 7-year-old child will be
    1. higher than in an adult.
    2. lower than in an adult.
    3. the same as for an adult.
    4. twice that of an adult.

13. If a patient's blood pressure measures 146/92 on the left arm and 138/84 on the right arm, what would you do?
    1. retake the pressure on both arms.
    2. retake the pressure on the left arm.
    3. record both pressures on the chart.
    4. wait 30 minutes and take the pressures again.
14. When performing an assessment on a patient, you should
    1. check that all peripheral pulses are present.
    2. compare peripheral pulses from one side to the other.
    3. check peripheral pulses on the dominant side of the body.
    4. only check the radial and dorsalis pedis pulses.
15. Your patient's blood pressure measures 15 points higher than on her last visit. She has no history of hypertension. What would you do?
    1. Wait 15 minutes and take the pressure again.
    2. Just record the pressure.
    3. Ask if something upsetting has happened.
    4. Inquire when the last meal was eaten.
16. Interference with accurate measurement of body temperature occurs if the patient
    1. has been chewing gum.
    2. just came in from the cold.
    3. rushed getting to the office.
    4. has been speaking before the temperature is measured.

CRITICAL THINKING ACTIVITIES

1. Take the respiratory rate of a healthy individual and a patient with a lower respiratory infection. List the possible physiological reasons for the difference in the respiratory rate.
2. Explain the mechanisms by which the body elevates temperature to combat a pyrogen.
3. Why do you think that taking a major class examination might raise your pulse rate?

MEETING CLINICAL OBJECTIVES

Directions: The following suggested activities will help you meet the stated clinical practice objectives for the chapter. Review your school's clinical objectives for the week and outline a plan of activities that will help you meet them. If unsure as to how to meet them, consult with your instructor at the beginning of the clinical day.

1. Practice taking the temperature by the various routes and with a glass thermometer and an electronic thermometer.
2. Practice taking blood pressure on as many patients as possible. Have an experienced nurse check your readings on a few people to be certain you are accurate.
3. Try to correlate each vital sign with what is happening in the patient's body to explain changes in vital signs.
4. Work with a classmate and check the respiratory rate on five people. You should both have the same results.
5. Practice taking the radial pulse on ten different people. Have a classmate check the pulse by counting at the same time on at least three people to be certain that you are accurate.
6. Take an apical pulse on five different people. Have a classmate or instructor check your results. You should be within a couple of beats of each other.

STEPS TOWARD BETTER COMMUNICATION

VOCABULARY BUILDING GLOSSARY

Term	Pronunciation	Definition
A. Individual Terms		
abatement	a BATE ment	lessening, decreasing
alter	AL ter	to change
blunt	blunt	not sharp, with a flattened end
calibrated	CAL i BRAT ed	marked with measurements
clockwise	CLOCK wise	in the direction of the hands of the clock move
contraindicated	con tra IN di ca ted	shows treatment is not desirable
distract	dis TRACT	bring attention elsewhere
flared	flared	wide, opened
impaired	im PAIR ed	damaged
mode	mode	method
occlusive	oc CLU sive	closing off or obstructing
prone	prOne	likely; lying face down
peripheral	per IPH er al	outside the main area, to the edge
propelled	pro PELL ed	pushed with strong force
readily	READ i ly	quickly and easily
secrete	se CRETE	to manufacture and produce a substance
simultaneously	si mul TAN e ous ly	occurring at the same time
superficial	su per FI cial	on the surface, shallow
unobtrusively	un ob TRU sive ly	quietly, without bringing attention to one's own action
B. Phrases		
defining characteristics	de FIN ing char ac ter IS tics	signs or symptoms that explain an illness or nursing diagnosis
in conjunction with	in con JUNC tion with	together with, two or more things used together
jot down	JOT down	to make a written note
keep pace with	keep PACE with	to keep up with, to maintain equal position
owing to	OW ing to	because of, due to
"restore the unit"	re STORE the unit	put things in the room back in their original or correct places

COMPLETION

Directions: Fill in the blank(s) with the correct term(s) from the Vocabulary Building Glossary to complete the sentence.

1. The antibiotics were bringing about an abatement of the patient's symptoms.
2. The wrong size blood pressure cuff will alter the reading.

3. If the patient is allergic to the sulfonamides, those drugs are contraindicated for treatment of his upper respiratory infection.
4. Pushing the plunger on the syringe caused the medication to be propelled into the patient's body.
5. Because the patient was having difficulty breathing, his nostrils were flared.
6. It is easy to measure the temperature and the pulse mode.
7. It is wise to distract the patient when counting respirations.
8. To begin measuring blood pressure with an aneroid or mercury sphygmomanometer, you must turn the valve clockwise to close it before beginning to squeeze the bulb.
9. A rectal temperature is measured with a thermometer that has a blunt end.
10. When assessing circulation, besides measuring the radial pulse, you should also check the peripheral pulses.

VOCABULARY EXERCISE

Blunt and *superficial* are not medical terms, but are used in the textbook for explanation of medical information. In the following sentences they are used to describe a person's conversation. Can you describe what the words mean in both cases? You may need to use a nonmedical dictionary.

His conversation is very blunt. If he thinks you are boring, he says so.

Her conversation is superficial. She never talks about anything important.

	Meaning in text	Meaning in conversation
blunt	not sharp, flattened end	short + to the point
superficial	on the surface, shallow	not true

WORD ATTACK SKILLS

Directions: Break these words into their parts and see if you can figure out the definition. Underline the accented syllable. Check your answer in the dictionary.

1. hemodynamics (Skill 20-5)
   surrounding energy—forceful
2. antecubital space (Skill 20-7)
   less than 18 m. in length, cubal Area

PRONUNCIATION SKILLS

Directions: Underline the stressed syllable in these words, then practice saying them aloud to yourself or with a partner. The accent for the first word is underlined as an example.

<u>ap</u> ne a	bra dyp ne a	ta chyp ne a	eup ne a	dysp ne a
hy pox i a	ar rhyth mi a	tach y car di a	di as tol ic	a scul ta tory
feb rile	py rex i a	def er ves ence	di a phor e sis	
sphyg mo man o me ter				

COMMUNICATION EXERCISE

Directions: Read and practice the dialogue with a partner.

SAMPLE DIALOGUE A

Nurse: "I'm going to take your vital signs and then I will look at your incision. Did you sleep well last night?"

Mr. S. "I slept O.K., except they woke me up twice to check me over."

Nurse: "I'm going to take your blood pressure first. Can you hold your pajama sleeve up for me?"

Mr. S.: "Sure; like this?"

Nurse: "That's fine. This may be a little uncomfortable as I pump up the cuff. (Measures BP.). It's 142/86 this morning. That's better than it was yesterday."

Mr. S.: "I'm glad to hear that!"

Nurse: "Now let's take your temperature and count your pulse rate."

Directions: Fill in the blanks in the conversation to complete the sentences for Sample B; read and practice this with a partner.

SAMPLE B

Nurse: "Slip this probe under the tongue. The thermometer will 'beep' when it is done. Turn your face over for me, so I can feel your pulse more easily."

Mr. S.: "OK."

Nurse: (Places fingers over artery.) "There it is. It is regular at 76 beats per minute."

Review the chapter highlights, answer the study questions, and complete the critical thinking activities at the end of the chapter in the textbook.

TWENTY-ONE

Assessing Health Status

TERMINOLOGY

A. MATCHING

Directions: Match the terms in column I with the correct definitions in column II.

Column I			Column II	
1.	k	auscultation	a.	Tissue elasticity
2.	i	cerumen	b.	Fluid in the interstitial spaces
3.	b	edema	c.	Tissue damage or discontinuity of normal tissue
4.	f	kyphosis	d.	Involuntary fine movement of the body or limbs
5.	c	lesion	e.	Exaggerated lumbar curve
6.	e	lordosis	f.	increased curve in the thoracic area of the spine
7.	L	olfaction	g.	Pronounced lateral curvature of the spine
8.	m	palpation	h.	Tapping on the body surface to produce sounds
9.	h	percussion	i.	Ear wax
10.	j	quadrant	j.	One-quarter of an area
11.	G.	scoliosis	k.	Listening for sounds within the body with a stethoscope
12.	d	tremors	l.	Smelling for distinctive odors
13.	a	turgor	m.	Touch used to feel various parts of the body

B. COMPLETION

Directions: Fill in the blank(s) with the correct word(s) from the terms list in the chapter in the textbook to complete the sentence.

1. Normal breath sounds heard over the central chest or back are called bronchovesicular; they are equal in length during inspiration and expiration.
2. Soft, rustling sounds heard in the periphery of the lung fields are vesicular breath sounds.

3. The croaking sound of stridor indicates a partial obstruction of an upper air passage.
4. When auscultating the lungs, listen for any adventitious sound by learning the normal breath sounds.
5. A musical, whistling, high-pitched sound produced by air being forced through a narrowed airway is termed a wheeze.
6. The Rinne hearing test compares bone and air conduction of sound and is performed with a tuning fork.
7. The weber hearing test checks conduction of sound through bone.
8. An abnormal accumulation of serous fluid within the peritoneal cavity is called ascites.
9. Fluid is present in the lungs when sounds are auscultated.
10. The term pallor refers to paleness of the skin.

IDENTIFICATION

Directions: For each of the following problems, identify the correct form of assessment technique.

1. b excessive air in the abdominal area	a.	inspection
2. d difficulty breathing	b.	palpation
3. d hyperactive bowel sounds	c.	percussion
4. b pain in the abdomen	d.	auscultation
5. e alcohol ingestion	e.	olfaction
6. a rash on the skin		
7. a presence of wound infection		
8. b presence of muscle spasm		
9. a laceration on forearm		
10. b temperature elevation		

SHORT ANSWER

Directions: Write a brief answer for each question.

1. The physical examination generally includes the following major areas:
   a. Social Data
   b. Head + Neck
   c. Chest
   d. Abdomen
   e. Genitourinary
   f. Extremeties + Muscoskelatal
   g. Endocrine
2. Give examples of examinations for which the following positions are used:
   a. lithotomy pelvic exam
   b. knee-chest rectal examination
   c. Sims' sigmoidoscopy examination

3. The areas and responses assessed during the neurological examination or "check" are:
 consensual
 a. _pupil size measured - pupils should get small when exposed to light_
 b. _vital signs - diseases in intracranial pressure affect these_
 c. _EOMS checked - eye muscles - using finger_
 d. _accommodation - pupil should dilate when viewing far object_

4. Assessment information pertinent to daily care of the patient includes:
 a. _Elimination Safety + Security Nutritional needs_
 b. _Rest + Activity needs Hygiene + grooming (bathing_
 c. _Psychosocial Circulations peri-care_
 toileting

5. ✓ A nursing assessment of the areas of basic needs would include:
 a. _Resting + Activity needs_
 b. _Nutritional, Fluid + electrolyte needs_
 c. _Safety + Security_
 d. _Hygiene + Grooming_
 e. _Oxygenation + Circulation needs_
 f. _Psychosocial needs_
 g. _Elimination_

6. Topics for patient teaching regarding preventive health care are:
 a. _need for regular physical examinations_
 b. _recommended periodic diagnostic tests_
 c. _need for immunizations_
 d. _warning signs of cancer_
 e. _teach breast examination_
 f. _teach self-testicular exam_

COMPLETION

Directions: Fill in the blank(s) with the correct word(s) to complete the sentence.

1. Olfaction may be used to detect a ___sweetish___ odor to the breath that may indicate diabetic acidosis.

2. When weighing an infant, you must keep ___close___ hovering to prevent a fall while adjusting the scale weights.

3. Blood pressure is never taken on an extremity containing a ___dialysis shunt___ or on the side where a ___dissection___ or lymph node dissection has occurred.

4. The heart valve sounds are heard best with the ___bell___ of the stethoscope.

5. To check for dehydration in the elderly patient it is best to check the ___mucous membranes___.

6. When checking peripheral pulses, they should be ___compared bilaterally___

7. When assessing for dependent edema, press the fingers into the tissue over the ___tibia___ just above the ___ankle___.

8. The planning phase of the nursing process requires that ___appropriate goals or expected outcomes___ be written for each nursing diagnosis.

9. One way to remember the areas to assess concerning basic needs is to recall the acronym ___RNSHOPE___.

10. Patients should be assessed from head to toe at least once each shift.

11. When assessing patients, it is important to instruct the patient about the purpose of diagnostic tests that are ordered.

12. The purpose of properly draping the patient for the physician's examination is to prevent embarrassment during the exam.

APPLICATION OF THE NURSING PROCESS

Directions: Write a brief answer for each question.

1. After gathering patient assessment data, what is the next step?
ex. nursing diagnosis, answer questions
pschosocial & cultural assessment

2. The main purpose of assessing for cultural preferences and health beliefs is so that an individualized care plan can be formulated.

3. The most important method for gathering data upon physical assessment is observe behavior, & appearance - then make judgement of health status.

Head to Toe Assessment

4. How is the data obtained during assessment used to choose appropriate nursing diagnoses?
Ht & Wt Temp.
Vital signs pulse
Basic physical examination respiration

5. Although writing goals or expected outcomes occurs during the planning step of the nursing process, other planning tasks might include:
Rest & Activity, nutrician, hygeine, elimination
Safety & security

6. After the initial assessment, additional assessments should be made
history of any complaints, vital signs taken
and patient prepared for examination

7. Evaluation of the assessment process is based on:
thouroughness of data collection - communication
skills, sight hearing, smell, touch

MULTIPLE CHOICE

*Directions: Choose the **best** answer to each of the following questions. Some of these questions require synthesis of information with previously acquired knowledge and critical thinking.*

Situation: J.T., a 62-year-old male, presents with abdominal pain, nausea, feelings of malaise, and fatigue.

1. While collecting assessment data, an important question to ask J.T. is
   1. "What is your occupation?"
   2. "Are you experiencing shortness of breath?"
   3. "When did you have your last bowel movement?"
   4. "Do you have a headache?"

2. In order to determine the location of the abdominal pain you would use which one of the following techniques?
   1. inspection
   2. percussion
   3. auscultation
   4. palpation

3. While exploring the symptom of nausea, an appropriate question to ask is
   1. "What did you eat prior to the onset of nausea?"
   2. "How many hours are you sleeping each night?"
   3. "Is your vision blurred?"
   4. "Do you vomit easily?"

4. A very pertinent part of the physical examination on J.T. is
   1. inspection of the extremities.
   2. auscultation of bowel sounds.
   3. auscultation of the lungs.
   4. percussion of the flank areas of the back.

Situation R.S., a 46-year-old female, presents with menstrual difficulties, fatigue, and mood swings.

5. A pelvic examination is ordered. You would place the patient in the lithotomy position with the feet in the stirrups and ask her to
   1. move her buttocks to the edge of the table.
   2. let her knees fall together.
   3. tense her abdominal muscles.
   4. hold her breath during the exam.

6. When gathering a history from R.S. for this problem you would ask
   1. "When was the first day of your last period?"
   2. "How much water are you drinking daily?"
   3. "When was your last bowel movement?"
   4. "Are you experiencing any indigestion?"

Situation P.R., a 16-year-old male, sustained a head injury while playing soccer.

7. When performing a neurological check on P.R., you look at each pupil to determine
   1. if the shape is regular.
   2. if they have become smaller.
   3. the state of consciousness.
   4. whether one pupil is larger than the other.

8. When checking extraocular movements, you ask the patient to follow an object as it is moved into different positions and watch to see if
   1. the pupils constrict when focusing on the object.
   2. the pupils dilate when focusing on the object.
   3. the eyes move in a normal coordinated manner.
   4. there is blinking while trying to focus on the object.

9. To check extremity strength, you ask the patient to
   1. touch his finger to his nose.
   2. raise the left leg.
   3. push the soles of the feet against your hands.
   4. bend the right knee.

10. You check P.R.'s mental orientation by asking
    1. where he is right now.
    2. who the current president of the U.S. is.
    3. how the injury occurred.
    4. where his parents are.

CRITICAL THINKING ACTIVITIES

1. Describe the steps in a focused cardiovascular assessment.
2. Teach a family member about the recommendations for periodic diagnostic testing. Points to cover:
3. From memory, list the equipment that would be needed for the physician to perform a physical examination on an adult male or female.

MEETING CLINICAL OBJECTIVES

Directions: The following suggested activities will help you meet the stated clinical practice objectives for the chapter. Review your school's clinical objectives for the week and outline a plan of activities that will help you meet them. If unsure as to how to meet them, consult with your instructor at the beginning of the clinical day.

1. Practice performing an initial physical and psychosocial assessment on classmates and family members. Organize your approach so that it will be in a consistent order each time you perform such an assessment. Make up index cards to guide you; use an outline format. Use the cards when you are in the clinical setting.
2. Practice the neurological "check" on at least four people.
3. When assigned to the clinical setting where a proctosigmoidoscopy examination, a pelvic examination, and pap smear may be done, review the procedure for setting up and assisting the physician with each exam.
4. Teach a female about self breast examination and teach a male about self testicular examination.

STEPS TOWARD BETTER COMMUNICATION

VOCABULARY BUILDING GLOSSARY

Term	Pronunciation	Definition
acronym	AC ro nym	a word made from initials of other words, (e.g., BP = blood pressure)
appraising	ap PRAI sing	evaluating
ascertaining	as cer TAIN ing	finding out information
astute	a STUTE	intelligent
holistic	ho LIS tic	relating to the total being (body, mind, and spirit)
opacity	o PAC i ty	not allowing light to pass through
patent	PA tent	open, unobstructed
patency	PA ten cy	amount of openness
sluggishly	SLUG gish ly	slowly
subsides	sub SIDES	goes down, becomes less strong

COMPLETION

Directions: Fill in the blank(s) with the correct word(s) from the Vocabulary Building Glossary to complete the sentence.

1. Performing a physical assessment is part of the process used when ascertaining the patient's condition.
2. A cataract causes an opacity of the lens in the eye.
3. Nurses are taught to provide holistic care to patients, considering body, mind, and spirit.
4. While appraising information from the chart, the nurse discovered that the patient previously had a hip fracture.
5. A fever usually subsides when the patient is given acetaminophen.
6. PT is an acronym for physical therapy.
7. Normal bowel sounds indicate that the bowel is patent.
8. When all assessment data has been gathered, an astute decision about the care needed for the patient can be made.

VOCABULARY EXERCISE

Directions: Complete the statement with one of the following words.

a. occluded b. abnormal c. sluggish d. a word made from the initials of other words

1. Adventitious means abnormal.
2. An acronym is a word made from initials of other words.
3. The opposite of patent is occluded.
4. Brisk is the opposite of sluggish.

WORD ATTACK SKILLS

PRONUNCIATION OF DIFFICULT TERMS

A. Directions: Practice pronouncing the following words. (The stressed syllable is written in capital letters, the "long mark" or macron (-) indicates that the sound of that letter is the same as the name of the letter.)

A SCĪ tes	ech chy MŌ sis	er y THĒ ma
GUAĪ ac	LĒ sion	nys TĀG mus
PĀ tent	pe TĒ chē aē	RhON chus/RhON chī
RIN nē test	san GWIN ē ous	STRĪ dor
tin NĪ tous	Weber (VĀ ber) test	

B. Directions: Divide the following two words into syllables and put a line under the accented syllables; practice pronouncing the words with a partner.

1. sphygmomanometer checks BP

otoscope—checks ear

2. ophthalmoscope ____ checks the eye

ABBREVIATIONS

Directions: Write the meaning for the following abbreviations.

1. PMI point of maximum impulse
2. PERLA pupils, equal, round, reactive to light, accommodation
3. BSE breast self examination
4. PCA patient controlled analgesia
5. ADL Activities of daily living
6. TSE testicular self examination
7. EOMS extraocular movements for the eyes
8. GI gastrointestinal
9. DRE Digital Rectal exam

COMMUNICATION EXERCISE

Interviewing and communication skills include:

- Maintaining a relaxed, pleasant manner.
- Maintaining the correct degree of formality.
- Being respectful of the person and his or her privacy.
- Speaking carefully and distinctly where the patient can see your lips.
- Using correct pronunciation.
- Asking the person to repeat if you do not understand.
- Repeating the information received to make sure you understood it correctly.
- Saying so when you do not know something and then finding out the answer.

Here is a communication example for performing the beginning of a basic needs assessment (Table 21-5):

Nurse: "Good morning, Ms. T., I'm Diane, your student nurse today. I need to gather some information about you and perform an examination. Is there anything you need before we begin?"

Ms. T.: "I just need to turn and get out of this position first."

Nurse: Let me help you to turn and sit up. Is that better?"

Ms. T.: "Yes, I'm fine now."

Nurse: (Visually assessing the patient) "Did you have any problems with mobility or muscle strength before this surgery?"

Ms. T.: "I'm always stiff first thing in the morning, but after I'm up a while I can move around just fine. I'm not as strong as I used to be, but that is expected at 78 years old. I do have some arthritis in my hands and that makes it difficult to do some things, especially when it flares up."

Nurse: "Does the arthritis prevent you from managing to bathe, groom, and dress?"

Ms. T.: "No, I can do those things; it just takes me longer sometimes."

Nurse: "What about cooking, eating, or cleaning up?"

Ms. T.: "I can manage to cook O.K. with my electric can opener and large-handled knives and utensils. My daughter helps me clean really well once a month."

Nurse: "How many hours a night do you usually sleep?"

Ms. T.: "It varies; most of the time I'm in bed by 10:00, but sometimes I'll watch a movie that runs later. I usually wake up about 6:30. If I'm short on sleep, I'll nap after lunch."

Nurse: "Do you awaken at night much?"

Ms. T.: "I have to get up once during the night to use the bathroom, but I only awaken more when I have been out to dinner and had more liquid than usual."

Nurse: "Does pain interfere with your usual activities or sleep?"

Ms. T.: "Well, right now it does, but then I just had the surgery yesterday. When my arthritis flares up I have to take a lot of ibuprofen and sometimes something stronger or I have trouble sleeping."

A. Directions: Practice obtaining the rest of the information needed for the basic needs assessment with a partner. Ask the questions and have the partner supply the answer. Continue with the assessment depending on the answer given.

B. Directions: Fill in what you would say in the following dialogue regarding the psychosocial assessment of Ms. T.:

Nurse: "Do you belong to a church or a spiritual group?"

Ms. T.: "Yes, I'm a member of the Presbyterian church. I go most Sundays."

Nurse: "What about your support system. Who can you count on when ___your sick___?"

Ms. T.: "My daughter is very helpful, but she lives an hour away. My friend, Betty, will help me and my neighbor, Jim, is available if I call him."

Nurse: "How would you describe your mental outlook? Are you ever ___depressed___? How do you handle upsetting events?"

Ms. T.: "I'm usually fairly happy, but I get lonely sometimes. I wouldn't really call it depressed, except when I was told I had to have this surgery. I'm glad that's over.

I talk with my friend Betty when I have a problem. If I feel down, I remind myself of how lucky I am to have so few health problems and to still be in my own place.

I find music will cheer me up too."

Nurse: "Will you be able to have someone care for you at home while you recover, or would you like to speak with the ___social worker___ to arrange your convalescence?"

Ms. T.: "My daughter is taking some time off of work and I will go to her house to recover."

Nurse: "Will you be able to obtain your ___meds___ and ___dressings___ without a problem?"

Ms. T.: "Yes, my insurance will cover what I need. I have a supplemental policy from my years of employment."

Nurse: "What are your ___goals___ at this point in time?"

Ms. T.: "My biggest fear is that this lump was malignant and I will have to undergo chemotherapy. I worry about who will take care of me if I get really sick. My daughter works full time and she has three small children."

Nurse: "Let's wait and see what the Social worker/Home Healthcare. Now, considering your discharge tomorrow, let's see what you need to know. How will you shower, cook, get meds, change dressings medications?"

S.T: "How often should the dressing be changed? How do I clean the wound? Will it hurt?"

C. Directions: Write a short dialogue for a home health visit to a patient you have visited before. Include a quick assessment of general condition.

CULTURAL POINTS

Think about what foods, practices, and beliefs from your culture might seem unusual to a nurse who grew up in a different culture. What suggestions can you make for how the nurse could deal with the differences? How will you deal with such differences when you have a patient from a culture different from your own? Do you think you will have an advantage in understanding how the patient might feel?

Review the chapter highlights, answer the study questions, and complete the critical thinking activities at the end of the chapter in the textbook.

TWENTY-TWO

Admitting, Transferring, and Discharging Patients

TERMINOLOGY

A. MATCHING

Directions: Match the terms in column I with the definitions in column II.

Column I		Column II	
1. f	MSW	a.	Health maintenance organization
2. e	deductible	b.	The amount the patient pays for each service before insurance pays
3. c	autopsy	c.	Examination of remains by a pathologist to determine cause of death
4. a	HMO	d.	County medical officer responsible for investigating unexplained deaths
5. d	coroner	e.	Amount per calendar year a patient pays before insurance begins to pay for care
6. b	co-pay	f.	Master's degree in social work

B. COMPLETION

Directions: Fill in the blank(s) with the correct term(s) from the terms list in the chapter in the textbook to complete the sentence.

1. The discharge Planner is the RN or social worker who coordinates home care after hospitalization when the patient needs it.
2. Prior authorization is not needed for an emergency admission, such as might occur after an automobile accident.
3. Most patients over 65 years of age are covered by medicare, government health insurance for the elderly.
4. medicaid is a state insurance program for the poor who cannot afford health insurance.
5. A Routine Admission admission would occur for a patient who was scheduled to have a hip replacement surgery.
6. health Maintenance organization is a system of health care that was designed to lower the costs of health care.

SHORT ANSWER

Directions: Write a brief answer for each question.

1. The role of the admitting department is to collect personal and insurance info. + verify authorization for admission

2. You would cover the following points when orienting a patient to the patient unit.
   a. show location of call bell + how to use it
   b. location of bathroom + use of emergency bell
   c. how to operate TV and Telephone
   d. explain visiting hours
   e. fill water pitcher or explain NPO
   f. Show patient where belongings are kept
   g. introduction with a smile

3. When a patient is transferred to another facility, the five types of information which must be sent with the patient are:
   a. primary + secondary diagnosis
   b. current orders
   c. med. including dosage, route, frequency + time
   d. physician names + phone numbers
   e. brief synopsis of hospital stay

4. Types of information to be included in the patient's discharge instructions when going home are:
   a. list of meds.
   b. activity restrictions
   c. special diet instructions
   d. name + phone # of physician
   e. ordered follow-up appointments
   f. transportation

5. When it appears that a patient has died, the nurse must: provide support for significant others, document time of death, contact physician to pronounce death, provide privacy

6. If a patient brings valuables to the hospital they should be sent home or locked away.

7. The nurse who notes that orders have been transcribed is legally responsible for their accuracy.

8. Orders are signed off by nurse.

9. When a patient is transferred to another unit or facility it is important to also notify family members.

10. Discharge planning begins at admission.

11. Discharge orders are written by the physician.

12. The nurse is responsible for seeing that all belongings accompany the patient at discharge.

13. Home health services may include skilled nursing such as wound care diabetic care + teaching, IV medication, personal care, respiratory care.

14. Other home health services include long-term planning, counseling community services, financial planning.

15. If a patient decides to leave before he or she is discharged, the nurse must immediately notify physician immediately.

16. Responsibilities of the nurse when a patient wishes to leave against medical advice are assist patients to understand any risks of their well-being should they leave.

17. Patients who consider leaving against medical advice need to know that sometimes insurance companies will refuse to pay.

18. List four ways you may be able to assist a significant other when a patient has died.
   a. offer to call a priest or spiritual advisor
   b. listen
   c. offer to make phone calls
   d. Allow adequate time to say goodbyes

19. Three reasons an autopsy may have to be done are:
   a. patient has died of unknown causes
   b. at the hands of another
   c. patient hasn't been seen by a physican—a specific time frame

MULTIPLE CHOICE

*Directions: Choose the **best** answer for each of the following questions.*

1. A priority during orientation to the patient unit is how to
   1. work the TV.
   2. call the nurse.
   3. use the telephone.
   4. obtain meals.

2. When a patient brings medications from home the nurse should
   1. allow the family to administer them.
   2. make a list of the medications and send them home with the family.
   3. ask the physician to write an order for each medication so they can be administered to the patient.
   4. place them in the bedside drawer and ask the patient to refrain from taking them.

3. Nursing duties at the time of discharge include
   1. ordering medications to be discontinued.
   2. arranging transportation home.
   3. making certain the patient understands discharge instructions.
   4. helping the patient with arrangements to take care of the hospital bill.

4. Obtaining prior authorization for admission to the hospital is usually the responsibility of the
   1. nurse assigned to the patient.
   2. nursing unit to which the patient is assigned.
   3. admitting office of the hospital.
   4. the admitting physician's office.

5. When a patient is to be transferred to another facility, transportation by ambulance is arranged by the
   1. nurse assigned to the patient.
   2. hospital discharge planner.
   3. attending physician.
   4. patient's family.

6. An autopsy would most likely be necessary in which one of the following incidences?
   1. A patient dies while recovering from a myocardial infarction (heart attack).
   2. A 91-year-old patient who was being treated for congestive heart failure dies at home.
   3. A patient with long-term diabetes dies while being treated for end-stage renal disease.
   4. A patient dies while being treated for injuries sustained in an assault.

7. M.A. is admitted after sustaining a fall from a ladder at home. He has fractured his femur. He is assigned to you and you start his admission process. You appropriately say to him **first**
   1. "So you fell off a ladder, M.A."
   2. "Welcome to the unit. We'll take good care of you."
   3. "My name is S.D., LPN/LVN. I will be your nurse for this shift"
   4. "If you will put on the gown, I will be back in a bit."

8. M.A. tells you "This is the first time I have ever been in a hospital as a patient." He appears apprehensive. Your best response would be
   1. "We'll take good care of you here. Don't you worry."
   2. "This must be very scary for you, M.A."
   3. "Your wife, here, will watch out for you, won't you E.A.?"
   4. "I'll be happy to answer any questions or address your concerns, M.A."

9. M.A. is ready for discharge. When preparing to send him home, it is most important to include on his discharge instruction sheet
   1. your name and home phone number.
   2. whether each medication should be taken with food or not.
   3. the social worker's name and phone number.
   4. a list of specific foods he is to eat.

10. D.O. is being transferred from your unit to the convalescent unit. It is most important that you
    1. notify his family of the transfer before moving him.
    2. check all drawers, the closet, and bed linens for his personal possessions.
    3. transfer him by stretcher to the other unit.
    4. provide time for him to say goodbye to his roommate who has been there for several days.

11. A.T. has been transferred to your unit. The transferring nurse has given you a report on his condition and helped you settle him in bed. Your next priority would be to
    1. perform a head-to-toe assessment.
    2. read all the orders the physician has written.
    3. check his MAR to see what medications he is receiving.
    4. document the transfer in the chart.

12. There are no available beds on your unit. The ER has called up wanting to transfer a patient up and is inquiring if there is anyone who can be discharged. You know that T.C. is ready to go home, but he has no discharge order. You know that
    1. the admitting office would have to call the physician.
    2. the unit secretary would need to contact the insurance company to verify the discharge.
    3. you would need to call the physician to see if he will order the patient discharged.
    4. you must check with the patient to see if he feels ready to go home.

CRITICAL THINKING ACTIVITIES

1. What information would be important for you to know when you enter a hospital as a patient?
2. How would you obtain needed information upon admission for a patient who is comatose?
3. What could you do to help an elderly patient who is worried about leaving his wife home alone when he is admitted to the hospital?

MEETING CLINICAL OBJECTIVES

Directions: The following suggested activities will help you meet the stated clinical practice objectives for the chapter. Review your school's clinical objectives for the week and outline a plan of activities that will help you meet them. If unsure as to how to meet them, consult with your instructor at the beginning of the clinical day.

1. Review the admission forms and then assist a staff nurse who is admitting a new patient. Orient the patient to the unit.
2. Help a nurse transfer a patient to another unit; listen carefully to the report given to the new nurse.
3. Collaborate with the social worker regarding discharge needs of an assigned patient. Describe the patient's home needs to the social worker.
4. Role play a situation in which a patient seeks to leave against medical advice.
5. Outline how you would interact with a family of one of your assigned patients should that patient suddenly expire.

STEPS TOWARD BETTER COMMUNICATION

VOCABULARY BUILDING GLOSSARY

Term	Pronunciation	Definition
alleviate	al LEV i ate	to make less difficult; relieve
bereaved	be REAVed	a person whose loved one has died
deterioration	de TER i or A tion	going into a worse condition
devastating	DEV as ta ting	overwhelming; causing great emotional stress
in general	in GEN er al	usually
lethargic	le THAR gic	showing little energy or interest, tired
protocols	PRO to cols	rules for action under certain conditions
significant other	sig NIF i cant OTH er	any close friend, partner, or family member who has as special relationship with the patient
synopsis	syn OP sis	summary
verified	VER i fIEd	checked to make sure it is correct

COMPLETION

Directions: Fill in the blank(s) with the correct word(s) from the Vocabulary Building Glossary to complete each sentence.

1. The patient's significant other was her male companion of 15 years.
2. Each nurse must follow the accepted protocols when allergies are identified during assessment.
3. The medication list of a confused patient should be verified with the family.
4. When transferring a patient to another unit within the hospital, a synapsis is given of the patient's condition and current treatment.
5. Orienting the patient to the unit and hospital routine will alleviate some anxiety.
6. Valuables must be treated with care as the loss of a prized piece of jewelry can be devastating to the patient.
7. The patient was very lethargic upon admission and wouldn't respond very well to questions.
8. In General, the patient is welcomed to the unit before beginning the assessment process.

VOCABULARY EXERCISE

Choose a family member, friend, or classmate, and write an assessment of the person from what you can perceive visually. If possible, take and record vital signs. Use the vocabulary in Table 22-1 in the textbook.

WORD ATTACK SKILLS

Directions: Write the opposite of the given term.

1. alert ____________________
2. lethargic ____________________
3. oral ____________________
4. labored ____________________
5. shallow ____________________
6. sighted ____________________

COMMUNICATION EXERCISE

Directions: Choose a partner and perform the following role plays; switch roles between "patient" and "nurse."

- Role play introducing a patient to the unit.
- Now do the same role play in an unfriendly, impolite, or impatient manner. How does it feel when you are playing the role of the patient?

- Practice comforting or being available to listen to someone whose loved one has just died. What to say in case of death:

  "I am sorry for the death of your loved one."

  "I am sorry for your loss."

  "I am sorry."

  "I am so sorry."

  "You have my sympathy."

CULTURAL POINTS

In some religions, such as Islam, it is often considered the duty of the nearest relative of the same sex to prepare the body for burial. This may be by washing it in a certain ritual way. When death is approaching for such a person, try to find out what would be usual for this culture to do so that you can accommodate the family after the death. If there is a conflict between family wishes and hospital rules, you will need to be very careful how you explain it to the family or ask the physician to talk to them.

Review the chapter highlights, answer the study questions, and complete the critical thinking activities at the end of the chapter in the textbook.

TWENTY-THREE

Diagnostic Tests and Specimen Collection

TERMINOLOGY

Directions: Fill in the blank(s) with the correct term(s) from the terms list in the chapter in the textbook to complete the sentence.

1. The technique of ____________________ is used to obtain a sample of bone marrow for diagnostic testing.
2. A breast ____________________ is often performed to determine whether a lump in the breast needs to be removed.
3. An ____________________ is usually flexible, contains a fiberoptic light, and is used to view the interior of body structures.
4. Pressure must be placed over the site of insertion of the catheter used for an angiogram, or a ____________________ may form.
5. One sign of liver disorders is ____________________, with yellow skin and mucous membranes.
6. Blood chemistry tests are usually combined into a ____________________ where many tests are performed sequentially at one time.
7. A colonoscopy is performed to detect ____________________ in the colon which might become malignant.
8. ____________________ are taken of genitourinary secretions for the detection of sexually transmitted diseases.
9. A ____________________ is passed over the upper right quadrant of the abdomen to conduct an ultrasound study of the gallbladder.

MATCHING

Directions: Match the tests in column I with the descriptions in column II.

Column I

1. ______ angiography
2. ______ MRI
3. ______ culture
4. ______ CT scan
5. ______ cystoscopy
6. ______ EEG
7. ______ IVP
8. ______ lumbar puncture
9. ______ Pap smear
10. ______ proctosigmoidoscopy
11. ______ thoracentesis
12. ______ venipuncture

Column II

a. Examination of the rectum and sigmoid colon with a proctoscope
b. Computed tomography scan
c. Magnetic resonance imaging
d. Insertion of a needle into the subarachnoid space between the lumbar vertebrae to withdraw cerebrospinal fluid
e. Electrical recording of brain waves
f. Radiography of an artery after injection with a contrast medium into the bloodstream
g. Growing organisms in a laboratory culture medium
h. Examination of the bladder through a cystoscope
i. Intravenous pyelogram
j. Laboratory test to determine cervical (or other) cancer
k. Insertion of a needle into a vein to withdraw blood
l. Insertion of a needle into the pleural space to withdraw fluid or air or to instill medication

COMPLETION

Directions: Fill in the blank(s) with the correct word(s) from the textbook chapter to complete the sentence.

1. Diagnostic tests are performed to aid in the ___________________ of disease.
2. Magnetic resonance imaging is a ___________________ method of visualizing parts within the body without the use of contrast media or ionizing radiation.
3. Sonography uses ___________________ to outline structures.
4. ___________________ is the study of blood and its ___________________.
5. An increase in leukocytes is termed ___________________ and often indicates ___________________.
6. The ___________________ test is used to monitor anticoagulant drugs such as sodium warfarin.
7. Inflammatory conditions cause an increase in the erythrocyte ___________________ rate.
8. Food and drink are withheld for ___________________ hours prior to some blood chemistry tests.
9. Whenever obtaining blood for a diagnostic test, the nurse must ___________________ to prevent contamination.

10. The blood of the diabetic patient is frequently tested using capillary blood and a ____________________.

11. Blood urea nitrogen (BUN) and creatinine levels are important indicators of ____________________ function.

12. Because urine ____________________, specimens should be analyzed soon after collection.

13. Tissues obtained by biopsy are examined by a ____________________.

14. Fluoroscopy is used to examine ____________________ in the GI system.

15. Radionuclide studies are performed in the ____________________ department.

16. KUB stands for ______________, ______________, ______________.

17. When preparing the patient for an MRI, all ____________________ must be removed from the body.

18. The ECG represents the ____________________ of the cardiac cycle.

19. Cardiac catheterization determines the function of the ____________________, ____________________, and ____________________ circulation.

20. Pulmonary function tests provide information about ____________________ function, lung ____________________, and ____________________ of gases.

21. Common x-rays of the GI system include an ____________________ and a ____________________.

22. After any diagnostic test that utilizes a contrast medium or dye of some sort, the patient is encouraged to ____________________ a lot of ____________________.

23. A gastroscopy is usually performed in the ____________________ laboratory.

24. Colonoscopy examines the entire ____________________ for polyps, areas of inflammation, and malignant lesions.

25. ERCP, ________________________________, is used to identify a cause of biliary obstruction such as ________________, ________________, ________________, or tumor.

MULTIPLE CHOICE

*Directions: Choose the **best** answer to each of the following questions.*

1. Teaching for the patient undergoing an upper GI in the morning would include
   1. why a bowel prep is necessary.
   2. the need for a liquid dinner.
   3. the reason an IV line will be started.
   4. not to take anything by mouth (NPO) after midnight.

2. Post-test nursing care specific to the patient who has had an arteriogram includes
   1. taking vital signs periodically.
   2. checking pulses distal to the catheter insertion site.
   3. keeping the patient NPO for four hours.
   4. ambulating the patient every two hours.

3. H.T.'s CBC revealed a Hgb of 11.8 gm/dL, a platelet count of 320,000/mm^3, and a WBC of 7,500/uL. These results indicate
   1. a low platelet count.
   2. a high leukocyte count.
   3. normal platelets and low WBCs.
   4. normal WBCs and a low hemoglobin.

4. One of the nurse's main responsibilities in assisting with a lumbar puncture is to
   1. hand the physician the instruments.
   2. help the patient maintain the correct position.
   3. sterilize the equipment after use.
   4. maintain pressure on the puncture site afterwards.

5. To prepare a Pap smear for the laboratory,
   1. it must be "fixed" on the slide.
   2. it has to be sent to the lab immediately.
   3. a stain is applied to the slide.
   4. the secretions must be kept moist.

6. Fluoroscopy is done during x-ray examination of the
   1. liver.
   2. extremities.
   3. GI system.
   4. lungs.

7. Pretest preparation for a colonoscopy that is not necessary for a barium enema includes
   1. NPO after midnight.
   2. colon prep.
   3. increasing fluid intake.
   4. pretest sedation.

8. One difference for the patient between an x-ray and an MRI study is that for the MRI the patient must
   1. hold very still for an extended period.
   2. remove normal clothing.
   3. drink several glasses of water beforehand.
   4. refrain from breathing for two minutes at a time.

9. Which one of the following diagnostic procedures requires a signed consent?
   1. chest x-ray
   2. gallbladder sonogram
   3. cardiac catheterization
   4. pulmonary function test

10. A part of the preparation for the colonoscopy that differs from other GI tests is that the patient must
    1. take laxatives the day before the test.
    2. be NPO for 12 hours before the test.
    3. have an enema the morning of the test.
    4. have a liquid diet for 2–3 days prior to the test.

APPLICATION OF THE NURSING PROCESS

Directions: Write a brief answer for each question.

1. Four assessment factors to be considered when a diagnostic test is to be performed on a patient are:
   a. ______________________________
   b. ______________________________
   c. ______________________________
   d. ______________________________

2. A nursing diagnosis that is appropriate for any patient who is not familiar with a diagnostic test to be performed is ______________________________.

3. An expected outcome for the above nursing diagnosis might be
   ______________________________.

4. A very important part of nursing intervention prior to diagnostic tests is
   ______________________________.

5. An important part of nursing intervention after a diagnostic test has been performed is
   ____
   ______________________________.

6. A part of the evaluation process when serial diagnostic tests are being performed is to
____
____

CRITICAL THINKING ACTIVITIES

1. Make an outline of the teaching points you would cover for the patient undergoing a cardiac catheterization.
2. How would you prepare the patient who is to undergo an MRI of the brain?
3. If a patient asks how sonography works, what would you say?

MEETING CLINICAL OBJECTIVES

Directions: The following suggested activities will help you meet the stated clinical practice objectives for the chapter. Review your school's clinical objectives for the week and outline a plan of activities that will help you meet them. If unsure as to how to meet them, consult with your instructor at the beginning of the clinical day.

1. Outline pretest and post-test nursing care for patients undergoing three different diagnostic tests or procedures.
2. Interact with a patient who has fears regarding a diagnostic procedure. Plan ahead by reviewing therapeutic communication techniques.
3. While in clinical, tell the staff you would like opportunities to perform finger-stick blood glucose tests using a glucometer. Remember to wear gloves.
4. Seek opportunities to assist with a lumbar puncture, thoracentesis, paracentesis, bone marrow aspiration, or liver biopsy, or prepare to assist with these procedures. Outline your duties and the supplies you would need to gather. You might role play a simulated situation with a peer.
5. Prepare to calm and soothe a patient who is very anxious about having her first pelvic exam and Pap smear performed.
6. Teach a patient about an MRI diagnostic test. Place an outline on a card to help you review the points to cover.

STEPS TOWARD BETTER COMMUNICATION

VOCABULARY BUILDING GLOSSARY

Term	Pronunciation	Definition
ampule	am PULE	a small, sealed, glass or polyethylene container of a measured amount of medication
deteriorates	de TER i or ates	loses quality
diagnostic	di ag NOS tic	an analysis made to find the cause or source of a problem or illness

shunt (noun)	SHUNT	a passage between two natural channels, either a natural irregularity or manmade
shunt (verb)	SHUNT	to turn to one side; to bypass
titer	TI ter	the strength or concentration of one substance mixed with others
troubleshoot	TROU ble SHOOT	to look for a way to fix a problem

COMPLETION

Directions: Fill in the blank(s) with the correct term(s) from the Vocabulary Building Glossary to complete the sentence.

1. It was hoped that the __________________ test would show what was wrong with the patient.
2. The blood test showed a rise in the __________________ of Rocky Mountain spotted fever antibodies.
3. Urine must be sent to the lab right away as it __________________ when allowed to sit for any length of time.
4. When the machine would not turn on, the nurse had to __________________ to find the problem.

WORD ATTACK SKILLS

Directions: In this chapter there are a number of suffixes (a word part at the end of the word) used to describe procedures. Look at the meanings of these suffixes. Find examples in the textbook and write them in the blanks.

1. -scope means an instrument to visually examine.

   ____

2. -scopy means a process of visual examination, using a -scope

   ____

3. -graph means a recording instrument showing relationships by using a diagram

   ____

4. -graphy means a process of recording

   ____

PRONUNCIATION OF DIFFICULT TERMS

Directions: Divide the following words into syllables and put a line under the accented syllables. Practice pronouncing the words.

1. angiography
2. cholangiopancreatography
3. cystoscopy
4. electroencephalogram
5. gastroscopy

6. myocardial infarction
7. paracentesis
8. proctosigmoidoscopy
9. radiopaque
10. radioimmunoassays
11. thoracentesis

COMMUNICATION EXERCISE

Directions: Practice this dialogue with a partner.

A nurse explains to her patient, Mr. F., how to prepare for a exercise stress test, and what will happen.

Nurse:	"Good morning, Mr. F. The doctor has ordered an exercise stress test for you."
Mr. F.:	"Is that with a treadmill? Is that where I have to walk on one of those moving platforms?"
Nurse:	"That's right. He wants to measure your heart performance and blood pressure while you exercise."
Mr. F.:	"What will happen?"
Nurse:	"The technician will attach wires to your skin with stick-on electrodes and place a blood pressure cuff on your arm. They will show the heart rate and pattern of electrical activity in your heart and your blood pressure while you exercise. The platform may move at a steady pace, or they may increase the speed or incline it gradually to see how exercise affects your heart."
Mr. F.:	"I guess I can handle that OK."
Nurse:	"I don't think it will be too difficult for you. You must not smoke or eat for at least four hours before the test."
Mr. F.:	"Uh oh! Can I eat breakfast before the test?"
Nurse:	"You can have a light breakfast as the test isn't scheduled until 1:00 P.M."
Mr. F.:	"Well, that's good."
Nurse:	"You can take your heart and blood pressure medications as usual."
Mr. F.:	"O.K."
Nurse:	"I need you to sign this consent form, please."
Mr. F.:	"OK, it doesn't sound too bad. Where do I sign?"
Nurse:	"Here on this line. I hope the test shows your heart is O.K."

Review the chapter highlights, answer the study questions, and complete the critical thinking activities at the end of the chapter in the textbook.

TWENTY-FOUR

Fluid, Electrolyte, and Acid-Base Balance

TERMINOLOGY

A. MATCHING

Directions: Match the terms in column I with the definitions in column II.

Column I		Column II	
1. ______	acidosis	a.	A mineral or salt dissolved in body fluid
2. ______	ascites	b.	Degree of elasticity of tissue
3. ______	alkalosis	c.	Abnormal accumulation of fluid within the peritoneal cavity
4. ______	dehydration	d.	Decrease in pH
5. ______	edema	e.	Condition of severe muscle cramps, carpal pedal spasms and laryngeal spasm
6. ______	electrolyte	f.	Removal of water from a tissue
7. ______	interstitial	g.	Increase in pH
8. ______	intracellular	h.	Excessive accumulation of interstitial fluid
9. ______	stridor	i.	Shrill, harsh sound upon inspiration
10. ______	tetany	j.	Fluid in spaces surrounding the cells
11. ______	transcellular fluid	k.	Fluid within the cells
12. ______	turgor	l.	Gastrointestinal secretions

COMPLETION

Directions: Fill in the blank(s) with the correct term(s) from the terms list in the textbook chapter to complete the sentence.

1. A young man involved in an auto accident sustained a severe cut to his leg and lost a lot of blood; he is suffering from __________________.
2. A patient's lab work shows a low potassium value. This patient has __________________.
3. The electrolyte imbalance __________________ can cause tetany.
4. The process by which substances move back and forth across the membrane until they are evenly distributed is called __________________.

5. ____________________ refers to the movement of pure solvent across a membrane.
6. When solute and water are of equal concentration, a solution is ____________________.
7. When a substance is introduced into the blood that makes the fluid in the vascular compartment ____________________, fluid will be drawn from the cells into the vascular compartment.
8. If a patient is hydrated too quickly with isotonic solution, the vascular fluid becomes ____________________ and fluid will move into the tissues.
9. The movement of fluid outward through a semipermeable membrane is termed ____________________.
10. Substances, regardless of their electrical charge, may be moved from an area of lower concentration to an area of higher concentration by ____________________.
11. A state of dehydration often causes the electrolyte imbalance ____________________.
12. Burn patients often develop the electrolyte imbalance ____________________.
13. The electrolyte imbalance, ____________________, usually only occurs in the presence of kidney failure.
14. Respiratory acidosis occurs from an increase in ____________________.
15. Metabolic acidosis often occurs in the ____________________ patient.

IDENTIFICATION

A. Directions: Indicate whether each of the following laboratory values is normal or if an electrolyte imbalance is present. If an imbalance is present, indicate what that imbalance is.

1. K^+ 3.2 mEq/L ____________________
2. Na^+ 148 mEq/L ____________________
3. Ca^{++} 9.6 mg/dL ____________________
4. HCO_3^- 24 mEq/L ____________________
5. K^+ 4.9 mEq/L ____________________
6. Na^+ 132 mEq/L ____________________

B. Directions: For each of the following sets of blood gases, tell what type of problem exists: respiratory acidosis, metabolic acidosis, respiratory alkalosis, metabolic alkalosis.

1. pH 7.32, pCO_2 47 mmHg, HCO_3 23 mEq/L ____________________
2. pH 7.48, pCO_2 33 mmHg, HCO_3 26 mEq/L ____________________
3. pH 7.30, pCO_2 38 mmHg, HCO_3 20 mEq/L ____________________
4. pH 7.50, pCO_2 45 mmHg, HCO_3 28 mEq/L ____________________

SHORT ANSWER

Directions: Write a brief answer for each question.

1. List the four main functions of water within the body:
   a. ______________________________
   b. ______________________________
   c. ______________________________
   d. ______________________________
2. List the primary location of these electrolytes:
   a. sodium ______________________________
   b. potassium ______________________________
3. Which two factors help to keep the fluid in the vascular compartment?
   ____
   ____
4. Intake and output records are evaluated to determine if there is
   ______________________________.
5. Another way to assess for alterations in fluid balance is to keep a record of
   ______________________________.
6. An early sign of decreased vascular volume from fluid volume deficit is
   ______________________________.
7. When imbalances in calcium or magnesium are suspected, assessment of
   ____________ should be performed.
8. To assess for Chvostek's sign, you would ______________________________
   ______________________________.

APPLICATION OF THE NURSING PROCESS

Directions: Write a brief answer for each question.

1. When assessing for signs of hypokalemia in the patient who is taking a digitalis preparation, you would ask about:
   ____
   ____
2. When assessing for fluid volume deficit in the elderly patient, you would assess:
   ____
   ____
3. The patient who is known to have a fluid volume deficit from loss of blood may also have the nursing diagnosis of:
   ____
4. Appropriate expected outcomes for the patient with the nursing diagnosis Fluid volume deficit related to severe diarrhea would be:
   ____
   ____

5. Actions to assist the patient who has severe diarrhea to regain and maintain fluid balance might be:

____

____

____

____

6. To evaluate the effectiveness of actions to combat fluid volume deficit, you would check:

____

____

____

____

MULTIPLE CHOICE

*Directions: Choose the **best** answer for each of the following questions.*

1. J.S., age 76, is admitted with vomiting and diarrhea of three days' duration. Besides assessing skin condition when looking for signs of dehydration, you would look for
   1. dull eyes.
   2. brittle nails.
   3. dry mucous membranes.
   4. dry hair.

2. Dehydration may occur more quickly for J.S. than for a younger person because
   1. there is less subcutaneous fat in the older adult.
   2. the thirst mechanism is more active in the older adult.
   3. there is a decrease in the urine-concentrating ability of the kidney in the older adult.
   4. more antidiuretic hormone is produced in the older adult.

3. J.S. is started on IV therapy. A sign that he is receiving too much or too rapid IV fluid, when compared with previous data, would be
   1. full, bounding, pulse.
   2. very rapid pulse rate.
   3. decreasing urine output.
   4. sudden vomiting.

4. When assessing J.S., you look for signs of electrolyte imbalance. A sign of hypokalemia would be
   1. hypertension.
   2. muscle weakness.
   3. mental confusion.
   4. oliguria.

5. A sign that J.S. has developed hypernatremia would be
   1. abdominal cramps.
   2. low urine output.
   3. cardiac arrhythmia.
   4. nausea and vomiting.

6. J.S.'s condition improves and he is started on oral nourishment. The following amounts were entered on his I and O sheet: juice 120 mL, cereal 180 mL, tea 150 mL, urine 380 mL, IV fluid 1050 mL, emesis 50 mL. J.S.'s oral intake was
   1. 450 mL.
   2. 350 mL.
   3. 830 mL.
   4. 1450 mL.

7. C.P., age 46, is admitted with decreased level of consciousness and symptoms of influenza. He is a diabetic. His blood gases are pH 7.32, CO_2 36, HCO_3 20. You would determine that his acid-base imbalance is
   1. respiratory acidosis.
   2. metabolic alkalosis.
   3. respiratory alkalosis.
   4. metabolic acidosis.

8. You would expect C.P.'s breathing to be
   1. deep and rapid.
   2. shallow and rapid.
   3. shallow and slow.
   4. regular rate and depth.

9. Because of the excess glucose in C.P.'s system, water is drawn from the cells into the vascular system and then excreted. An appropriate nursing diagnosis for him would be
   1. Fluid volume overload.
   2. Alteration in tissue perfusion.
   3. Fluid volume deficit.
   4. Ineffective breathing pattern.

10. One method of tracking fluid balance status in patients such as C.P. and J.S. in addition to recording I and O is to
    1. determine acid-base status.
    2. encourage intake of oral liquids.
    3. check electrolyte laboratory values.
    4. compare weight from day to day.

11. W.O. has hyponatremia. A nursing intervention appropriate for him is
    1. encourage the intake of milk.
    2. restrict his fluid intake.
    3. administer the ordered diuretic.
    4. give foods high in potassium.

12. Osmosis differs from diffusion in that it refers to
    1. movement of solutes from the cells to the interstitial fluid.
    2. movement of solvent across a membrane.
    3. substances moved across a membrane with the use of energy.
    4. movement of fluid out of the vascular system.

13. One cause of calcium imbalance is
    1. diabetes mellitus.
    2. congestive heart failure.
    3. arteriosclerosis.
    4. cancerous bone metastasis.

14. When teaching patients about calcium intake, you include that the absorption of dietary calcium is enhanced by
    1. vitamin B complex.
    2. vitamin C.
    3. vitamin D.
    4. iron.

15. A.C. is admitted with elevated blood pressure, rapid weight gain, edema, and restlessness. An appropriate nursing diagnosis for him would probably be
    1. Fluid volume excess.
    2. Fluid volume deficit.
    3. Risk for fluid volume deficit.
    4. Altered urinary elimination.

CRITICAL THINKING ACTIVITIES

1. Prepare a teaching plan for the patient with kidney disease who needs to decrease his intake of potassium. What foods should be avoided?

2. Prepare a teaching plan for the Hispanic-American patient who has hypertension. He will need to decrease the sodium in his diet. Outline the plan:

MEETING CLINICAL OBJECTIVES

Directions: The following suggested activities will help you meet the stated clinical practice objectives for the chapter. Review your school's clinical objectives for the week and outline a plan of activities that will help you meet them. If unsure as to how to meet them, consult with your instructor at the beginning of the clinical day.

1. Make a list of the food and drink containers used by the dietary department in your clinical facility and the amounts each holds.
2. Practice calculating intake for each patient assigned regardless of whether the patient is on intake and output recording.

3. Practice calculating the IV intake for each patient assigned who has an IV for the hours you are in clinical.
4. For each assigned patient, figure out what you would need to include in calculating output if it was to be recorded.
5. Assess each assigned patient for signs of hypokalemia, fluid volume deficit, or fluid volume excess.
6. Scan each assigned patient's laboratory values for abnormalities of electrolytes and acid-base balance.

STEPS TOWARD BETTER COMMUNICATION

VOCABULARY BUILDING GLOSSARY

Term	Pronunciation	Definition
buffer	BUF fer	a cushion; used to protect something from outside harm or irritation
compensatory	com PEN sa to ry	balancing a lack of one thing with more of another
considerable	con SID er a ble	large or lengthy
constituents	con STI tu ents	parts of a whole
deplete	de PLETE	use up or empty out
gradient	GRA di ent	a rate or degree of change
ingestion	in GES tion	the process of eating and drinking or taking something into the body orally
lethargic	le THAR gic	sleepy, tired, with little energy
obligatory	o BLIG a tory	necessary, required
pit	PIT	an indentation or small hollow
tented	TENT ed	coming to a point, like a tent
tracking	TRACK ing	keeping a record of; keeping track of
twitch	TWITCH	slight contraction or quiver

COMPLETION

Directions: Fill in the blank(s) with the correct term(s) from the Vocabulary Building Glossary to complete the sentence.

1. It takes ___________________ time for the kidneys to adjust pH when the body becomes acidic.
2. The lungs blow off excess carbon dioxide as a ___________________ mechanism when the body becomes too acidic.
3. When ever the patient is receiving intravenous fluids, ___________________ intake and output is important.
4. When the body is in a state of alkalosis, muscles may ___________________.
5. The patient experiencing ketoacidosis may become very ___________________ and may go into a coma.

6. Sodium bicarbonate is a ________________ and is given when acidosis needs to be corrected.
7. When the patient is taking a potassium depleting diuretic, ________________ of extra potassium is necessary.

VOCABULARY EXERCISE

Adjectives are often used to describe signs and symptoms.

irritable	scanty	weak	thready
moist	full	bounding	pale
dry	faint	sticky	
slow	elevated	rapid	

Directions: List the adjectives that might be used for signs and symptoms for the following:

1. lung sounds: ________________
2. pulse: ________________
3. blood pressure: ________________
4. mucous membranes: ________________
5. urine: ________________
6. skin: ________________

WORD ATTACK SKILLS

Directions: Opposites are often used when documenting assessment changes. Write the opposites for these words:

Words		Opposites
1. shallow	________________	active
2. rapid	________________	decrease
3. passive	________________	deep
4. moist	________________	dry
5. attraction	________________	excess
6. gain	________________	repellent
7. increase	________________	slow
8. deficit	________________	loss

Prefixes and suffixes are word parts with specific meanings that are attached to words to change their meaning in some way. Recall that prefixes are added to the beginning of the word, suffixes to the end.

Negative prefixes meaning *no* or *not*: im-balance dis-orientation un-usual
Medical and scientific terms often use prefixes and suffixes.

Prefix	Meaning	Example	Meaning
hyper-	excessive, above	hypercalcemia	calcium excess/high calcium
hypo-	deficient, below	hypocalcemia	calcium deficiency/low calcium
ab-	away from	absorb	draw away from
ex-, extra-	out, outside	excrete	throw out/eliminate
		extracellular	outside of the cell
re-	again, behind	reabsorb	absorb again
intra-	within	intracellular	within/inside a cell
inter-	between	interstitial	between the parts of a tissue
trans-	across, through	transport	carry across
iso-	equal, same	isotonic	equal tension

Suffix	Meaning	Example	Meaning
-tonic	tension	hypertonic	greater tension/concentration
-emia	blood condition	hypercalcemia	excess calcium in the blood
-osis	abnormal condition	acidosis	abnormal amount of acid

PRONUNCIATION OF DIFFICULT TERMS

Directions: Practice pronouncing the following words.

interstitial = in ter STISH ial

turgor = TUR gor (compare with turgid = TUR gid)

COMMUNICATION EXERCISE

Directions: With a partner, write and practice a dialogue explaining to a patient why you will be measuring intake and output and what the patient will need to do (use the call light, remember what he or she eats and drinks, etc.).

Review the chapter highlights, answer the study questions, and complete the critical thinking activities at the end of the chapter in the textbook.

TWENTY-FIVE

Concepts of Basic Nutrition and Cultural Considerations

TERMINOLOGY

A. MATCHING

Directions: Match the terms in column I with the definitions in column II.

Column I	Column II
1. ______ amino acid	a. Processes of taking in nutrients and absorbing and using them
2. ______ cholesterol	b. Process of converting food into substances that can be absorbed and utilized
3. ______ carbohydrate	c. Essential substance for the building of cells
4. ______ digestion	d. Body's main source of energy
5. ______ fat	e. Metabolized form of sugar in the body
6. ______ fiber	f. Table sugar
7. ______ fructose	g. Sugar found in fruit
8. ______ glucosc	h. Sugar found in milk
9. ______ lactose	i. Carbohydrate that is not broken down by digestion
10. ______ mineral	j. Substance that supplies nine calories per gram consumed
11. ______ nutrition	k. A component of fat
12. ______ obesity	l. Essential nutrients taken in through food or supplements
13. ______ protein	m. Inorganic substances contained in animals and plants
14. ______ sucrose	n. Excessive accumulation of body fat
15. ______ vitamin	o. Building blocks of protein

COMPLETION

Directions: Fill in the blank(s) with the correct term(s) from the terms list in the chapter in the textbook to complete the sentence.

1. A __________________ contains all nine essential amino acids and are of animal source.

2. Plant sources of protein are ____________________ because they do not contain all essential amino acids.
3. Proteins from plant sources that are combined in the diet to achieve complete protein intake are called ____________________.
4. Nine amino acids are considered ____________________ because they must be consumed through food sources.
5. The liver can manufacture eleven ____________________ amino acids.
6. A disorder of malnutrition that results from severe starvation is ____________________.
7. A condition of severe protein deficiency that occurs in infants after weaning from breast milk in countries where food is scarce is ____________________.
8. The ____________________ diet excludes all sources of animal food.
9. Most ____________________ are unsaturated fat, with the exception of coconut oil and palm oil.
10. Animal food sources provide the most ____________________ fats.
11. When the fat soluble vitamins A, D, E, and K are ingested in excessive quantities they can cause ____________________.
12. Foods prepared in the ____________________ manner are prepared for use according to Jewish law.

REVIEW OF STRUCTURE AND FUNCTION

Directions: Match the structures in column I with the functions in column II.

Column I		Column II
1. ______ tongue	a.	Absorbs nutrients
2. ______ salivary glands	b.	Assists in changing food to a semiliquid state
3. ______ stomach	c.	Absorbs fluid and electrolytes
4. ______ small intestine	d.	Secrete saliva containing enzymes
5. ______ liver	e.	Secretes bile for the digestion of fats
6. ______ gallbladder	f.	Secretes digestive enzymes and insulin
7. ______ large intestine	g.	Stores and concentrates bile
8. ______ pancreas	h.	Manipulates food, mixing it with saliva

SHORT ANSWER

Directions: Write a brief answer for each question.

1. Fat's main function in the body is to____.
   Four other functions of fat are:
   a. ____
   b. ____
   c. ____
   d. ____

2. The three essential fatty acids important to good nutrition are ______________________________.

3. The recommended daily allowance of fat is __________% of total calories.

4. Protein is essential for rebuilding ______________ and ______________.
   Other functions of protein are:
   ____
   ____
   ____

5. Protein intake should be __________% of the total daily calories.

6. Carbohydrates should make up about __________% of the daily diet. Each gram of carbohydrate supplies ______________ calories.

7. Functions of carbohydrates include:
   a. ______________________________
   b. ______________________________
   c. ______________________________
   d. ______________________________
   e. ______________________________

8. Minerals are necessary for proper ______________ and ______________ function and act as catalysts for many cellular functions.

9. Other functions of minerals include:
   a. ______________________________
   b. ______________________________
   c. ______________________________

10. A general rule regarding water requirements is that the patient needs to take in an amount equal to the recorded fluid output plus ______________.

11. Give one example of how each of the following factors might influence nutrition.
    a. Age: ______________________________
    b. Illness: ______________________________
    c. Emotional status: ______________________________
    d. Economic status: ______________________________
    e. Religion: ______________________________
    f. Culture: ______________________________

12. By ______________ months of age, the birth weight of the infant should ______________. By the end of the first year the birth weight should ______________.

13. It is often difficult to get ______________ to eat much.

14. School-age children often desire ______________ more than other foods and parents must set a good example of proper nutrition.

15. Adolescents tend to consume many ______________ and may not eat a balanced diet.

16. Often adults only eat the ______________ meal at home and this often leads to inadequate nutrition and ______________.

17. The group most at risk for inadequate nutrition is the ______________.

IDENTIFICATION

A. *Directions: Indicate the vitamin responsible for each function.*

1. ______ Maintenance of epithelial cells and mucous membranes
2. ______ Promotes bone and teeth mineralization
3. ______ Needed for carbohydrate metabolism
4. ______ Helps regulate energy metabolism
5. ______ Necessary for blood clotting
6. ______ Metabolism of amino acids
7. ______ Formation of red blood cells
8. ______ Helps maintain normal cell membranes
9. ______ Essential for certain enzyme systems
10. ______ Aids in hemoglobin synthesis

B. *Directions: List a primary function in the body of each of the following minerals and one consequence of deficiency.*

1. Calcium ______________________________
   Deficiency causes: ______________________________
2. Chloride ______________________________
   Deficiency causes: ______________________________
3. Magnesium ______________________________
   Deficiency causes: ______________________________
4. Phosphorus ______________________________
   Deficiency causes: ______________________________
5. Potassium ______________________________
   Deficiency causes: ______________________________
6. Sodium ______________________________
   Deficiency causes: ______________________________
7. Chromium ______________________________
   Deficiency causes: ______________________________
8. Fluorine ______________________________
   Deficiency causes: ______________________________
9. Iodine ______________________________
   Deficiency causes: ______________________________
10. Iron ______________________________
    Deficiency causes: ______________________________
11. Zinc ______________________________
    Deficiency causes: ______________________________

APPLICATION OF THE NURSING PROCESS

Directions: Write a short answer for each question.

1. While assessing E.O., you find she weighs 142 lbs. and is 64" tall. What is her BMI?
____

2. E.O. has just been diagnosed with colon cancer and is preparing to undergo surgery and then chemotherapy. What is a probable nursing diagnosis for this patient related to her nutritional needs? ______________________________

3. Write two expected outcomes for the above nursing diagnosis.
   a. ______________________________
   b. ______________________________

4. Indicate two nursing interventions to assist E.O. to meet each of the expected outcomes.
   a. ______________________________
   b. ______________________________
   c. ______________________________
   d. ______________________________

5. Indicate an evaluation statement for each of the above expected outcomes that would indicate that they are being met.
   a. ______________________________
   b. ______________________________

6. What type of data found on assessment might indicate that these outcomes are not being met?
____

7. If the outcomes are not being met, what would you do?
____
____

MULTIPLE CHOICE

*Directions: Choose the **best** answer for each of the following questions.*

1. D.R. is 76 years old and has arthritis in her hands. When performing a nutritional assessment for D.R. you would particularly want to know
   1. if her family eats with her often.
   2. if she can easily prepare her own food.
   3. if she eats only one hot meal a day.
   4. whether she has any food dislikes.

2. J.H. is 46 years old. He is 5’8" tall and weighs 158 lbs. He has the intestinal flu and is suffering from severe nausea, vomiting, and diarrhea. An appropriate nursing diagnosis for this patient would be
   1. Nutrition, altered: less than body requirements
   2. Nutrition, altered: more than body requirements
   3. Fluid volume excess
   4. Fluid volume deficit

3. F.B., a 64-year-old female who is recovering from hip surgery, has little appetite. In order to encourage her to eat you would
   1. remind her that protein is essential to healing.
   2. create an attractive and pleasant environment and encourage family to sit with her while she eats.
   3. offer to feed her some extra bites after she is finished.
   4. cut up her food for her to make eating easier.

4. From the following evaluation statements, which statement would indicate that the expected outcome of "Patient will gain 1 lb. per week" is being met?
   1. Made appropriate food choices from a 2500 calorie menu.
   2. Consumed 60% of food and fluids at dinner.
   3. Gained 0.5 lb. since day before yesterday.
   4. Lost 3 lbs. during chemotherapy treatment.

5. A.R. is 30 lbs. overweight. You are discussing a weight loss plan with him. You explain that the only way to realistically lose weight is to cut calories or
   1. revise the amount of fat consumed.
   2. eat only high-protein foods.
   3. revise the amount of carbohydrates eaten.
   4. increase the daily activity level.

6. You use the Food Guide Pyramid to help A.R. construct an appropriate balanced diet. You explain that the greatest number of servings of food per day should come from the
   1. grain group.
   2. meat group.
   3. fruit group.
   4. vegetable group.

7. Because A.R. also has a high cholesterol level, you recommend that he reduce red meat to two times a week and obtain adequate protein in the diet by eating
   1. fish or poultry several times a week.
   2. two eggs each morning for breakfast.
   3. protein fortified cereal for two meals a day.
   4. pasta with tomato sauce several times a week.

8. You explain to A.R. that the most effective way to lose weight—other than cutting calories—and keep it off is to
   1. eat more fruits and vegetables.
   2. drink 6–8 glasses of water a day.
   3. exercise for at least 30 minutes 3–5 times a week.
   4. totally abstain from alcoholic beverages.

9. A.R. eats a lot of Mexican dishes. In trying to cut down on his fat intake, he should
   1. refrain from eating any Mexican dishes.
   2. eat soft tacos rather than fried tacos.
   3. ask for meat enchiladas rather than cheese enchiladas.
   4. use extra hot peppers on food to "cut the fat."

10. N.Y. is an 82-year-old widow who lives alone and lives on a very limited income. Her arthritis makes it difficult for her to shop and prepare her meals. In order to improve N.Y.'s nutritional intake, you might suggest she try
    1. taking her noon meal at the corner Senior day-care center.
    2. asking a neighbor to shop for fresh foods for her twice a week.
    3. buy a microwave oven and cookware and learn to use it.
    4. buy a freezer so her daughter can prepare meals for her on the weekends for the rest of the week.

11. N.Y. checks a frozen dinner her daughter put in her freezer. She sees it contains 9 grams of fat and 396 calories. She understands that this means that
    1. 36 calories come from fat.
    2. 27 calories come from fat.
    3. 9% of the meal is fat.
    4. 81 calories come from fat.

12. A lacto-vegetarian will eat
    1. any food except for eggs.
    2. plant foods only.
    3. Plant and dairy foods.
    4. poultry and plant foods.

13. Vitamin supplements should be taken only as recommended because if taken in large quantities fat-soluble vitamins can cause
    1. gastric irritation.
    2. diarrhea.
    3. weight gain.
    4. toxicity.

14. A mainstay of the Asian diet that is a good source of protein is
    1. mushrooms.
    2. rice.
    3. soybeans.
    4. bamboo shoots.

15. If baby Dan weighed 8 lbs. at birth, at one year of age he should weigh
    1. 24 lbs.
    2. 32 lbs.
    3. 16 lbs.
    4. 20 lbs.

16. When solid foods are introduced into baby Dan's diet, they should
    1. begin with puréed meat dishes.
    2. start with cooked fruits.
    3. be sweetened with honey.
    4. be introduced gradually, one food at a time.

17. A guideline that is helpful in getting a toddler to eat more is to
    1. eat with him or her.
    2. keep foods from touching each other on the plate.
    3. serve only one food at a time.
    4. feed him or her each bite yourself.

18. A good snack for a school-age child is
    1. peanut butter on apple slices.
    2. buttered popcorn.
    3. cookies and milk.
    4. chocolate-covered ice cream bar.

19. When considering the nutritional needs of the elderly adult, you know that
    1. nutrient requirements do not change with age.
    2. more calories are needed for tissue repair.
    3. the taste for sweets decreases with age.
    4. preferences for foods often change.

20. Iodine is necessary in the diet for the function of
    1. formation of tooth enamel.
    2. building of strong bones.
    3. maintenance of hair follicles.
    4. the thyroid gland.

CRITICAL THINKING ACTIVITIES

1. Your friend wants to go on a high-protein diet, cutting out carbohydrates in the form of grain products and sweets. If a multivitamin tablet is not taken daily, what possible disorders might this friend develop from vitamin B-group deficiencies?

2. J.L., a 16-year-old neighbor, leads a very active teen life. She rarely eats meals at home. She is concerned about weight gain. How could you counsel her about managing her diet while eating at fast-food restaurants?

3. A.R., age 2, will not eat much of anything but Cheerios and milk. What teaching could you do for her mother to assist her to improve Annie's diet?

4. Analyze your own diet. Is the calorie intake appropriate to maintain a normal weight? Is the diet well balanced? What changes should be made?

MEETING CLINICAL OBJECTIVES

Directions: The following suggested activities will help you meet the stated clinical practice objectives for the chapter. Review your school's clinical objectives for the week and outline a plan of activities that will help you meet them. If unsure as to how to meet them, consult with your instructor at the beginning of the clinical day.

1. Find and look through the diet manual for the clinical facility to which you are assigned.
2. Perform a nutritional assessment on a patient from a different culture. Work with the patient to plan an appropriate balanced diet that contains sufficient protein, but is low fat.
3. Teach a patient about foods needed to increase potassium intake when the patient is on furosemide (Lasix), a potent diuretic.

STEPS TOWARD BETTER COMMUNICATION

VOCABULARY BUILDING GLOSSARY

Term	Pronunciation	Definition
child rearing	CHILD REARing	caring for and educating children
comprise	com PRISE	include, form
compromised	COM pro MISEd	endangered
consume	con SUME	eat
finicky	FIN ick y	very particular, with definite likes and dislikes
Meals on Wheels	MEALS on WHEELS	a program where a meal is prepared and delivered to an elderly person's home by volunteers
peer	PEER	a person of similar age, ability, social status
sparingly	SPAR ing ly	in small amounts

VOCABULARY EXERCISE

Directions: Underline the Vocabulary Building Glossary words used in the sentences below.

1. Child rearing comprises feeding, clothing, nourishing, training, loving, and educating a child.
2. Finicky eaters consume some foods sparingly.
3. The lack of green vegetables in his diet compromised his health.
4. Many volunteers for the Meals on Wheels program are retired and enjoy helping their peers.

COMMUNICATION EXERCISE

Often in English speech, especially informal conversation, words are left out and certain sounds are omitted between words, within a word, or even changed, depending on the sounds that follow. English learners need to understand these omissions when they hear them. They may even choose to use some of them in order to sound more like a native speaker.

Directions: In the following conversation, see where the omissions occur. Draw a line under them and write the words as they would be spoken and written in formal speech.

Nurse:	"Morning, Ms. A. How're you today?"
Ms. A.:	"I'm OK, but I wish they'd gimme a better breakfast!"
Nurse:	"Whaddaya mean? What'd you have?"
Ms. A.:	"Just some lukewarm watery tea, an' cold oatmeal 'n' milk—with no salt. An' the toast was dry 'n' cold."
Nurse:	"Doesn't sound very appetizing. I'll speak to dietary. Didya call the nurse 'n' ask fer hot tea?"
Ms. A.:	"Naw. 't wasn' worth it. I'm goin' home today anyway."
Nurse:	"That's good news. But ya' know you're on a low-sodium diet. That means your not 'sposed to have salt added to your food."
Ms. A.:	"Not even a little in cooking?"
Nurse:	"Not if ya want to follow doctor's orders and keep your blood pressure down. We don't want to see you back in here again."
Ms. A.:	"No offense, but I don' wanna BE back here again. I'll jus' hafta try ta get usta it, I guess."
Nurse:	"That's the spirit. Now let me take your vital signs."

Words that should be used:

1. ____________________
2. ____________________
3. ____________________
4. ____________________
5. ____________________
6. ____________________
7. ____________________
8. ____________________
9. ____________________
10. ____________________
11. ____________________
12. ____________________

CULTURAL POINTS

1. When planning a diet for any patient, it is good to find out what they like to eat and suggest a diet that includes as many of their preferred foods as is healthy and look at ways to modify those foods so they can be kept in the diet. However, if a person really loves salty french fries, they might prefer mashed potatoes to baked fries with no salt!
2. With patients from other cultures, you may want to ask about their usual diet and see if there are ways it can be modified to meet their current dietary needs. Another consideration is that the ethnic group may have special types of foods it believes will aid in healing, such as hot

and cold (temperature or character). Vietnamese women may fear losing heat during labor and delivery and prefer a special diet of salty, hot foods. North Americans usually look at soups, especially chicken soup, hot drinks like tea, and puddings as comforting and healing foods when they are sick.

Review the chapter highlights, answer the study questions, and complete the critical thinking activities at the end of the chapter in the textbook.

TWENTY-SIX

Diet Therapy and Assisted Feeding

TERMINOLOGY

A. COMPLETION

Directions: Fill in the blank(s) with the correct term(s) from the terms list in the chapter in the textbook to complete the sentence.

1. Eating a high-fat diet increases the risk of ___________________ and narrowing of the arteries.
2. It is recommended that people who have ___________________ decrease their sodium intake to decrease edema.
3. Excessive blood glucose is a problem in people who have ___________________.
4. More young women than young men develop ___________________ ___________________, a disorder in which as few calories as possible are eaten in an effort to remain very thin.
5. The diagnosis of ___________________ requires that a person have an excessive accumulation of fat tissue as determined by the body mass index (BMI) rating.
6. The disorder in which a person induces vomiting to control weight gain is called ___________________.
7. Diet and exercise are recommended to control the high blood pressure that occurs with the disorder ___________________.
8. To be diagnosed with ___________________, a patient must have a blood pressure above 140/90 on at least three occasions.
9. A ___________________ tube is inserted percutaneously with the aid of an endoscope inserted into the stomach.
10. Most feeding solutions have ___________________ when compared to water or saline because of the concentration of solutes.
11. A(n) ___________________ tube is used for either evacuation of stomach contents or the instillation of feedings.

IDENTIFICATION

Directions: Identify foods that are allowed on a clear-liquid and full-liquid diet. Mark the foods only allowed on a full-liquid diet with an "F" and foods that are allowed on both diets with a "B." Mark foods not included in either diet with an "N" for not allowed. (See Appendix 4 in the textbook to verify answers.)

1. ______ orange juice
2. ______ tea
3. ______ vegetable beef soup
4. ______ eggnog
5. ______ Cream of Wheat cereal
6. ______ mashed potatoes
7. ______ Jell-O
8. ______ popsicles
9. ______ custard
10. ______ margarine
11. ______ milk
12. ______ ice cream

SHORT ANSWER

Directions: Write a brief answer for each question.

1. The nurse's role in promoting the goals of diet therapy is to:
   a. ______________________________
   b. ______________________________
   c. ______________________________
2. Postoperative patients progress from being NPO to
   ______________________________.
3. For the disorders of anorexia nervosa and bulimia, both ______________ and ______________ counseling are necessary.
4. Appropriate weight gain during pregnancy is ______________ lbs. during the first trimester and ______________ per week during the second and third trimesters.
5. Alcoholism often causes a ______________ deficiency.
6. Obesity is thought to contribute to the risk of
   ____
   ______________________________.
7. Diet therapy for cardiovascular disease focuses on the reduction of
   ______________________________.
8. In order to help patients with cardiovascular disease plan an appropriate diet, you teach them that one teaspoon of salt contains ______________ of sodium.
9. The difference between type I diabetes and type II diabetes is that in type II diabetes, insulin is
   ____
   ______________________________.
10. Patients with diabetes are at higher risk for:
    a. ______________________________
    b. ______________________________
    c. ______________________________
    d. ______________________________
    e. ______________________________

11. The goal of diabetes treatment is to keep the blood glucose between ____________ mg/dL.

12. Dietary considerations for the HIV/AIDS patient include:
    a. ____________
    b. ____________
    c. ____________
    d. ____________
    e. ____________
    f. ____________

13. Feeding tubes are often used to increase nutrition in patients at risk of malnutrition from the effects of:
    a. ____________
    b. ____________
    c. ____________
    d. ____________

14. When a patient has an nasogastric or small-bore feeding tube in place it is essential to check tube placement when ____________.

15. Advantages of the PEG tube over the nasogastric or small-bore feeding tube are:
    ____
    ____________.

16. To check the placement of the PEG tube—which must be done before each feeding or the administration of medication—you would
    ____
    ____________.

17. The normal amount of formula given at one feeding is _____ ounces.

18. Tube feeding solutions should be administered slowly to prevent ____________ and ____________.

19. What might happen if feeding tube placement is not checked before administering a feeding?
    ____
    ____
    ____________.

20. Four principles to follow when administering a tube feeding are:
    a. ____________
    b. ____________
    c. ____________
    d. ____________

APPLICATION OF THE NURSING PROCESS

Directions: Write a short answer for each question.

1. J.K. is suffering from malnutrition due to inflammatory bowel disease. She is started on TPN. Four assessments you must make regarding her nutritional status and safety with this treatment are:
    a. ____________
    b. ____________
    c. ____________
    d. ____________

2. T.P. has AIDS. He has sores in his mouth that make eating painful. He has frequent diarrhea and is rapidly losing weight. He is depressed about his diagnosis and has little appetite. He is started on tube feedings. In planning care for him you determine that appropriate nursing diagnoses related to nutrition problems are:

____

____

____

____

3. Appropriate expected outcomes for these nursing diagnoses might be:

____

____

____

____

4. Four actions to be implemented to decrease the risk of injury to the patient receiving a tube feeding are:
   a. _______________
   b. _______________
   c. _______________
   d. _______________

5. Indicate the correct order for actions in administering a feeding via feeding tube.
   a. ______ Unclamp the tube.
   b. ______ Flush the tube with water.
   c. ______ Check the placement of the tube.
   d. ______ Elevate the patient's head and upper body.
   e. ______ Prepare the feeding bag.
   f. ______ Check for residual feeding in the stomach.
   g. ______ Start the feeding.
   h. ______ Irrigate the tube.

6. Three evaluation statements that would indicate that tube feeding is a successful intervention for the nursing diagnosis of Nutrition, altered: less than body requirements for the above patient would be:
   a. _______________
   b. _______________
   c. _______________

MULTIPLE CHOICE

*Directions: Choose the **best** answer to each of the following questions.*

1. M.R., like several of her co-workers, is gaining weight. Besides reducing fat in the diet, she (like most Americans) should reduce the intake of
   1. ice cream.
   2. prepared foods.
   3. refined sugar.
   4. soft drinks.

2. A patient condition that greatly increases caloric need and causes a need for nutritional creativity is
   1. healing joint replacement.
   2. severe burns.
   3. infection with fever.
   4. inflammatory bowel disease.

3. B.C. is receiving tube feedings. If he has a stomach residual of 85 mL at the time the next tube feeding is due, you should
   1. hold the feeding and notify the physician.
   2. go ahead and give the next feeding.
   3. check the patient for constipation.
   4. mix the next feeding at 2x strength ordered.

4. After giving B.C.'s intermittent tube feeding, you would
   1. immediately clamp the tube.
   2. leave the tube open for ten minutes.
   3. flush the tube with a small amount of water.
   4. instill 30 mL of air to clear the tube.

5. B.C. has a small-bore feeding tube in place. Care for him related to this tube would include
   1. cleansing the abdomen around the insertion site each shift.
   2. auscultating for bowel sounds each shift.
   3. repositioning the tube in the nostril every eight hours.
   4. cleansing the nare with a moist cotton-tipped stick every shift.

6. The rationale for leaving B.C. in an elevated position after each feeding is
   1. to prevent nausea.
   2. to prevent reflux.
   3. to decrease the chance of diarrhea.
   4. for gravity flow into the intestine.

7. S.N., age 18, has type I diabetes. She is trying to adjust her diet and exercise to maintain her blood glucose within normal limits. Her blood glucose is 142 mg/dL at 4 P.M. This reading is
   1. within normal limits.
   2. high.
   3. low.
   4. not important.

8. The purpose of trying to maintain S.N.'s blood glucose within normal limits is to
   1. prevent complications of diabetes.
   2. help her to feel better.
   3. assist with the maintenance of a normal diet.
   4. prevent further weight loss.

9. S.N. is placed on an 2000 calorie diabetic diet. If she eats 64 grams of carbohydrates, 4 grams of fat, and 8 grams of protein for breakfast, she has already consumed how many calories of the day's allotment?
   1. 624
   2. 324
   3. 364
   4. 304

10. S.N. becomes nauseated and starts vomiting. You recommend that she stick to a clear-liquid diet and take plenty of fluids. A food that she could have on this diet is
    1. milkshakes.
    2. chicken noodle soup.
    3. orange juice.
    4. beef broth.

CRITICAL THINKING ACTIVITIES

1. Make out a diet plan for a patient with hypertension that is balanced and contains no more than 2000 calories a day. Include snacks.
2. Outline ways to assist a home care cancer patient to increase calorie and protein intake.
3. Plan ways to assist an African-American patient with hypertension and atherosclerosis to adapt his diet to low-fat based on cultural eating patterns and food preferences.

MEETING CLINICAL OBJECTIVES

Directions: The following suggested activities will help you meet the stated clinical practice objectives for the chapter. Review your school's clinical objectives for the week and outline a plan of activities that will help you meet them. If unsure as to how to meet them, consult with your instructor at the beginning of the clinical day.

1. Seek assignment to a patient who is receiving tube feedings; outline the assessment and care needed for this patient.
2. Seek assignment to a patient who is receiving TPN. List the signs and symptoms of complications that you must watch for in this patient.
3. Develop a diet teaching plan for a new diabetic patient.
4. Review laboratory results on each assigned patient checking nutritional parameters.

STEPS TOWARD BETTER COMMUNICATION

VOCABULARY BUILDING GLOSSARY

Term	Pronunciation	Definition
binge	BINGE	extreme activity, to excess
bland	BLAND	mild, having little taste or seasoning
collaboration	co LAB o RA tion	working together
differentiate	dif fer EN ti ate	explain how several things are different from each other
discrepancies	dis CREP an cies	disagreements in facts or figures (in a chart or record)
exacerbation	ex A cer BA tion	increase; worsening
instilled	in STILLed	put into
malabsorption	mal ab sorp tion	not properly absorbing food from the intestines
nares	NAR es	nostrils, the two openings in the nose
prevalent	PREV a lent	commonly found
prior to	PRI or to	before
purging	PURG ing (purj ing)	causing bowel evacuation
rationale	ra tion Ale	the reason why something is done
resection	RE sec tion	cutting out a piece of an organ (such as the bowel)
trimester	TRI mes ter	three months

COMPLETION

Directions: Fill in the blank(s) with the correct term(s) from the Vocabulary Building Glossary to complete the sentence.

1. There were some ____________________ between what the patient said he usually ate and what the family indicated he ate that would explain his weight gain.

2. A low-sodium diet is very ____________________ but can be improved with the use of other herbs when cooking.
3. Colon cancer often requires ____________________ of the bowel.
4. The person with bulimia often tends to be a ____________________ eater.
5. The nurse often works in ____________________ with the dietitian when trying to change a person's dietary habits.
6. The first ____________________ of pregnancy is a time of very rapid fetal growth.
7. Eating hot, spicy food or caffeine often causes an ____________________ of gastritis.
8. After giving a tube feeding, water must be ____________________ into the tube to clear the formula so that clumping and clogging does not take place.

PRONUNCIATION EXERCISE

Directions: The sound "L" is difficult for some people to pronounce. Compare how the sounds "N," "L," and "R" are made.

First make the sound "N" by placing the tongue against the roof of the mouth, touching the teeth all around with the sides of the tongue. Use your voice, and the sound "N" will come through your nose.

Practice: nice no never nutrition nurse anorexia nares

To make the sound "L," keep the tip of the tongue against the roof of the mouth, but narrow and lower the tongue so the sides of the tongue are not touching the teeth. Use your voice to say "L." The sound and the air goes over the sides of your tongue and out of your mouth. glucose cell "tolerate oral fluid"

Practice alternating the sounds: no/low night/light knife/life knock/lock need/lead ten/tell nab/lab nook/look snow/slow connect/collect never/lever

To make the sound "R," drop the tip of the tongue so it does not touch the roof of the mouth. The sides of your tongue should touch your back teeth. The air flows out over the tip of the tongue through the middle of the mouth. radiation rationale prior rapid residual

Practice: lay/ray long/wrong gleam/green glass/grass laser/razor illustrate/irrigate flee/free tell/tear

To Review:

"N"—The tongue touches the roof of the mouth and the teeth on all sides. Sound goes out the nose.
"L"—The tip of the tongue touches the roof of the mouth and the air flows out the sides
"R"—The tip of the tongue does not touch the roof of the mouth and the air flows out the middle.

Now practice the words with "L," "R," and "N" in the Vocabulary Building Glossary and the Terms List.

PRONUNCIATION OF DIFFICULT TERMS

Directions: Practice pronouncing the following words with a peer.

anorexia nervosa	an o REX i a ner VO sa
atherosclerosis	ATH er o scler O sis
diabetes mellitus	DI a be tis mel LI tis
esophageal	e soph a GE al (ee sof ah jee al)

hyperosmolality	HY per os mo lal i ty
lipoprotein	li po PRO tein
percutaneous	per cu TAN e ous
endoscopic gastrostomy	EN do SCOP ic gas TROS to my
triglycerides	tri GLI cer ides (tri gliss er ides)

COMMUNICATION EXERCISE

1. Here is an example of a therapeutic communication with a patient who needs to alter his diet.

   Mr. H. has hypertension. Although he has been started on medication, his blood pressure has not come down as much as desired. It is necessary to find out if he is following diet and exercise guidelines that were given to him a few weeks ago.

Nurse: "Mr. H., your blood pressure is not coming down as much as we would like. You are still in the hypertensive range. Have you looked at the diet and exercise guidelines we gave you?"

Mr. H.: "Yes, I read them over. I'm taking a walk as often as I can. I'm not adding any salt at the table anymore either."

Nurse: "Let's look more closely at the foods you are eating and the way they are prepared. What did you have for breakfast today?"

Mr. H.: "I had bacon and eggs with an English muffin and orange juice for breakfast. Oh, and coffee, of course."

Nurse: "How often do you eat that type of breakfast?"

Mr. H.: "About three or four times a week, I guess."

Nurse: "Bacon in particular has a lot of sodium in it. Would it be possible to leave off the bacon all but one or two of those days?"

Mr. H.: "I guess I could try that."

Nurse: "Now, tell me about yesterday's lunch and dinner."

Mr. H.: "For lunch we went to the deli and I had a pastrami sandwich and a dill pickle, cole slaw, and iced tea. For dinner, we had ham and sweet potatoes, peas, cottage cheese and fruit salad, and iced tea. For dessert there was ice cream."

Nurse: "O.K., let's see, the pastrami and dill pickle are loaded with sodium. A green salad with oil and vinegar dressing is usually lower in sodium than cole slaw because of the type of dressing that is on that. Ham is preserved and is very high in sodium. Peas and cottage cheese also have some sodium in them as do all milk products like ice cream. From the reading of the guidelines you did do you recall other things that might be substituted for these foods?"

Mr. H.: "I think that fresh fish seemed lower in sodium than ham or pastrami. An apple might have less sodium than a dill pickle. A sorbet bar might have less sodium than ice cream and still satisfy my sweet tooth. I don't recall much else."

Nurse: "Why don't you and your wife go over the guidelines again and we will talk about it when you come in to have your blood pressure checked again next week?"

Mr. H.: "I guess we could do that. I'll try to think more about what I am eating."

2. Practice this conversation using "L" with a partner.

Nurse: "Hello, Mr. M. How are you feeling?"

Mr. M.: "Less good than last night. My left leg is a little sore."

Nurse: "Let's look at it."

Mr. M.: "I can't lift it even a little."

Nurse: "Dr. Lincoln should look at it. I'll leave a call for her to drop by on her rounds."

Mr. M.: "Can I have my lunch now? I'm awfully hungry."

Nurse: "It's a little early. It's only eleven o'clock. Would you like me to order you some lemonade and a light snack?"

Mr. M.: "Only a little lemon and a lot of sugar. That's the way I like it."

Nurse: "I'll leave your request with the kitchen help. See you later."

Review the chapter highlights, answer the study questions, and complete the critical thinking activities at the end of the chapter in the textbook.

TWENTY-SEVEN

Assisting with Respiration and Oxygen Delivery

TERMINOLOGY

A. MATCHING

Directions: Match the terms in column I with the definitions in column II.

Column I	Column II
1. ______ anoxia	a. Adhesive, sticky
2. ______ apnea	b. Machine that measures oxygen saturation of the blood
3. ______ cannula	c. Device supplying moisture to air or oxygen
4. ______ dyspnea	d. Above-normal level of carbon dioxide in the blood
5. ______ cyanosis	e. Tube for insertion into a cavity or vessel
6. ______ expectorate	f. Device that dispenses liquid in a fine spray
7. ______ humidifier	g. Difficulty breathing
8. ______ hypercapnia	h. Absence of breathing
9. ______ hypoxia	i. Bluish color around lips and of mucous membranes from lack of oxygen
10. ______ nebulizer	j. Cough up and spit out secretions
11. ______ oximeter	k. Low level of oxygen in the blood
12. ______ retraction	l. Muscles move inward upon inspiration
13. ______ stridor	m. Condition of being without oxygen
14. ______ tachypnea	n. Shrill, harsh sound made when breathing is obstructed
15. ______ tenacious	o. Rapid breathing

B. COMPLETION

Directions: Fill in the blank(s) with the correct term(s) from the terms in the chapter in the textbook to complete the sentence.

1. In the emergency or short-term situation, an ________________ tube is often used to maintain a patent airway.

2. For longer-term assisted ventilation, a ____________________ is performed.
3. An ____________________ is needed to insert a tracheostomy tube.
4. The process of ____________________ uses the respiratory muscles and diaphragm to draw air into the lungs.
5. The passive relaxation of the respiratory muscles causes ____________________ and air flows out of the lungs.
6. When there is a lower level of oxygen in the blood than normal, the patient has ____________________.
7. The exchange of air between the lungs and the atmosphere is called ____________________.
8. ____________________ is the exchange of oxygen and carbon dioxide between the atmosphere and the body cells.

REVIEW OF STRUCTURE AND FUNCTION OF THE RESPIRATORY SYSTEM

Directions: Identify the correct structure to match the function performed by the respiratory system.

chemoreceptors	central nervous system (CNS)
mucous membranes	alveolar membrane
bronchi	upper airway passages
alveolar macrophages	blood

1. ________________________________ controls respiration.
2. ________________________________ channel air to and from the lungs.
3. ________________________________ phagocytize inhaled bacteria and foreign particles.
4. ________________________________ sense changes in oxygen or carbon dioxide and signal the brain stem.
5. ________________________________ secrete mucous to assist cilia to cleanse respiratory tract of foreign particles.
6. ________________________________ allows diffusion of oxygen and carbon dioxide from alveoli into the bloodstream.
7. ________________________________ transports oxygen to the cells and carbon dioxide to the lungs.
8. ________________________________ warm and humidify air on its way to the lungs.

SHORT ANSWER

Directions: Write a brief answer for each question.

1. Three causes of hypoxemia are:
   a. ________________________________
   b. ________________________________
   c. ________________________________
2. List one advantage of each of these oxygen delivery methods.
   a. Nasal cannula ________________________________
   b. Simple mask ________________________________
   c. Partial rebreathing mask ________________________________

d. Non-rebreathing mask ______________________________
e. Venturi mask ______________________________
f. Tracheostomy collar ______________________________
g. T-bar ______________________________

3. List four safety precautions to be observed when patients are receiving oxygen therapy.
   a. ______________________________
   ____
   b. ______________________________
   ____
   c. ______________________________
   ____
   d. ______________________________
   ____

4. Five symptoms that indicate the patient should be assessed for possible hypoxia are:
   a. ______________________________
   b. ______________________________
   c. ______________________________
   d. ______________________________
   e. ______________________________

5. Nursing responsibilities for the patient undergoing pulse oximetry are:
   ____
   ____
   ____
   ____

6. List four reasons an artificial airway may be used.
   a. ______________________________
   b. ______________________________
   c. ______________________________
   d. ______________________________

SEQUENCING

Directions: Place the following actions in correct sequential order (1, 2, 3, etc.) for the following situation: You are waiting in line at the grocery store when the person in front of you collapses.

______ Check the carotid pulse (which is absent).
______ Call for help.
______ Shake and shout name or "Are you O.K.?" (No response.)
______ Give two breaths.
______ Position hands for chest compressions.
______ Give two quick, short breaths.
______ Give 15 chest compressions.
______ Tilt head and open airway.
______ Form seal around nose and mouth with your mouth.
______ Check for presence of respiration (none).
______ Continue CPR sequence.

APPLICATION OF THE NURSING PROCESS

Directions: Write a brief answer for each question.

1. G.C. is one day post-op from gallbladder surgery. She says she "doesn't feel right" and seems a bit short of breath after being up for her bath. What would you do to assess her respiratory status?

____

____

____

____

____

2. You find that G.C. has diminished breath sounds in the right lower lobe, a respiratory rate of 24, pulse of 92, and some shortness of breath upon exertion. What would be the appropriate nursing diagnosis for her, relevant to her respiratory status?

____

3. Write an expected outcome for the chosen nursing diagnosis.

____

4. What nursing actions would assist G.C. in meeting the expected outcome?

____

____

____

____

5. How would you determine if the nursing interventions are effective in helping G.C. meet the expected outcome?

____

____

____

____

MULTIPLE CHOICE

*Directions: Choose the **best** answer for each of the following questions.*

1. I.D., age 72, has developed hypostatic pneumonia while recovering from extensive trauma from a motor vehicle accident. He is started on oxygen via nasal cannula. He has no preexisting respiratory disease. You know that a normal rate of oxygen flow for him would be
   1. 1–2 L/min.
   2. 2–3 L/min.
   3. 4–6 L/min.
   4. 7–10 L/min.

2. I.D. is beginning to show signs of restlessness and irritability. A nursing action that might help is to have him
   1. turn, cough, and deep breathe.
   2. take a good nap.
   3. submit to a back rub.
   4. take some pain medication.

3. An important nursing action for I.D. while undergoing oxygen therapy is to
   1. restrict oral fluid intake.
   2. cleanse nares frequently.
   3. increase calorie intake.
   4. place the head of the bed at 30 degrees.

4. The physician has ordered postural drainage for I.D. The best time to perform this procedure is
   1. mid-morning.
   2. after breakfast.
   3. mid-afternoon.
   4. before meals.

5. Another nursing action to assist patients with pneumonia to obtain better oxygenation is to
   1. have them up in a chair as much as possible.
   2. ambulate them three times per day.
   3. insist they stay as quiet as possible.
   4. keep them on a full-liquid diet.

6. A factor in keeping I.D.'s secretions thinned so they can be coughed up—other than using a humidifier—is to
   1. use chest percussion treatments.
   2. encourage a sitting position while awake.
   3. increase his fluid intake.
   4. suction him once every two hours.

7. F.P., age 64, has an endotracheal tube in place. She suffered a head injury six days ago in a fall and is comatose. The endotracheal tube should be replaced by a tracheostomy tube, if an airway is still needed, after
   1. 10 days.
   2. 2 weeks.
   3. 1 week.
   4. 3–5 days.

8. F.P. remains comatose and in need of ventilation. A tracheostomy tube is inserted. When suctioning the tracheostomy, the suction pressure should be set between
   1. 60–80 mm Hg.
   2. 80–120 mm Hg.
   3. 100–140 mm Hg.
   4. 20–60 mm Hg.

9. For proper technique in suctioning F.P.'s tracheostomy, you would
   1. rotate and use intermittent suction while introducing the catheter into the bronchus.
   2. suction for 20 seconds at a time.
   3. rotate the catheter and use suction while pulling the catheter out of the bronchus.
   4. suction for five seconds at a time.

10. F.P. is receiving positive-pressure ventilation. This means that her cuffed tube must be
   1. inflated for ventilation to be most effective.
   2. deflated for suctioning procedure.
   3. replaced every three days.
   4. repositioned each shift to prevent ulceration.

CRITICAL THINKING ACTIVITIES

1. How could you help the patient who has sustained fractured ribs and is having difficulty deep breathing and coughing perform these needed exercises?

2. What would you say to the patient who has a chest tube about what to expect when the tube is taken out?

3. Outline a teaching plan to explain to a patient about the purpose of pulse oximetry and how it works.

MEETING CLINICAL OBJECTIVES

Directions: The following suggested activities will help you meet the stated clinical practice objectives for the chapter. Review your school's clinical objectives for the week and outline a plan of activities that will help you meet them. If unsure as to how to meet them, consult with your instructor at the beginning of the clinical day.

1. Find a preoperative patient to whom you can teach the techniques for proper deep breathing and coughing.
2. Assist a patient to correctly use an incentive spirometer.
3. Help a patient assume positions for postural drainage of the lungs. If a patient is not available, practice the positioning with a family member.
4. Ask to be assigned to a patient who is receiving oxygen. Practice adjusting the flow rate and correctly applying the delivery device.
5. Go with another nurse to perform tracheostomy care, then ask to be assigned to a tracheostomy patient so that you can perform the needed care.
6. Practice tracheostomy suctioning in the skill lab if possible with a peer observing your technique.
7. Review chest tube care and then ask to be assigned to a patient with a chest tube.

STEPS TOWARD BETTER COMMUNICATION

VOCABULARY BUILDING GLOSSARY

Term	Pronunciation	Definition
ambient	AM bi ent	surrounding; "ambient light" means the light that is around, available
brink	BRINK	edge, almost occurring
combustion	com BUS tion	the process of burning; "supports combustion" means it enables the process of burning
copious	COP i ous	a very large amount, abundant
intertwined	in ter TWINed	twisted together, connected

COMPLETION

Directions: Fill in the blank(s) with the correct word(s) from the Vocabulary Building Glossary to complete the sentence.

1. The patient was coughing and producing ____________________ sputum.
2. The patient's respiratory illness was worsening and he was on the ____________________ of respiratory failure.
3. Oxygen administration was discontinued and the patient was observed for a while on ____________________ oxygen in the room air.
4. It is dangerous to cause a spark in a room where oxygen is being used because oxygen will support ____________________.

WORD ATTACK SKILLS

Directions: Note the use of these prefixes and suffix.

-pnea = breathing
a- = not
dys- = difficult, poor
tachy- = rapid
brady- = slow

Even though the following words have the same root, the prefixes change the accent and therefore the pronunciation:

AP ne a
bra dy NE a (the p is silent)
dysp NE a
ta chyp NE a

(Note: hypercapnia is spelled with an i; it has a different meaning than pnea. -capnia refers to carbon dioxide.)

PRONUNCIATION OF DIFFICULT TERMS

Directions: Practice pronouncing the following words.

alveolar macrophages	AL ve O lar MAC ro PHAG es
atelectasis	AT e LEC ta sis
chemoreceptors	CHE mo re CEP tors
endotracheal	en do TRACH e al
hypercapnia	hy per CAP ni a
obturator	ob tu RA tor
oximeter	ox IM e ter
tracheostomy	trach e OS to my

GRAMMAR POINTS

Usually, the verb tense called the "present continuous" or "present progressive" is used when an action is happening right now: You are reading these words and you are answering the questions. It is used to answer the question "What are you doing?" "I am taking vital signs." It is formed by using the simple present form of be + verb + -ing.

This same verb tense may be used to describe activities that stop and start during a longer period that includes the present time. You can use this form when you interview patients to learn about symptoms they are having:

Are you coughing? (Not this minute, but today, or over the past few days continuing until now.)

Are you wheezing?

Are you experiencing shortness of breath?

How are you feeling? (This can mean "now," or in general over recent days.)

How much are you smoking?

Are you drinking a lot of water?

Are you getting any exercise?

COMMUNICATION EXERCISE

1. With a partner, write a dialogue describing to a patient who has a chest tube what to expect when the tube is taken out (Critical Thinking Activity #2 above). Practice the dialogue with your partner.
2. With a partner, practice the guidelines for interviewing the patient with a respiratory problem, Table 27-5.

Review the chapter highlights, answer the study questions, and complete the critical thinking activities at the end of the chapter in the textbook.

TWENTY-EIGHT

Promoting Urinary Elimination

TERMINOLOGY

A. MATCHING

Directions: Match the terms in column I with the definitions in column II.

Column I		Column II	
1. ______	anuria	a.	Needing to urinate at night during sleep hours
2. ______	cystitis	b.	Pus in the urine
3. ______	dysuria	c.	Narrowing, usually of a tube or opening
4. ______	hematuria	d.	To urinate
5. ______	nocturia	e.	Absence of urine
6. ______	oliguria	f.	Inflammation of the bladder
7. ______	polyuria	g.	Decreased urine output
8. ______	pyuria	h.	Blood in the urine
9. ______	stricture	i.	Painful urination
10. ______	void	j.	Excessive urination

B. COMPLETION

Directions: Fill in the blank(s) with the correct term(s) from the terms list in the chapter in the textbook to complete the sentence.

1. When it is too tiring for a patient to walk to the bathroom, toileting may be done with the __________________ chair.
2. Sometimes running water in the sink will help a patient initiate __________________.
3. Urine left in the bladder after urination is called __________________.
4. Various medications cause urine __________________ as a side effect, particularly in the male.
5. When the patient is unable to control the bladder sphincter, urinary __________________ occurs.
6. A __________________ is an artificially created opening on the abdomen for the discharge of urine.

7. Urinary ________________ is performed when the patient is unable to eliminate urine from the bladder.

8. A ________________ is only suitable for use on the male patient.

REVIEW OF STRUCTURE AND FUNCTION OF THE URINARY SYSTEM

Directions: Match the structures in column I with the functions in column II.

Column I		Column II	
1. ______	kidney	a.	Carries urine from the bladder to the outside of the body
2. ______	bladder	b.	Extracts metabolic waste
3. ______	ureter	c.	Manufactures urine
4. ______	nephron	d.	Carries urine from the kidney to the bladder
5. ______	urethra	e.	Controls the release of urine from the bladder
6. ______	sphincter	f.	Holds 1000–1800 mL of urine

IDENTIFICATION

Directions: Mark the items from a urinalysis report with an "X" if they are abnormal. (Answer requires synthesis and application of knowledge.)

1. ______ Color: dark amber
2. ______ Character: slightly cloudy
3. ______ Specific gravity: 1.025
4. ______ pH: 6.0
5. ______ Glucose: 1+
6. ______ Protein: 0
7. ______ Ketones: 0
8. ______ Leukocytes: moderate
9. ______ Erythrocytes: 0
10. ______ Bilirubin: slight
11. ______ Pyuria: trace

SHORT ANSWER

Directions: Write a brief answer for each question.

1. Describe three nursing measures to assist patient to urinate normally.
   a. ________________________________
   b. ________________________________
   c. ________________________________

2. List four reasons urinary catheterization may be ordered.
   a. ________________________________
   b. ________________________________
   c. ________________________________
   d. ________________________________

3. When catheterizing a patient you accidentally contaminate the catheter. You must ________________________________.

4. Intermittent catheterization is used for patients who ________________.

5. Three reasons bladder irrigation may be ordered are to:
   a. ________________
   b. ________________
   c. ________________

6. An important principle to be applied when irrigating the bladder is ________________.

7. Urinary incontinence can be managed by ________________
____
____

8. Symptoms of cystitis are ________________.

COMPLETION

Directions: Fill in the blank(s) with the correct word(s) to complete the sentence.

1. The average adult voids from ________________ times a day.
2. Foul-smelling urine may indicate ________________.
3. Each patient should void at least every ________________ hours.
4. Urine specimens should be tested immediately, because after ________________ of standing the urine changes characteristics.
5. When instructing the patient on how to collect a 24-hour urine specimen you would tell him or her to void and ________________ the specimen at the beginning of the test.
6. Urine is strained when it is suspected that the patient has a urinary ________________.
7. A fracture pan is used when the patient is unable to ________________ on a regular bedpan.
8. Men generally have an easier time voiding when in the ________________ position.
9. A ________________ catheter is curved and is easier to insert into the male when the prostate is enlarged.
10. A bladder ________________ may be used to soothe irritated bladder tissues and promote healing.
11. The lighter the shade of urine, the more ________________ it is.
12. When placing a fracture pan, the wide lip goes ________________.
13. When catheterizing a female, it is wise to identify the location of the ________________ and the ________________ before opening the catheter kit.
14. Suprapubic catheters are often used after gynecologic surgery so that ________________ can be reestablished before the catheter is removed.
15. When performing a bladder irrigation, you must be careful not to exert ________________ which might damage the bladder and cause pain.

APPLICATION OF THE NURSING PROCESS

Directions: Write a brief answer for each question.

1. If V.O., age 72, states that he has been experiencing a very frequent need to urinate, what questions would you ask to further assess the situation?

2. If the assessment data indicates V.O. seems to be having trouble with an enlarged prostate, what would be three possible nursing diagnoses for him? Place a "*" next to the most appropriate one.

3. Write two expected outcomes for the starred nursing diagnosis.
   a. __________
   b. __________

4. A tendency for a man who is experiencing frequent urination is to decrease fluid intake. What would you tell V.O. about his fluid intake?

5. Treatment for V.O.'s problem takes time to be effective. How would you evaluate progress toward meeting the expected outcomes?

MULTIPLE CHOICE

*Directions: Choose the **best** answer for each of the following questions.*

1. T.Y. is to undergo tests to determine the status of his kidney function. One test used to see if the kidney is concentrating urine correctly is a
   1. urine culture.
   2. specific gravity.
   3. 24-hour urine test.
   4. microscopic exam of urine.

2. Continued urine retention can eventually damage the kidneys. If that happens, the kidneys will not be able to remove waste materials from the body or
   1. regulate fluid balance.
   2. absorb nutrients for cellular growth.
   3. help regulate body temperature.
   4. secrete hormones needed for growth.

3. You obtain a urine specimen for urinalysis from T.Y. Which characteristic of the specimen is abnormal?
   1. aromatic odor
   2. slightly acidic pH
   3. cloudy appearance
   4. straw color

4. When collecting T.Y.'s 24-hour urine specimen, it is important to
   1. limit fluids to less than 1000 mL per day.
   2. start the test with a full bladder.
   3. add the voiding at the end of the test to the container.
   4. force fluids to at least 3000 mL per day.

5. Data that would indicate that T.Y. was experiencing retention of urine would be
   1. voiding 15 times a day.
   2. cloudy urine.
   3. low specific gravity of urine.
   4. palpation reveals a distended bladder.

6. A Foley catheter is ordered for T.Y. to relieve his symptoms until treatment can correct the situation. When a urinary catheter is left in place for more than a couple of days in a male, it should be
   1. taped to the leg.
   2. taped to the abdomen.
   3. looped on the upper thigh.
   4. replaced every three days.

7. When inserting the catheter into the penis of T.Y., if resistance is felt, an appropriate action is to
   1. have T.Y. bear down and apply pressure to the catheter.
   2. remove the catheter and try a smaller one.
   3. tell him to take a deep breath and twist the catheter while inserting it.
   4. call a urologist to insert the catheter.

8. P.R., age 68, is recovering from a hip fracture and pinning. She has a Foley catheter in place. You know that it is **most** important to
   1. encourage fluid intake of 3000 mL a day.
   2. be certain the catheter and drainage tubing are free from kinks.
   3. empty the Foley bag when it is 3/4 full.
   4. assess the output every two hours.

9. The first step in beginning a urine continence training program is to
   1. toilet the patient every two hours.
   2. increase fluid intake to dilute the urine.
   3. collaborate with other health care workers.
   4. assess when voidings are occurring.

10. Besides scheduled toileting, one action that may assist P.R. to regain bladder control is to
   1. teach her Kegel exercises.
   2. ambulate her regularly.
   3. use absorbent panty liners to prevent wetness.
   4. restrict fluids to 1000 mL per day.

CRITICAL THINKING ACTIVITIES

1. Write an outline for a specific teaching plan for a multiple sclerosis patient who has lost nerve control over the bladder and needs to learn to self-catheterize.
2. Write a specific teaching plan for a newly married woman who is having recurrent cystitis.
3. Explain to an older male family member why symptoms of prostate enlargement and urinary retention should be treated as soon as possible. Outline the points you would cover:

MEETING CLINICAL OBJECTIVES

Directions: The following suggested activities will help you meet the stated clinical practice objectives for the chapter. Review your school's clinical objectives for the week and outline a plan of activities that will help you meet them. If unsure as to how to meet them, consult with your instructor at the beginning of the clinical day.

1. With a peer, practice comfortably placing a bedpan under a patient. Use water to partially fill the pan and practice removing it without spilling.
2. Practice catheterization procedure until you can do it efficiently and aseptically five times in the skill lab or simulated at home. Have a peer check your technique as you do the procedure.
3. Ask to observe catheterization procedures on your assigned unit before attempting to perform one.
4. Seek opportunity to obtain a sterile specimen from a Foley catheter.
5. Teach a patient how to obtain a mid-stream urine specimen.
6. Seek opportunity to remove a Foley catheter.

STEPS TOWARD BETTER COMMUNICATION

VOCABULARY BUILDING GLOSSARY

Term	Pronunciation	Definition
bulbous	BUL bous	shaped like a lightbulb, with a larger rounded end
dependent	de PEN dent	1) relying on someone or something else; 2) hanging down
deficit	DEF i cit	below the normal or desired level
diversion	di VER sion	an alternative way, going a different way
distal	dis tal	away from the center of the body or point of attachment
hypertrophy	hy PER tro phy	increase in volume of a tissue or organ, caused by enlargement of existing cells
impede	im PEDE	get in the way of, block, slow down
instillation	in STIL LA tion	addition, putting into
invalid	in VAL id	not correct, not able to be used
invalid	IN val id	a person who is ill, or weakened by ill health or injury
patency	PA tent cy	having a clear passage
prone	PRONE	1) likely to do or have something; 2) lying face down
pucker	PUCK er	to draw together in small wrinkles, tighten in a circle
stasis	STA sis	a slowing or stopping of the normal flow of a bodily fluid

COMPLETION

Directions: Fill in the blank(s) with the correct term(s) from the Vocabulary Building Glossary to complete the sentence.

1. Some people have a very ____________________ nose.
2. A stone can ____________________ urine flow from the kidney if it lodges in a ureter.
3. Older adults often develop ____________________ of urine in the bladder because they do not empty it completely.
4. One treatment for bladder cancer may be an ____________________ of chemotherapy agents into the bladder.
5. Many women are very ____________________ to bladder infections induced by bacteria entering the urethra during intercourse.
6. The urinary meatus will ____________________ if it is touched with a swab when preparing to catheterize the female patient.
7. A urinary catheter must remain ____________________ or urine will back up into the kidney and may cause tissue damage.

VOCABULARY EXERCISE

Directions: Make six sentences using the different meanings of the three words dependent, invalid, and prone (two sentences for each word).

1. ____
2. ____
3. ____
4. ____
5. ____
6. ____

PRONUNCIATION OF DIFFICULT TERMS

Directions: Practice pronouncing the following words.

catheterization	CATH e ter i ZA tion
erythrocytes	e RY thro cytes
hypertrophy	hy PER tro phy
leukocytes	leu ko cytes
micturition	mic tu ri tion
reagent	re AG ent
urostomy	ur OS to my

COMMUNICATION EXERCISE

Directions: With a peer, practice your pronunciation by role playing the "Communication Cue" in the chapter in the textbook.

Review the chapter highlights, answer the study questions, and complete the critical thinking activities at the end of the chapter in the textbook.

TWENTY-NINE

Promoting Bowel Elimination

TERMINOLOGY

A. MATCHING

Directions: Match the terms in column I with the definitions in column II.

Column I		Column II	
1. ______	ostomy appliance	a.	Waste eliminated from the colon
2. ______	constipation	b.	Opening from the abdomen into the intestine
3. ______	diarrhea	c.	Expel feces
4. ______	defecate	d.	Entrance of ostomy
5. ______	excoriation	e.	Passage of hard, dry feces
6. ______	flatus	f.	Enlarged veins inside or outside the rectum
7. ______	hemorrhoids	g.	Partially digested blood in the stool
8. ______	melena	h.	Stool having high fat content
9. ______	ostomy	i.	Gas
10. ______	steatorrhea	j.	Abrasion of the skin
11. ______	stool	k.	Diversion of intestinal contents from the normal path
12. ______	stoma	l.	Device to gather and contain ostomy output
		m.	Frequent, watery stools

B. COMPLETION

Directions: Fill in the blank(s) with the correct term(s) from the terms list in the chapter in the textbook to complete the sentence.

1. When an elderly person is on bed rest and is receiving narcotic pain medications, ____________________ may occur as constipation worsens.
2. Another term for stool is ____________________.
3. Bowel ____________________ is extremely upsetting to patients and not much fun for nurses either.
4. When there is a small amount of bleeding in the intestine it often appears as ____________________ blood in the stool.

5. A ___________________ occurring when an impaction is being removed can cause cardiac dysrhythmia and an alteration in blood pressure.
6. Intra-abdominal pressure is created by performing the ___________________ and is used to initiate defecation.
7. A ___________________ may be performed when the bowel has been invaded by cancerous tumor.
8. The intestinal villi ___________________ with aging and nutrient absorption may decrease in some elderly patients.
9. An ___________________ is an opening into the small intestine for the diversion of intestinal contents.
10. Whenever the patient has an ostomy, meticulous ___________________ care is needed to keep the skin around the stoma in good condition.
11. The material discharged by an intestinal ostomy is called ___________________.

REVIEW OF STRUCTURE AND FUNCTION OF THE INTESTINAL SYSTEM

Directions: Match the structures in column I with the functions in column II.

Column I		Column II	
1. ______	small intestine	a.	Reabsorbs water, sodium, and chloride
2. ______	large intestine	b.	Absorb food substances
3. ______	sigmoid colon	c.	Attaches transverse colon to rectum
4. ______	rectum	d.	No known digestive function
5. ______	rectal sphincter	e.	Controls movement of substances into the large intestine
6. ______	veriform appendix	f.	Allows passage of feces to outside of body
7. ______	intestinal muscle layers	g.	Processes chyme into a more liquid state
8. ______	villi	h.	Controls release of feces
9. ______	anus	i.	Expand and contract to move chyme and feces
10. ______	ileocecal valve	j.	Stores feces for expulsion

SHORT ANSWER

Directions: Write a brief answer for each question.

1. Four factors that can interfere with normal bowel elimination are:
   a. ___________________
   b. ___________________
   c. ___________________
   d. ___________________

2. Give the possible cause for each of the following abnormal stool characteristics:
   a. Melena: ___________________
   b. Occult blood: ___________________
   c. Pale colored stool: ___________________
   d. Mucus: ___________________

e. Foul-smelling stool that floats in water: ______________________
f. Liquid stool: ______________________
g. Hard, dry stool: ______________________

3. Preoperative assessment of the patient who is to undergo an ostomy may reveal fear of:
a. ______________________
b. ______________________
c. ______________________
d. ______________________

4. One intervention that can be helpful to the patient who is to have an ostomy is
____
____

5. Three types of intestinal diversions are:
a. ______________________
b. ______________________
c. ______________________

6. Four ways to prevent constipation are:
a. ______________________
b. ______________________
c. ______________________
d. ______________________

7. Rectal suppositories work to promote bowel movements by:
a. ______________________
b. ______________________
c. ______________________

8. Conditions that may require a bowel ostomy are:
a. ______________________
b. ______________________
c. ______________________
d. ______________________

APPLICATION OF THE NURSING PROCESS

Directions: Write a brief answer for each question.

1. When assessing for normal bowel function you would:
____
____
____

2. R.M., age 56, is hospitalized due to trauma from a fall off of a ladder. He is receiving narcotic pain medication. He is normally a very active man. From this data, you know that he should have which nursing diagnosis related to bowel function?
____

3. Write an expected outcome for the above nursing diagnosis.
____

4. Interventions to prevent bowel problems for R.M. would be:
____
____

5. To evaluate whether the expected outcome is being met, you would evaluate:

____

____

MULTIPLE CHOICE

*Directions: Choose the **best** answer for each of the following questions.*

1. K.M. has developed constipation. The physician orders a rectal suppository to stimulate defecation. When inserting a rectal suppository, you should
   1. freeze the suppository so it is rigid.
   2. squirt lubricant into the rectum first.
   3. place it 2-3 inches above the outer sphincter.
   4. use two fingers to correctly position it.

2. The suppository does not work and an enema is ordered for K.M. When giving an enema to a patient in bed, the best patient position for instilling the solution is
   1. left Sims'.
   2. right lateral.
   3. supine.
   4. prone.

3. When administering the enema to K.M., you would position the solution container no higher above his buttocks than
   1. 6 inches.
   2. 18 inches.
   3. 12 inches.
   4. 22 inches.

4. Restricting the height of the solution container prevents
   1. bubbling and flatus from occurring in the bowel.
   2. the solution from running much too slowly.
   3. the solution from going too high in the colon.
   4. the solution from entering at too high a pressure.

5. The amount of solution you would use for K.M.'s enema is
   1. 300–500 mL.
   2. 1500–2000 mL.
   3. 400–800 mL.
   4. 500–1000 mL.

6. The amount of soap you would add to the water for a soapsuds enema for K.M. is
   1. 30 mL per 1000 mL.
   2. 10 mL per 500 mL.
   3. 5 mL per 1000 mL.
   4. 2 mL per 500 mL.

7. K.M. needs diet counseling to prevent further constipation. You would explain that he should
   1. drink lots of fluid with meals.
   2. eat cold cereal every morning.
   3. eat lots of nuts.
   4. increase vegetable and whole grain intake.

8. D.Z., age 82, has a new colostomy because of colon cancer. Sometimes an elderly patient cannot manage self-care due to pre-existing problems with
   1. fragile skin.
   2. arthritis.
   3. back problems.
   4. transient dizziness.

9. D.Z. is very concerned about odor from his colostomy. You might teach him that one way to prevent excessive unpleasant odor is to
   1. eat lots of fresh fruit.
   2. avoid gas-forming foods.
   3. eat only cooked vegetables.
   4. avoid too much fresh fruit.

10. When planning for teaching D.Z. about his colostomy care, you explain that he should report to the doctor if the
    1. effluent is always formed.
    2. effluent is very soft.
    3. stoma is pale in color.
    4. appliance needs emptying several times a day.

CRITICAL THINKING ACTIVITIES

1. E.D. is a 36-year-old executive who eats on the run for most meals. She is having difficulty with increasing constipation. Outline a teaching plan for her to combat this problem. Consider her lifestyle.
2. Prepare to instruct a clinic patient how to collect a stool specimen at home for testing for occult blood. Outline your points of instruction:
3. Prepare a teaching plan for a patient who needs to learn to self-catheterize a continent diversion. Plan outline:

MEETING CLINICAL OBJECTIVES

Directions: The following suggested activities will help you meet the stated clinical practice objectives for the chapter. Review your school's clinical objectives for the week and outline a plan of activities that will help you meet them. If unsure as to how to meet them, consult with your instructor at the beginning of the clinical day.

1. If a skill lab is available, practice giving an enema to a mannequin with a peer to observe technique. Practice until you are comfortable with the equipment and the procedure.
2. Work on a bowel training program with a patient or relative who has a long-standing problem with constipation.
3. Ask for an opportunity to obtain and test a stool specimen for occult blood.
4. Seek clinical opportunities to give various types of enemas.
5. Contact the agency enterostomal therapist and ask to go along on patient visits and teaching sessions.
6. Attend the local ostomy society meeting.
7. Obtain a copy of the literature available for ostomy patients from the local chapter of the American Cancer Society.
8. In the clinical setting, seek opportunity to assist with colostomy, ileostomy, and urostomy care.

STEPS TOWARD BETTER COMMUNICATION

VOCABULARY BUILDING GLOSSARY

Term	Pronunciation	Definition
commode	com MODE	a toilet seat
compromised	COM pro mised	affected by exposing to danger or problems
distension	dis TEN sion	swelling, or pushing out because of internal pressure
heed	HEED	pay attention to
induced	in DUCEd	caused; brought on by
longitudinal	lon gi tud in al	lengthwise; along the long part of something

oblique	o blique (o BLEEK)	slanting; not straight across, but at a sharp angle
scanty	SCAN ty	a slight or small amount
tepid	TEP id	slightly warm
triggering	TRIG ger ing	starting a reaction
wafer	WA fer	a thin, flat, round disc

COMPLETION

Directions: Fill in the blank(s) with the correct term(s) from the Vocabulary Building Glossary to complete the sentence.

1. Patients who are prone to constipation need to learn to ____________________ the urge for defecation.
2. Constipation often causes abdominal ____________________, making the patient quite uncomfortable.
3. A tap water enema distends the bowel ____________________ defecation.
4. A karaya ____________________ is often used on the skin to protect it when an ostomy appliance is applied to the stoma.
5. The appliance plate had to be trimmed to an ____________________ angle in order to fit properly on the abdomen.
6. A portable ____________________ is often used for bed rest patients and is placed beside the bed.
7. When a patient has an impaction, ____________________ amounts of liquid stool may be passed intermittently.

WORD ATTACK SKILLS

Directions: If an ostomy is an opening into the intestine, where specifically are the following located?

1. colostomy ____
2. ileostomy ____
3. urostomy ____

PRONUNCIATION OF DIFFICULT TERMS

Directions: Practice pronouncing the following words.

chyme	CHYME (kime)
ileocecal	il e o CE cal
longitudinal	lon gi TUD in al
oblique	o BLIQUE (o BLEEK)
sphincter	SPHINC ter (sfink ter)
steatorrhea	STE a tor rhe a
villi	VIL li (VIL eye)

COMMUNICATION EXERCISES

1. Read and practice the following dialogue.

Nurse: "Good morning, Mr. H. How are you feeling today?"

Mr. H.: "Oh, not so good."

Nurse: "Why? What's the matter?"

Mr. H.: "I'm having my surgery today."

Nurse: "That does make you nervous, I know. Is there anything in particular you are worried about?"

Mr. H.: "I suppose they think I will pull through the surgery or they wouldn't do it."

Nurse: "Of course they do. Did the doctor talk to you about the risks?"

Mr. H.: "Yeah, and I guess that is OK. I'll pull through. It is just that they are going to put in an os-something."

Nurse: "An ostomy. They will make a small hole in your abdominal wall that connects to your intestine."

Mr. H.: "And then they will put on that bag thing. I won't even be able to go to the bathroom and I'll have a bulge under my clothes."

Nurse: "It can be adjusted so it hardly shows. We'll show you how."

Mr. H.: "But it's full of crap and I'll smell and nobody will want to be around me—especially my girlfriend!"

Nurse: "Why don't I schedule you for a visit with someone from the Ostomy Association. They can help you with your questions and your feelings. It helps to talk to someone who has been through it."

Mr. H.: "OK. I think I am going to need all the help I can get!"

2. A. Here is a dialogue concerning assessment of bowel function.

Ms. D., age 56, has begun having considerable abdominal bloating and some hard, dry stools. She has come to see the doctor because of this problem.

Nurse: "Ms. D., I need to ask you some questions about your bowel function."

Ms. D.: "O.K."

Nurse: "When did you first notice this abdominal bloating?"

Ms. D.: "It started about eight months ago, but has become progressively worse."

Nurse: "Have you noticed any particular relationship between the bloating and what you eat?"

Ms. D.: "I would say there is, but I can't pin down what foods seem to make it worse. I suspect wheat, tomato, sugar, wine, and who knows what else. Spicy food affects me too."

Nurse: "So, you have more bloating when you eat any of these foods?"

Ms. D.: "It seems that way, but then now I seem to bloat up if I eat anything."

Nurse: "Tell me about your usual diet and fluid intake. Do you eat enough fiber?"

Ms. D.: "I have cereal and fruit juice for breakfast during the week. For lunch I eat yogurt, an apple, and some crackers. I have a couple of low-fat, fruit-filled cookies for dessert. For dinner we eat salad every night as well as some fresh fruit as an appetizer. I fix a casserole with pasta or we have chicken or stir fry. We eat a piece of meat on the weekends. Once in a while we will have a grilled pork chop during the week. We havc bread with dinner. Our portions are very moderate. I have a piece of hard candy for dessert later in the evening and light ice cream or frozen yogurt once or twice a week. I drink decaf for breakfast and mid-morning, lots of water during the day, and a diet coke mid-afternoon. We eat some peanuts or pretzels at cocktail time and I drink tonic with lime—once in a while with a capful of gin in it. I have wine with dinner about three times a week. No more than one or two glasses though."

Nurse: "It seems like you are eating pretty well. You could use more vegetables though."

Ms. D.: "Oh, I use raw vegetables in the salad every night. My husband doesn't like cooked vegetables other than potatoes very much. We do eat potato several times a week and I eat the skin."

Nurse: "That sounds pretty good. What about your bowel movements?"

Ms. D.: "I have small, harder stools, sometimes three or four a day, sometimes every other day. The pattern isn't consistent."

Nurse: "Do you ever have alternating constipation and diarrhea?"

Ms. D.: "Not really. I'll have a loose stool sometimes if I eat really spicy food or drink a lot of wine."

Nurse: "What about pencil-thin stool?"

Ms. D.: "Occasionally after a severe episode of bloating, I will have soft, pencil-like stool. It quickly returns to normal."

Nurse: "Have you ever noticed blood in your stool?"

Ms. D.: "No, I have only ever had blood if I had a hemorrhoid flare-up. I developed one hemorrhoid during the last week of pregnancy."

Nurse: "What about abdominal cramping?"

Ms. D.: "I do have intermittent cramping, especially in the middle of the night. It is diffuse but seems to start somewhere around my belly button."

Nurse: "About how often does this happen?"

Ms. D.: "It varies; it may occur several nights in one week and then not again for two or three weeks."

Nurse: "O.K., Ms. D. The doctor will examine you and then will probably order some tests. We can probably find some medication that can help you with this problem."

2. B. Using the example above, write a dialogue evaluating an elderly patient who lives alone and has been experiencing constipation. Make dietary recommendations.

3. Write out a dialogue for contacting the enterostomal therapist as suggested for a clinical activity. Explain who you are, why you want to go on patient visits, and make arrangements for the time and place to meet. Practice the dialogue, then make the contact. (If possible, have a peer whose first language is English critique your dialogue and help you practice the pronunciation.)

Review the chapter highlights, answer the study questions, and complete the critical thinking activities at the end of the chapter in the textbook.

THIRTY

Pain, Comfort, and Sleep

2/17/04

TERMINOLOGY

A. MATCHING

Directions: Match the terms in column I with the definitions in column II.

Column I

1. __F__ acupressure
2. __d__ acupuncture
3. __h__ analgesic
4. __L__ bolus
5. __C__ chiropractic
6. __B__ endorphins
7. __i__ insomnia
8. __e__ meridian
9. __K__ narcolepsy
10. __g__ non-steroidal anti-inflammatory drugs (NSAIDs)
11. __A__ pain
12. __J__ sleep apnea

Column II

a. Feeling of distress or suffering
b. Naturally occurring, opiate-like peptides
c. Manipulation of the joints and adjacent tissues of the body
d. Insertion of fine sterile needles into various points on the body
e. Line or passageway of energy that passes through the body
f. Pressure applied to various points on the body
g. Non-opioid pain medications that have no steroidal effect
h. Drug that relieves pain
i. Difficulty in getting to sleep or staying asleep
j. Periods when breathing stops during sleep
k. Uncontrollable falling asleep during usual waking hours
l. Concentrated dose given in a short period

SHORT ANSWER

Directions: Write a brief description of each of the following methods used to relieve pain and promote comfort.

1. Biofeedback technique: measures degree of muscle tension
Ice cold pk / heat pk, Dials, noises
Red – yel – green (calming

2. Distraction technique: purposefully focusing of attention away from undesirable pain

3. Epidural analgesia: anethesia used to

4. Guided imagery: Patient relaxed and was able to discuss comfort areas pain was at minimum

5. Hypnosis: trance-like state using focusing & relaxation giving the pt. suggestion - helpful to return to an alert state of consciousness

6. Meditation technique

7. Patient-controlled analgesia analgesia doses controlled by patient

8. Relaxation technique:

Breathing, Music

9. TENS:

10. The gate control theory is one view of pain transmission and ways to interrupt it. According to this theory, massage and vibration work to relieve pain by ______.

11. Engaging in interesting activity reduces pain perception by focusing one's attention away from pain.

12. Anxiety increases pain perception causing increase of focus of pain anger / depression / anxiety.

13. The three basic categories of medications for pain relief are: oral - PO
    a. nonopiod pain meds   PCA - pt control
    b. narcotics   IM
    c. adjuvant analgesics   topical - patch

14. PCA can be used via IV or subcutaneous.

15. The reason that objective assessment of pain is very difficult is because pain is can't be accurately measured.

16. Sleep and rest affect pain. A person who is rested shows both increased pain tolerance and a greater response to analgesic.

17. Sleep may be interrupted due to:
    a. pain
    b. fear
    c. stress
    d.

18. Lack of sleep can cause irritability and crabby stress.

19. The body receives the most rest during which phase of sleep?
REM sleep

20. Describe the stages of the sleep cycle.
   a. Stage 1: NREM Falls into light sleep - muscles relax
   Few minutes
   b. Stage 2: Falls into deeper sleep - Brain wave - larger activity
   20 minutes
   c. Stage 3: person enters delta sleep - slow wave
   Resp - slow - 30 min - 1 hour Body immobile
   d. Stage 4: deepest stage
   e. REM sleep: Sleep time in which you dream
   25% spent in REM

21. Lifestyle factors that affect sleep are:
   a. stress   lack of exercise
   b. caffeine   nicotine
   c. alcohol   illness
   d. family members   cold / hot
   e. school, employment

22. Environmental factors that affect sleep are:
   a. noise
   b. smells
   c. T.V., computer, telephone, bells, alarms

23. Obstructive sleep apnea can be successfully treated by dental appliance to reposition tongue & jaw.
C-PAP B-PAP machine

24. Snoring may be caused by:
   a. deviated septum   poor muscle tone
   b. obstructed airways

25. Heat for the relief of pain and swelling can be applied by:
   a. warm blanket
   b. warm water compress
   c. tub, whirlpool bath
   d. chemical heat pads
   e. aquathermia pads
   f. massage   icey hot creams

26. Three uses of cold for pain or discomfort are:
   a. Reduce swelling
   b. Calm muscle spasms
   c. Reduce pain in joints & muscles

27. Precautions when using ice packs are:
   a. not direct contact w/ skin (No-Red) - skin damage
   b. not left for more than 15 minutes

APPLICATION OF THE NURSING PROCESS

Directions: Write a brief answer for each question.

1. Your patient, L.F., age 36, was seriously injured in a motorcycle accident. He has multiple

fractures and is intubated and on a ventilator. How would you assess his need for pain medication? ↓ VeRBAl com. - PictuRe - pain scale

Body movements

Vents - SeT Rate = TOTAL Skin - sweats Diure

AleRT =

Non - AleRt - Restless, Facial expressions, tension - eyes/face

[margin: V/S ↑ Temp ↑ B/P ↑ Heart Rate Resp. same on vent]

2. Besides the obvious nursing diagnosis of "Pain," what other nursing diagnoses might be appropriate based on the above information? Risk FOR Fluid volume deficit NPO

Self care deficit

ImpAiRED Skin Integrity

ImpAiRED Social Interaction

3. Write one expected outcome for each of the above nursing diagnoses.

Skin - maintain Fluid volume - IV, CATH

Skin - " " Skin integrity

Self-care def. - encourage Independ.

Social - Family, communication - Speech M.H. - Depression

4. List four nursing actions that might be helpful in decreasing L.F.'s pain, based on the above information.

a. *PAin MEDS*

b. *Repositioning*

c. *MAssage*

d. *Communicate - their needs*

5. List one evaluation statement for each action above that indicates progress toward the expected outcomes.

a. *↓ Pain level*

b. *↓ Pain meds*

c. *Reposition - Skin Integrity*

d. *Comfort - Alt. ways Hot / Cold*

MULTIPLE CHOICE

*Directions: Choose the **best** answer for each of the following questions.*

1. M.G. has fallen and injured her elbow. It is not fractured, but there is considerable swelling and pain. She asks which over-the-counter analgesic would be best to take for the discomfort. You tell her that one with NSAID properties would be best. Which of the following would it be best to take?

 [margin: reduce swelling]

 1. acetaminophen
 2. aspirin
 3. ibuprofen ⟵ (circled)
 4. oxymorphone

2. M.G. asks what else she can do for the pain. You suggest the use of cold on the elbow because it will

 1. directly reduce swelling which will reduce pain. ⟵ (circled)
 2. distract from the pain.
 3. relax the muscles, reducing pain.
 4. focus attention to the area, stimulating healing.

3. In instructing M.G. how to apply ice packs, you would tell her that it is best to

 1. apply the ice directly to the skin.
 2. use the ice pack for 15 minutes several times a day. ⟵ (circled)
 3. alternate the ice pack with a heat pack.
 4. apply the ice pack for an hour at a time.

4. You would tell M.G. to use ____________________ as her ice for the elbow as it will conform to the area.
   1. ice cubes in a closed plastic bag
   2. ice water compresses
   3. frozen peas in a closed plastic bag
   4. ice water in a basin

5. M.G. tells you she is supposed to finish a work project this afternoon, but she probably cannot now. You tell her to go ahead and work because
   1. her elbow will heal anyway.
   2. the elbow is already swollen.
   3. using the arm will decrease the swelling.
   4. the distraction of work will decrease the pain.

6. G.H. comes to the clinic complaining of insomnia. In assessing the problem, you would ask her about
   1. her usual diet.
   2. what medications she takes in the morning.
   3. how she uses her leisure time.
   4. stresses and problems in her life.

7. G.H. lives right off the freeway in an apartment complex where many young people live. You wonder if her problem might be due to
   1. socializing.
   2. too much noise.
   3. loneliness.
   4. too little exercise.

8. One thing you would ask G.H. to do to try to locate the reason for her insomnia is to
   1. discuss the problem with her friends.
   2. review times in her life when she had no insomnia.
   3. keep a diary related to sleep and problems encountered.
   4. take a warm bath each time she cannot go back to sleep.

9. You would advise G.H. to
   1. get up at the same time each day and avoid naps.
   2. to eat a large snack before going to bed.
   3. to refrain from eating for six hours before bedtime.
   4. to totally eliminate alcohol and nicotine.

10. You suggest that G.H. snack on a dairy product at bedtime to promote sleep through
    1. warmth it produces in the body.
    2. filling the stomach and preventing hunger.
    3. analgesic effect of the protein in it.
    4. its L-tryptophan content.

CRITICAL THINKING ACTIVITIES

1. Write an imaging scenario to induce relaxation and reduce pain for a patient.
2. Look up the medications listed in Table 30-4 and list the potential side effects of each medication.
3. Write out and record a relaxation exercise that you can use for your own relaxation.

MEETING CLINICAL OBJECTIVES

Directions: The following suggested activities will help you meet the stated clinical practice objectives for the chapter. Review your school's clinical objectives for the week and outline a plan of activities that will help you meet them. If unsure as to how to meet them, consult with your instructor at the beginning of the clinical day.

1. Observe a nurse setting up a PCA pump and go with him or her to instruct the patient in its use.

2. Practice the use of alternative pain control techniques for a family member or friend for relief from a bad headache, muscle spasm, or other pain.
3. Use your own guided imagery "script" with patients to reduce pain.
4. Perform a sleep assessment on a patient. Assist the patient with methods that can be used to enhance sleep within the hospital environment.

STEPS TOWARD BETTER COMMUNICATION

VOCABULARY BUILDING GLOSSARY

Term	Pronunciation	Definition
A. Individual Terms		
adjuvant	ad ju vant	auxiliary; assisting
complementary	com ple MEN ta ry	a useful addition that makes something complete
divert	di VERT	move from one place to another
distraction	dis TRAC tion	focusing attention away from one thing to another
enhanced	en HANCed	made better
grimacing	GRIM a cing	twisting the facial muscles
induce	in DUCE	to gently cause; to make happen by gentle persuasion
jet lag	jet lag	a tired feeling caused by long distance travel into different time zones
pantomime	PAN to mime	to use hand, body, and facial movement without words to help someone understand what you are trying to say
perception	per CEP tion	the way a person sees or feels something
phantom	phan tom	a ghost; something unseen that comes and goes
stoic	STO ic	not showing feelings, especially pain
stressors	STRESS ors	things that cause stress
transient	TRAN si ent	temporary
verify	ver i fy	to prove something is true; to confirm
B. Phrases		
a fair degree	a FAIR de GREE	quite a bit; a lot
during the course of the night	dur ing the course of the night	over the whole time of the night
over-the-counter medications	O ver the COUN ter med i CA tions	medication available without a prescription
on occasion	on oc CAS ion	sometimes

VOCABULARY EXERCISE

Directions: Exercise I—Use Table 30-1, "Descriptive Terms for Pain," in the textbook in the following exercises. Work in pairs or small groups with a native English speaker and an English learner.

1. To express degree of pain, draw a line which goes from no pain to the worst degree of pain, and write the descriptive words on it in the order of the degree of the pain. Now pantomime (using gestures without speaking) that degree of pain for each word so that someone who does not understand English would know what you mean, and could indicate his or her own degree of pain.
2. Pantomime the meanings for the terms for quality of pain. Make sure the English learner understands the meaning of the word correctly, and that the partner can correctly identify the term being pantomimed.

COMMUNICATION EXERCISES

1. After practicing describing pain in the vocabulary Exercise above, take turns with a partner describing a pain nonverbally, and documenting it for the chart.
2. With a partner, role play questioning a patient about pain and writing the results on the chart. This time, ask and answer orally. Charting:

 ____

 ____

 ____

 ____

PRONUNCIATION OF DIFFICULT TERMS

Directions: Practice pronouncing the following words with a partner.

acupressure	AC u pres sure
acupuncture	AC u punc ture
analgesic	an al GE sic
anti-inflammatory	an ti- in FLAM a tor y
biofeedback	bi o FEED back
endorphins	en DOR phins
epidural	ep i DUR al
meridian	me RID i an
myocardial infarction	my o CARD i al in FARC tion
narcolepsy	NAR co lep sy

CULTURAL POINTS

What is the attitude toward pain in your native culture? Is it OK for some people to show pain (like women and children) but not others (like men and old people)? How are children treated when they cry? What are they told? How do you think this affects them when they are grown up? How could such cultural views affect their medical treatment? Talk about this with one of your peers.

Review the chapter highlights, answer the study questions, and complete the critical thinking activities at the end of the chapter in the textbook.

shift work	SHIFT work	when work is continuous over 24 hours and some people work in the day, some in the evening and some at night; each of these periods is a shift
to suffer from	to SUF fer from	to be ill with something or have a problem over a long period

COMPLETION

A. Directions: Fill in the blank(s) with the correct term(s) from the Vocabulary Building Glossary to complete the sentence.

1. An antidepressant is sometimes added along with analgesic medication as an ____________________ medication.
2. The person with serious ____________________ occurring in his or her life will often experience more pain from an injury.
3. Playing card games is one form of ____________________ used to reduce the sensation of pain.
4. When working with a person whose language you do not speak, you may need to use ____________________ to help them understand what you are trying to say.
5. Computer games can help ____________________ a patient's attention away from pain.
6. The effects of pain medication may be ____________________ by giving a soothing back massage.
7. Each patient's ____________________ of pain is different.
8. Men, in general, are more ____________________ regarding pain and do not show their feelings.
9. Chiropractic adjustment may be a ____________________ treatment to physical therapy for back pain.
10. The patient who has had an amputation may experience ____________________ pain seeming to be in the missing part.

B. Directions: Make sentences using the phrases above in the Vocabulary Building Glossary. Try to use at least two of the phrases in each sentence. Example:

<u>On occasion</u> I <u>suffer from</u> headaches.

1. ____
2. ____
3. ____
4. ____
5. ____
6. ____

THIRTY-ONE

Pharmacology and Preparation for Drug Administration

TERMINOLOGY

A. MATCHING

Directions: Match the terms in column I with the definitions in column II.

	Column I			Column II
1.	F anaphylaxis		a.	Drug name not protected by trademark
2.	I contraindications		b.	How drugs enter the body, are metabolized, reach the site of action, and are excreted
3.	C degrade		c.	Break down
4.	A generic		d.	Drug's effect on cellular physiology, biology, and its mechanism of action
5.	g noncompliance		e.	Results of drug action not related to intended action
6.	______ pharmacodynamics		f.	Severe allergic reaction
7.	______ pharmacokinetics		g.	Not taking drugs as prescribed
8.	e side effects		h.	Name protected by trademark
9.	h trade name		i.	Reasons not to administer
10.	J unit dose		j.	Single dose

B. COMPLETION

Directions: Fill in the blank(s) with the correct term(s) from the terms list in the chapter in the textbook to complete the sentence.

1. A drug such as an antibiotic is called an ____________________ because it produces a response.
2. A drug such as an antihistamine is called an ____________________ because it blocks a response.
3. A ____ occurs when one drug interferes with the way the other drug acts when taken alone.
4. Every drug administered in the agency is entered on the ____ after it is given.

5. Knowing the side effects of a drug and how it works helps nurses figure out the ______________________________ of the drug.

6. Alcohol causes a ______________________________ when consumed while taking a drug that depresses the central nervous system.

7. Some drugs have a very narrow ______________________________ and if a patient takes an extra pill, toxicity may develop.

8. Impaired hearing is a ______________________________ of several drugs, including furosemide, a diuretic.

SHORT ANSWER

Directions: Write a brief answer for each question.

1. Drugs are generally classified by:
   a. ______________________________
   b. ______________________________
   c. ______________________________

2. General action of drugs in the body is to ______________________________ ______________________________.

3. Patients are often noncompliant in taking their drugs because ______________________________ ______________________________ ______________________________.

4. Factors that affect how a drug works in a child's body are ______________________________.

5. List five things that should be considered when giving medications to an elderly patient:
   a. ______________________________
   b. ______________________________
   c. ______________________________
   d. ______________________________
   e. ______________________________

6. When medications are prescribed for the home care patient, the nurse should ______________________________ ______________________________ ______________________________

7. In the hospital the responsibility for the security of controlled drugs is ______________________________.

8. For a drug to receive approval of the FDA it must meet standards in these five areas: ______________________________ ______________________________

9. The five rights of drug administration are:
   a. ______________________________

b. ____________________

c. ____________________

d. ____________________

e. ____________________

10. Information the patient should be taught about each drug includes:
    a. ____________________
    b. ____________________
    c. ____________________
    d. ____________________
    e. ____________________
    f. ____________________

IDENTIFICATION

Directions: Identify the meaning of each of the following abbreviations and symbols. Write the correct letter in the blank provided for each one.

1. ______ ac
2. ______ DC
3. ______ gtt
4. ______ hs
5. ______ ID
6. ______ OS
7. ______ pc
8. ______ qod
9. ______ qs
10. ______ $\overline{s}$
11. ______ STAT
12. ______ tid

a. Every other day
b. Intradermal
c. Before meals
d. After meals
e. Left eye
f. Discontinue
g. Without
h. Drop
i. At bedtime
j. Immediately
k. Three times a day
l. Quantity sufficient

DRUG KNOWLEDGE

Directions: Using a drug handbook or a pharmacology textbook, look up the drug furosemide and fill in the information requested.

1. Classification: ____________________
2. Usual P.O. adult dosage: ____________________
3. Routes of administration: ____________________
4. One contraindication: ____________________
5. When it should be taken: ____________________

DRUG CALCULATIONS AND CONVERSIONS

Directions: Correctly convert or calculate the answer for each question.

1. 8 g = __________ gr
2. 180 gr = __________ g
3. 5 gr = __________ mg
4. 4.5 gr = __________ g
5. 180 mg = __________ gr
6. You are to give 10 cc of Robitussin. How many teaspoons would this be? __________
7. The patient weighs 54 lbs. You are to administer 70 mg Of drug per kg Of body weight. How many capsules will you give if each capsule contains 425 mg? __________
8. The order reads: 15 mEq KCl. You have available 30 mL of KCl with 2 mEq/mL. How many mL will you put in the patient's orange juice? __________
9. Vitamin E 400 U is ordered. You have on hand capsules with 200 U each. How many will you give? __________
10. You are to give 10 mg of morphine IM. The vial reads 15 mg/1 mL. How much will you give? __________

APPLICATION OF THE NURSING PROCESS

Directions: Write a brief answer for each question.

1. C.T. is admitted to your home care agency after her stay in the rehabilitation institute is finished. She has suffered a stroke and has hemiparesis. She has a history of heart disease with atrial fibrillation (arrhythmia) and congestive heart failure. She also has osteoarthritis of the knees and hands. What questions would you ask to establish a medication history and find out what medications she is currently taking?

2. What other information would you need in order to manage C.T.'s medication regimen?

3. The physicians believe that C.T. suffered the stroke because she was not taking her medications regularly. What would be the appropriate nursing diagnosis for C.T. regarding her use of medications?

4. Write an expected outcome for this nursing diagnosis.

____

5. What interventions might you use to assist C.T. in meeting the expected outcome?

____

____

____

____

____

6. How would you evaluate whether the expected outcome is being met? Write evaluation statements that would indicate the outcome is being met:

____

____

____

____

MEETING CLINICAL OBJECTIVES

Directions: The following suggested activities will help you meet the stated clinical practice objectives for the chapter. Review your school's clinical objectives for the week and outline a plan of activities that will help you meet them. If unsure as to how to meet them, consult with your instructor at the beginning of the clinical day.

1. Look up three drugs that your assigned patient is taking; pay particular attention to the nursing implications for each drug.
2. Accompany a nurse who is using the unit dose system to administer drugs.
3. Have a staff nurse show you how to correctly obtain and record a controlled substance drug.
4. Teach a patient about a new drug that has been prescribed.

MULTIPLE CHOICE

Directions: Choose the ***best*** *answer for each of the following questions.*

1. Which one of the following orders means to give the medication three times a day after meals?
    1. Ferrous sulfate 10 mg. P.O. bid ac.
    2. Ferrous sulfate 10 mg. P.O. qid pc.
    3. Ferrous sulfate 10 mg. P.O. tid pc.
    4. Ferrous sulfate 10 mg. P.O. tid ac.
2. Which one of the following forms of a drug will be absorbed the quickest?
    1. capsule
    2. tablet
    3. suspension
    4. ointment
3. A drug is only totally safe for a pregnant woman to take if it does not
    1. enter the mother's bloodstream.
    2. cross the placental barrier.
    3. enter the fetal brain.
    4. have any adverse effect on the mother.
4. Most drugs are mainly metabolized by the
    1. liver.
    2. kidneys.
    3. brain.
    4. bowel.

5. Sufficient fluid intake to eliminate drugs properly is at least
   1. 1000 mL/day.
   2. 1500 mL/day.
   3. 30 mL/kg/day.
   4. 50 mL/kg/day.
6. The "duration of action" of a drug is the time the drug
   1. takes to be metabolized.
   2. exerts a pharmacological effect.
   3. takes to be excreted.
   4. is O.K. to take before it is no longer effective.
7. Toxic effects of a drug are reached when
   1. the blood level reaches the therapeutic range.
   2. adverse effects occur.
   3. side effects appear.
   4. the blood level rises above the therapeutic range.
8. Although the physician orders the drug, before administering the drug the nurse is responsible for determining
   1. whether the patient will experience side effects.
   2. whether the patient takes the drug.
   3. the reason the drug is prescribed.
   4. whether the dose is within safe limits.
9. Elderly patients who have arthritis and are taking anti-inflammatory drugs must be monitored for
   1. gastrointestinal bleeding.
   2. orthostatic hypotension.
   3. rapid, irregular pulse.
   4. dehydration.
10. Unit dose drugs should be opened for administration
    1. at the bedside.
    2. after the second check of the medication.
    3. in the medication room.
    4. at the medication cart at the patient's door.

CRITICAL THINKING ACTIVITIES

1. Prepare to teach a patient about taking the drug digoxin. Outline points to cover:
2. Explain to a family member why it is illegal to share prescription tranquilizers with another family member. Outline the points you would make:
3. List the points of assessment that should be completed before a drug is administered to a patient:

STEPS TOWARD BETTER COMMUNICATION

VOCABULARY BUILDING GLOSSARY

Term	Pronunciation	Definition
categorize	CAT e gor ize	to put into categories, or similar groups
compliant	com PLI ant	willing to do as instructed
decree	de CREE	to make a rule
erroneously	er RON e ous ly	incorrectly, in error
incompatible	in com PAT i ble	do not work well together
readily	READ i ly	quickly and easily
susceptible	sus CEP ti ble	easily affected

tactful	TACT ful	polite, careful, indirect
to be knowledgeable about	to be KNOW ledge able (NAW lej a ble) a BOUT	to know about

COMPLETION

Directions: Fill in the blank(s) with the correct term(s) from the Vocabulary Building Glossary to complete the sentence.

1. Some drugs are ____________________, especially in the intravenous form, and may not be given together.
2. If a patient is not ____________________ with the medication schedule at home, you must be ____________________ when working with her on correcting the problem.
3. A liquid form of a drug is more ____________________ absorbed by the body.
4. If you do not perform the five rights and check the drug three times before administering it, you may give it ____________________.
5. If you can ____________________ an unfamiliar drug and know the action of that drug category, you will know most of the possible side effects of the unfamiliar drug.

WORD ATTACK SKILLS

Directions: Word Families—Look at the meanings of different forms of the words within a word family.

de VISE (dee vïze) (verb)	To think of or figure out a new method or system for doing something.
de VICE (dee vïs) (noun)	Something such as a piece of equipment designed for a special purpose.
com PLY (verb)	To do as instructed.
com PLI ance (noun)	Doing as instructed.
com PLI ant (adjective)	One who is doing as instructed.
NON com PLI ance (noun)	Not doing what is instructed, not following rules.

Kinetics means movement; therefore, **pharmacokinetics** means movement of drugs through the body.

Dynamics means actions and interactions; therefore, **pharmacodynamics** means the action and interaction of the drug in the body.

PRONUNCIATION OF DIFFICULT TERMS

Directions: Practice pronouncing the following words.

agonist	AG on ist
anaphylaxis	AN a phy LAX is (AN a pha LAX is)
antagonist	an TAG on ist
contraindications	CON tra in di CA tions
efficacy	ef FI ca cy

gastrointestinal	gas tro in TES tin al
noncompliance	NON com PLI ance
pharmacodynamics	PHAR ma co dy NAM ics
pharmacokinetics	PHAR ma co ki NET ics
synergistic	SYN er GIS tic

GRAMMAR POINTS

Various verb tenses: did you take/have you taken/are you taking

When you are communicating with a patient, it is often very important to know **when** something happens—when the pain or symptom occurs or when the medication was taken. To do this, both you and the patient must understand the time that you are talking about. If you are not sure, clarify by using time words such as yesterday, now, this morning, last night, three o'clock, etc.

Verb Tense or Time	Question	Answer
Simple Present (action is ongoing)	Do you take any medicine? Do you feel any pain?	I take ibuprofen every morning. My knee feels achy.
Present Progressive (action is happening now)	What over-the-counter medicines are you taking?	I am taking ibuprofen for my arthritis.
Simple Past (action completed)	What medicine did you take today?	I took my ibuprofen this morning.
Present Perfect (action has happened before this present time)	Have you taken your medicine this morning? Have you had any pain today?	Yes, I've already taken it. or Yes, I took it before breakfast. (Answer may be in the past) No, I haven't had any pain since yesterday.
Present Perfect Progressive (happening from the past up to this present time) Used for telling "how long a time."	How long have you been using ibuprofen? How long has your knee been hurting?	I've been using it for a couple of years now. It has been hurting for about a month.

COMMUNICATION EXERCISES

1. With a partner, prepare to assess an older adult's medication history. Use Question #1 in "Application of the Nursing Process" in this chapter to create a scenario dialogue about assessing what drugs and over-the-counter medicines this older, sometimes forgetful, person is taking. Practice the dialogue together.
2. Develop a script to assess what your patient knows about the drugs he or she is taking (why, when, how many, etc.) and any side effects he or she may be experiencing. Practice with a partner. Use three different common drugs for this exercise.
3. Develop a script that teaches the patient about furosemide.

CULTURAL POINTS

Think about your native culture's attitude toward drugs and medications and try to analyze it. Are the people afraid of medications, or do they expect the doctor to give them something every time they visit? Do they prefer herbal medicine, prescription pills, or injections? How does that compare with what you learned in this chapter?

In the U.S., there is a great reliance on prescription drugs, and belief—sometimes to an adverse degree—that they can cure anything. However, more people are turning to herbal remedies found in health food stores and pharmacies. Popular magazines and newspapers often have articles on the use of herbal medicine, as well as news about drugs being developed. One reason for this increased interest may be the very high cost of drugs in the U.S. as well as movement toward more natural and holistic methods. It should be remembered that herbal remedies may become toxic in high doses or interact with each other and with prescription medications. A drug history must include all types of herbs and medications the patient is taking.

Review the chapter highlights, answer the study questions, and complete the critical thinking activities at the end of the chapter in the textbook.

THIRTY-TWO

Administering Oral, Topical, and Inhalant Medications

TERMINOLOGY

A. MATCHING

Directions: Match the terms in column I with the definitions in column II.

Column I		Column II
1. ______	buccal	a. The base of the curvature of liquid medication in a container
2. ______	cerumen	b. Under the tongue
3. ______	douche	c. Through the skin
4. ______	fornices	d. Eye
5. ______	meniscus	e. Inner cheek
6. ______	ophthalmic	f. Ear
7. ______	otic	g. Vaginal irrigation
8. ______	sublingual	h. Archlike structures
9. ______	topical	i. Applied to the skin or mucous membrane
10. ______	transdermal	j. Ear wax

B. ABBREVIATIONS

Directions: Fill in the correct abbreviation or symbol for the indicated word in the following paragraph.

V.S. is being treated for asthma. Her medications are not adequately controlling her symptoms. The doctor orders a nebulizer treatment for her immediately (_________) to relieve her bronchospasm. He tells her to discontinue (_________) the antihistamine she has been taking as it does not seem to be helping. He prescribes oral (_________) montelukast sodium (Singulair) to be taken with water in the evening. He puts her on another metered dose inhaler (_________), triamcinolone acetonide (Azmacort), and tells her to use the new inhaler TID.

SHORT ANSWER

Directions: Write a brief answer for each question.

1. When administering medications, nurses are legally responsible for knowing:
   a. ______
   b. ______
   c. ______
   d. ______
   e. ______
   f. ______

2. When considering a written drug order's legality, you would check to see that it includes:
   a. ______
   b. ______
   c. ______
   d. ______
   e. ______
   f. ______
   g. ______

3. List the correct drug classification for each of the following drug actions:
   a. ______ inhibit clotting of blood
   b. ______ reduce congestion and allergic reactions
   c. ______ relieve anxiety and promote sleep
   d. ______ relieve cough
   e. ______ inhibit the growth of or kill microorganisms
   f. ______ relieve depression
   g. ______ increase mental alertness and function
   h. ______ reduce inflammation and pain

4. The reason the unit-dose medication administration system is considered safer than the prescription system of delivery is that ______ .

5. Medications that should not be crushed for administration via an enteral feeding tube are:
   a. ______
   b. ______
   c. ______

6. Three special considerations for administering oral and topical medications to an elderly patient are:
   a. ______
   b. ______
   c. ______

7. Describe the legal and professional responsibilities of the LPN/LVN related to medication administration. ______
   ______
   ______
   ______

8. One method that seems to help an elderly person who has difficulty swallowing to take a pill is to instruct the person to ______
   ______
   ______ .

COMPLETION

Directions: Fill in the blank(s) with the correct word(s) to complete the sentence.

1. Any medication order that is unclear, incomplete, or ambiguous must be ____________________.
2. The primary system of measuring medication dosage in the United States is the ____________________ system.
3. It is good practice to check any conversions and calculations for a divided dose with ____________________.
4. Topical medications are those applied to the ____________________ or ____________________.
5. When stat medication orders are written, the medication must be administered ____________________.
6. Medication orders are automatically canceled whenever a patient undergoes ____________________ or ____________________.
7. Medication orders written by the physician are transcribed onto the ____________________ which is used for the actual administration of each medication.
8. Medication cards are usually used only with a fixed system of medication administration such as when medications are dispensed from a ____________________ or ____________________.
9. Automated controlled dispensing systems are used to monitor and control ____________________.
10. Ointments are used to keep the medication in ____________________ contact with the skin.
11. The difference between a lotion and a liniment is that while a liniment is rubbed into the skin a lotion is ____________________ the skin.
12. The most common type of medicinal irrigation is the ____________________ irrigation.
13. Suppositories are a semisolid, cylinder-shaped medication inserted into the ____________________, ____________________ or ____________________, or ostomy ____________________ on the abdomen.
14. When pouring a liquid medication, always read the amount poured at the ____________________ of the fluid.
15. If a sublingual medication is swallowed rather than dissolved under the tongue, the medication becomes totally ____________________.

APPLICATION OF THE NURSING PROCESS

Directions: Write a brief answer for each question.

1. When administering medications, three assessments you should make in addition to following the five rights of medication administration are:
   a. ____
   b. ____
   c. ____
2. The patient who is suffering from extended nausea and vomiting would probably be given the nursing diagnosis ____.

3. The five goals of medication administration are:
   a. ______________________________
   b. ______________________________
   c. ______________________________
   d. ______________________________
   e. ______________________________

4. When implementing medication administration, it is best to follow the five rights of medication administration and to check each medication label ______________________________.

5. An evaluation statement indicating that antibiotic therapy for a wound infection has been effective might be ______________________________
____
______________________________.

MULTIPLE CHOICE

*Directions: Choose the **best** answer to each of the following questions.*

1. You are assigned to give medications to five patients during your shift. Each patient has more than one medication ordered. When checking each medication while using the unit dose system, you would
   1. verify the medication name and dosage and set the dose pack to one side.
   2. verify the date, time, medication name, dosage, and route.
   3. compare the medication administration sheet with the physician's order sheet before pulling out the medications.
   4. verify the medication name and dosage, open the package and place the pill in a medication cup.

2. When performing the necessary medication checks for your patients using the unit dose system, the third check is performed
   1. before returning the patient's medication bin or drawer to its place.
   2. just before going to the patient's bedside.
   3. after identifying the patient and before opening the package.
   4. before throwing away the package the pill came in.

3. Each time you administer medications to one of your patients, in addition to properly identifying the patient by comparing the name and number of the I.D. band to the imprint on the MAR, you would check the MAR sheet for
   1. known allergies.
   2. PRN medications.
   3. patient sex.
   4. next dose time.

4. One of your patients requests a PRN pain medication. When administering a PRN medication it is especially important to check
   1. drug interactions.
   2. date of the order.
   3. number of doses given.
   4. time last dose was given.

5. One of your patients needs a rectal suppository. You know to
   1. warm the suppository before insertion.
   2. chill the suppository before insertion.
   3. unwrap the suppository before insertion.
   4. place the patient in prone position for insertion.

6. One patient has been receiving an antibiotic for several days. You would evaluate its effectiveness by
   1. checking to see if at least 10 doses have been given.
   2. assessing for signs that the infection is subsiding.
   3. checking for the various side effects of the drug.
   4. checking the culture and sensitivity report for the drug's ability to kill the organism.

7. One patient requires instillation of eye drops. Two safety factors you check when administering eye medications are
   1. the medication does not blur the patient's vision or sting.
   2. the drops fall directly on the eye and do not run out.
   3. "ophthalmic" appears on the bottle and the medication is still in date.
   4. the eye is not red and does not have a discharge.

8. An order that reads "1 tablet subling prn chest pain" means
   1. administer one tablet orally.
   2. give one table sublingually each night.
   3. have patient place the tablet under the tongue when chest pain occurs.
   4. place one tablet on the tongue as needed for chest pain.

9. An order that is written, "Erythromycin 300 mg PO TID" means give erythromycin
   1. 300 mg orally three times a day.
   2. 300 mg orally twice a day.
   3. 300 mg at night for three days.
   4. 1 tablet orally three times a day.

10. An order that is written, "Mylanta 15 mL PO pc and HS" means give Mylanta
    1. 1 ounce before meals and at bedtime.
    2. 15 mL before meals and at bedtime.
    3. 2 ounces by mouth after meals and at bedtime.
    4. 15 mL by mouth after meals and at bedtime.

CRITICAL THINKING ACTIVITIES

1. What would you do if you poured up a dose of cough medicine and your patient then tells you she does not need it anymore and refuses to take it?
2. What would you do if your patient tells you that the pill you have for him to take does not look familiar and he wants to know why he is supposed to take it?
3. What would you do if the pill the patient is taking falls from the cup onto his covers as he is trying to put it in his mouth?

MEETING CLINICAL OBJECTIVES

Directions: The following suggested activities will help you meet the stated clinical practice objectives for the chapter. Review your school's clinical objectives for the week and outline a plan of activities that will help you meet them. If unsure as to how to meet them, consult with your instructor at the beginning of the clinical day.

1. Practice giving oral and topical medications using the five rights.
2. Actively seek experience in applying eye medications, transdermal patches, and topical ointments. Tell other nurses on your unit that you would like this experience.
3. Actively seek opportunity to administer a vaginal and rectal suppository or medication.
4. With a staff nurse or your instructor supervising, check out a scheduled (controlled drug) medication.

STEPS TOWARD BETTER COMMUNICATION

VOCABULARY BUILDING GLOSSARY

Term	Pronunciation	Definition
ambiguous	am BIG u ous	not clear, uncertain
deviation	DE vi A tion	a change, or doing something different than planned
potent	PO tent	powerful, strong

COMPLETION

Directions: Fill in the blanks with the correct terms from the Vocabulary Building Glossary above to complete the sentence.

This is a very ____________ drug. The directions for using it are ________________________, so we had better check with the doctor. I do not want to make any ____________ from his plans.

WORD ATTACK SKILLS

In English, there are many small words that have important functions in communication and meaning, but are not pronounced clearly or distinctly in conversation. They are often shortened and run together with other words. The non-native English speaker may not even hear the sound and may miss some important meaning. The native English speaker usually understands the meaning, but sometimes must ask for clarification.

Contractions of the negative and the verb "to be" are very common in informal speech and written communication. Common examples are:

I am = I'm, he is = he's, you are = you're, we are = we're

Common examples of negative contractions are:

cannot = can't, will not = won't, is not = isn't, did not = didn't

When native English speakers are not sure what they hear, they will say, "Did you say you can or cannot go?"

There are other contractions in sound that occur only with pronunciation and are not written. Because they are spoken so quickly and softly by the native speaker, the English learner often does not even hear them, but they are important to the meaning.

Following are some examples of short words and pronouns that are often reduced in sound, and the way they may sound in common speech:

and	I will have bread and butter.	I'll have bread 'n' butter.
	You are up bright and early!	You're up bright 'n' early!
or	Are you coming or going?	Are ya coming 'r'going?
	Do you want tea or coffee?	Do ya want tea 'r'coffee?
as	Your hands are as cold as ice!	They're 'z cold uz ice!

to	I need to go to the bathroom. Let's walk to the bed	I need t'go t'the bathroom. Le's walk t'th'bed.
can	Can you stand up? I don't think I can do it.	C'n ya stand up? I don't think I c'n do it.
will	You will feel better tomorrow. This will help you sleep.	You'll feel better t'morrow. This'll help ya sleep.
do	How do you do? Do you want me to raise the rail?	How d'ya do? D'ya want me t'raise the rail?
them	Where do you want them? I can't find them.	Where d'ya want 'em? I can't find 'em.
a, an	Could you help me give him a bath? It has only been an hour.	Could ya help me give'm 'bath? It's only been 'n hour.
have	You were supposed to have taken your medications an hour ago. What have you done with my clothes?	You're supposed to've taken y'r meds 'n hour ago. What've ya done with m'clothes?

When you are speaking with an elderly person, one who has a hearing loss, or a non-native English speaker, you will need to speak carefully, slowly, and distinctly to make sure they understand you. If you are a non-native English speaker, you will also need to listen carefully to know what the person is saying. You may have to ask them to repeat, or clarify by repeating what you think you understood them to say. They can correct you if you were wrong.

COMMUNICATION EXERCISES

1. Practice saying the sentences above with careful pronunciation and then with the contracted pronunciation. Can you hear and feel the difference?
2. Pick a spot where you can listen to people in conversation, like a seat in the cafeteria, near a telephone, or where friends are talking while waiting for class to begin. Listen carefully to what the native English speakers are saying, and see if you can tell what sounds are omitted or substituted. Can you understand what they are saying? Can you supply in your head the words that were reduced? Write five of the reduced words you heard here.

PRONUNCIATION OF DIFFICULT TERMS

Directions: Practice pronouncing the following words.

buccal	BUC cal (BUC cle)
cerumen	ce RU men
fornix, fornices	FOR nix, FOR ni CES (plural)

Review the chapter highlights, answer the study questions, and complete the critical thinking activities at the end of the chapter in the textbook.

THIRTY-THREE

Administering Intradermal, Subcutaneous, and Intramuscular Injections

TERMINOLOGY

A. MATCHING

Directions: Match the terms in column I with the definitions in column II.

Column I		Column II	
1. ______	ampule	a.	Small bottle
2. ______	bevel	b.	Formation of fibrous tissue
3. ______	bleb	c.	Scale of measurement
4. ______	cannula	d.	Visible elevation of the epidermis
5. ______	core	e.	Hollow shaft
6. ______	diluent	f.	Red, elevated wheals
7. ______	fibrosis	g.	Glass container of medication
8. ______	gauge	h.	Opening or interior diameter
9. ______	gluteal	i.	Solid material or particles
10. ______	lumen	j.	Fluid to dissolve solute
11. ______	solute	k.	Pertaining to the buttocks (muscle)
12. ______	urticaria	l.	Sticky or gummy
13. ______	vial	m.	Small circular piece at the center
14. ______	viscous	n.	Slanted part of needle tip

B. COMPLETION

Directions: Fill in the blank(s) with the correct word(s) to complete the sentence.

1. Skin testing for reaction to various substances is performed using an _________________ injection.
2. If a patient is allergic to the medication, an injection may cause _________________.
3. Medications that are given by injection are termed _________________ medications as they do not enter the gastrointestinal tract.
4. Medications such as hydroxyzine pamoate (Vistaril) should be given by the _________________ method of injection because it is very irritating to subcutaneous tissue.

5. Very small amounts of medication such as adrenalin (Epinephrine) are given with a ____________________ syringe.
6. Absorption time for the medication given by ____________________ injection is slower than that given intramuscularly.
7. When mixing two medications together in the same syringe, you must first check drug ____________________.
8. An ____________________ injection is administered at a 90 degree angle.

SHORT ANSWER

Directions: Write a brief answer for each question.

1. Parenteral routes are used for medication administration for the following three reasons.
   a. ____________________
   b. ____________________
   c. ____________________
2. When administering a parenteral injection, the nurse must take the following precautions:
   a. ____________________
   b. ____________________
   c. ____________________
   d. ____________________
3. The preferred sites for subcutaneous injections are ____________________ ____________________.
4. Heparin is given subcutaneously in the ____________________ sites.
5. When giving insulin and heparin, do not ____________________ before injecting the medication.
6. An intramuscular injection can be safely given in the following sites:
   a. ____________________
   b. ____________________
   c. ____________________
   d. ____________________
7. When patients are receiving repeated injections, you should ____________________.
8. To clear the needle of medication and to keep medication from flowing back up into the subcutaneous tissues, ____________________ technique is often used for intramuscular injections.
9. When giving injections to children it is important to provide ____________________ before, during, and after the injection.
10. Z-track method of injection is used for medications that are very ____________________ to the tissue.
11. Symptoms of anaphylactic shock include ____________________ ____________________ ____________________
12. When administering an intramuscular injection, it is essential to ____________________ before injecting to avoid ____________________.

13. When a 5/8" needle is used for a subcutaneous injection, the angle of injection should be ____________________.

14. Up to ____________________ mL of solution can be injected for an intramuscular injection safely.

15. When withdrawing medication from an ampule, a ____________________ needle should be used.

16. Tuberculin syringes are calibrated to measure ____________________ of a mL for giving very small doses.

17. Typical diluents for mixing drugs are ____________________ and ____________________.

18. Because injected medications are irretrievable, it is especially important to check for ____________________ before giving the injection.

19. Regarding absorption, ____________________ solutions are absorbed more rapidly than those in an ____________________ suspension.

20. Safety syringes are used to prevent ____________________ and the possibility of ____________________ illness.

21. Factors to consider when giving an intramuscular injection to an elderly patient are ____.

CORRELATION

Directions: Indicate the type of injection in column II that correlates with the item in column I.

		Column I		Column II
1.	______	1 1/2" 20 ga. needle	a.	Intradermal injection
2.	______	1/4" 27 ga. needle	b.	Subcutaneous
3.	______	TB syringe with 1/4" needle	c.	Intramuscular injection
4.	______	must form a bleb		
5.	______	placed in tissue above the muscle layer		
6.	______	may be placed in the gluteus medius		
7.	______	3 cc of medication		
8.	______	20 U of U 100 insulin		
9.	______	5,000 U of heparin sodium		
10.	______	tuberculin test		

APPLICATION OF THE NURSING PROCESS

Directions: Write a brief answer for each of the following questions.

1. Besides carefully checking the medication with the order before administration, give three patient assessments that should be made.
   a. ____
   b. ____
   c. ____

2. R.O. has vomited several times. The physician orders an antiemetic for him. What might be an appropriate nursing diagnosis for this patient related to this situation?

____

3. Write an expected outcome for the chosen nursing diagnosis.

____

4. Indicate three nursing interventions that could be implemented along with giving the antiemetic medication to ease R.O.'s nausea and prevent vomiting.
   a. ____
   b. ____
   c. ____

5. Write an evaluation statement that would indicate the expected outcome is being attained.

____

MULTIPLE CHOICE

*Directions: Choose the one **best** answer for each of the following questions.*

1. If the order reads "75 mg meperidine, 25 mg Promethazine IM on call," which syringe and needle would be the best choice for the injection if the patient is a normal-sized adult? Each medication is supplied with 50 mg/mL.
   1. 2 mL syringe with 23 gauge 1" needle
   2. 3 mL syringe with 20 gauge 2" needle
   3. 3 mL syringe with 22 gauge 1 1/2" needle
   4. 3 mL syringe with 23 gauge 5/8" needle

2. Heparin sodium 5,000 SC is ordered for the patient. Using a 25 gauge, 5/8" needle this medication should be injected
   1. at a 45 degree angle.
   2. at a 15 degree angle.
   3. at a 90 degree angle.
   4. at a 60 degree angle.

3. The proper technique for administering a Z-track injection is to
   1. insert the needle at a 45 degree slant.
   2. use a 3" needle at a 45 degree slant.
   3. insert the needle at a 90 degree angle and pull the tissue laterally before removing the needle.
   4. pull the tissue at the site laterally, then insert the needle at a 90 degree angle.

4. When drawing up medication from a vial, you would
   1. hold the vial at a 15 degree angle, stopper down.
   2. hold the vial absolutely vertically.
   3. Inject an equivalent amount of air into the vial for the medication to be withdrawn.
   4. with the vial stopper up, inject at least 1 mL of air before withdrawing the medication.

5. A sign that an intradermal injection has been successfully given is when
   1. a pale area 1/2" in diameter occurs at the site.
   2. a small bleb is evident at the injection site.
   3. a reddened wheal occurs at the injection site.
   4. an area of erythema occurs within 4 hours at the site.

6. When drawing medication from a glass ampule, a filter needle should be used because
   1. fragments of glass could be in the medication.
   2. ampules often contain precipitate material.
   3. the medication and the diluent may not be thoroughly mixed.
   4. the filter thoroughly mixes the medication upon injection.

7. If a patient begins to show signs of anaphylactic shock after an injection is given, you would call for help and immediately
   1. administer a corticosteroid injection.
   2. transfer the patient to the critical care unit.
   3. maintain an open airway and respiration.
   4. place the patient in an upright position.

8. When using the leg for an intramuscular injection, the area landmarks include
   1. the head of the greater trochanter.
   2. the posterior iliac spine.
   3. a hand's breadth below the end of the greater trochanter.
   4. a hand's breadth below the groin crease.

9. The advantage of a subcutaneous injection over an intramuscular injection is that
   1. there is less discomfort for the patient.
   2. the medication is injected more quickly.
   3. the medication is absorbed more slowly.
   4. the medication is absorbed more rapidly.

10. Besides changing color or forming a precipitate, incompatible drugs mixed in a syringe may
    1. increase the strength of the medication.
    2. render one or both medications inactive.
    3. cause severe burning when injected.
    4. cause inflammation at the injection site.

CRITICAL THINKING ACTIVITIES

1. If you are asked to give an injection to a patient at a place distant from a sharps biohazard container, what would you do with the syringe and exposed needle?

2. If you have drawn up a pain medication for a patient and then before you administer it the patient decides he does not want it after all (he wants pills instead), what would you do?

3. When do you perform the three checks of medication for your injectable medications? Be specific.

4. Describe how to correctly draw up two insulins in a syringe.

MEETING CLINICAL OBJECTIVES

Directions: The following suggested activities will help you meet the stated clinical practice objectives for the chapter. Review your school's clinical objectives for the week and outline a plan of activities that will help you meet them. If unsure as to how to meet them, consult with your instructor at the beginning of the clinical day.

1. Practice giving the various types of injections using a mannequin or injection pad in the skill laboratory if possible. If a skill laboratory is not available, practice drawing up and giving injections using an orange or rubber ball at home.
2. Practice palpating bony landmarks and correctly finding injection sites for all types of injections on five different people of varying sizes and weights.
3. Seek injection experience in the clinical setting by telling the nurses on the unit at the beginning of the day that you want injection experience.
4. Ask to be assigned to the out-patient surgery or ER department to obtain injection practice.
5. Correctly reconstitute drugs, draw up medications, and give all types of injections in the clinical area.
6. Combine two types of insulin and correctly administer the injection.
7. Follow standard precautions at all times.
8. Properly document injections administered.

STEPS TOWARD BETTER COMMUNICATION

VOCABULARY BUILDING GLOSSARY

Term	Pronunciation	Definition
A. Individual Terms		
aqueous	A que ous (À' kwee us)	watery; prepared with water
apprehensive	AP re HEN sive	concerned or worried about something that is going to happen
beveled	BEV eled	slanted
calibrated	CAL i bra ted	measured exactly
compatible	com PAT i ble	capable of working together
dexterity	dex TER i ty	skill with your hands
hasten	HAs ten (hÀ' sen)	to hurry, to make occur more quickly
induration	IN du RA tion	hardening; an abnormally hard spot
reconstituted	RE con sti TU ted	renewed; returned to its original state (by adding liquid)
scored	SCORed	marked with a line that allows accurate breaking apart
vial	VI al	a small bottle

B. Phrases

sloughing off	SLOUGH ing (SLUFF ing)off	shedding, falling off
needle stick	NEED le stick	process of sticking with a needle as in giving an injection; needle going through the skin

COMPLETION

Directions: Fill in the blank(s) with the correct term(s) from the Vocabulary Building Glossary above to complete the sentence.

1. Most injectable medications are prepared as an ________________ solution.
2. Many antibiotics come as a powder and must be correctly ________________.
3. Injection needles have a ________________ tip to make going through the skin smoother and less painful.
4. It requires a certain amount of ________________ to smoothly give an injection.
5. When medications are mixed in a syringe, they must be ________________.
6. Many injectable medications now come in a unit-dose ________________.
7. The majority of patients are at least a little ________________ when they are to receive an injection.
8. The nurse must be careful not to cause a ________________ to him- or herself when giving an injection to a patient.

Directions: Now for fun, substitute words from the Vocabulary Building Glossary for the underlined words in the following sentences.

1. The snake had <u>shed</u> its skin and the small boy picked it up <u>skillfully</u> and put it in a <u>small bottle</u> to keep it.
2. The woman was <u>worried</u> about drinking the <u>watery</u> lemonade, which had been <u>made</u> from a powder.
3. The pitcher had been <u>marked</u> and <u>measured</u> exactly.
4. The parents <u>hurried</u> to take the child to the doctor when they felt the <u>hard lump</u> on his leg.
5. The <u>slanted edge</u> of the mirrors <u>looked good</u> with the modern furniture in the room.

WORD ATTACK SKILLS

The words *vital, viable*, and *vial* look like they all come from the same root word. In fact, vital and viable do come from the same Latin roots (vitalis—of life, vita—life, vivere—to live), while vial comes from the Latin- and Greek-rooted word *phial*. (The "ph" and "v" sounds are very similar.) No wonder English is so difficult!

PRONUNCIATION OF DIFFICULT TERMS

Directions: Practice pronouncing the following words.

anaphylactic	an a phy LAC tic
diluent	DIL u ent
ecchymosis	EC chy MO sis
erythema	ER y THE ma
Mantoux	MAN toux (man' too)
parenteral	pa REN ter al
subcutaneous	SUB cu TA ne ous
tuberculin	tu BER cu lin
urticaria	UR ti CA ri a
viscous	VIS cous

COMMUNICATION EXERCISE

Write a script requesting experience in injection practice either from a nurse in a clinical setting or in out-patient surgery as suggested in the Clinical Activities 3 and 4 above. Be sure to clarify when and where you should go for the practice and whether you need to bring anything with you. Practice the dialogue with another student, then actually make the request. Were you satisfied with what you said and how you were understood? What would you do differently next time?

GRAMMAR POINTS

TIME CLAUSES

Sometimes it is necessary to explain a relationship in time between two events:

I was walking up the stairs when I fell.

This sentence is made up of a main (or independent) clause (I was walking up the stairs) and a dependent clause (when I fell).

- Time clauses begin with a time word such as when/while, before, and after.
- Time clauses have a subject and a verb like an independent clause.
- A time clause must be attached to a main clause to complete its meaning.

Main clause (can be used alone)	Time clause (must be used with a main clause)
1. I was walking up the stairs	when I fell.
2. D.M. learned to give himself injections	while he was in the hospital.
3. M.L. was eating	when her sister arrived.
4. The patient felt better	after she received the injection.
5. She was having a lot of pain	before the nurse gave her the injection.

- The time clause can come before or after the main clause. The meaning is the same.
- When the time clause comes first, it is followed by a comma.

Before she had lunch, she took her medication.

A. Use the five sentences above. Write the sentences putting the time clause first.

B. Write five sentences of your own using time clauses. Check with a native speaker to see if the sentences are correct.

CULTURAL POINTS

ASKING QUESTIONS

Teachers and employers in the United States are usually very happy to have their students and employees ask questions; in fact, they encourage it because it shows an interest in the subject or the job and a desire to understand, learn, and to do things correctly. The only time a superior or colleague might object to questions is when you have not studied or read the material or instructions and are taking the easy way to get the information by asking someone to give it to you. If you do not understand something, it is very important that you ask and people will usually be happy to help explain. It often will save a company time and money to have the employee understand the correct way to do something. In the health care field, it can often save lives as well.

Asking questions and double or triple checking is especially important when administering medications. If you do not understand how to measure or administer a medication, be sure to ask. Your supervisors and co-workers, and especially the patients, will appreciate your care and concern.

Review the chapter highlights, answer the study questions, and complete the critical thinking activities at the end of the chapter in the textbook.

THIRTY-FOUR

Administering Intravenous Solutions and Medications

TERMINOLOGY

A. MATCHING

Directions: Match the terms in column I with the definitions in column II.

Column I	Column II
1. ______ antineoplastic	a. Slow introduction of fluid into a vein
2. ______ autologous	b. Tube-like chamber that will hold 100 mL of fluid
3. ______ bore	c. Puncture of a vein
4. ______ burette	d. Introduction of blood components into the bloodstream
5. ______ embolus (catheter)	e. Channels within a tube
6. ______ infusion	f. Piece of catheter that has broken off and is obstructing blood flow
7. ______ lumens	g. Internal diameter
8. ______ transfusion	h. Related to self (own)
9. ______ venipuncture	i. Destroy or alter growth of malignant cells

B. COMPLETION

Directions: Fill in the blank(s) with the correct term(s) from the terms list in the chapter in the textbook to complete the sentence.

1. The IV solution $D_5$1/2NS is ________________ and will pull fluid into the vascular compartment.
2. The IV solution 0.45% saline is a ________________ solution and allows fluid to be drawn from the vascular space into the tissues.
3. Ringer's lactate IV solution is ________________ and keeps fluids stable within the body.
4. When the IV will not continue to flow, chances are that the site has ________________.
5. ________________ tubing is used to infuse viscous IV solutions and delivers 10 gtt/mL.
6. When an IV must run very slowly, ________________ tubing is used that delivers 60 drops per mL.
7. In order for intravenous fluids to be infused, a ________________ must be in place.

SHORT ANSWER

Directions: Write a brief answer for each question.

1. Four purposes for administering intravenous therapy are to:
   a. ____________________
   b. ____________________
   c. ____________________
   d. ____________________

2. List the seven guidelines related to intravenous therapy in order of priority from the most important to the least important.
   a. ____________________
   b. ____________________
   c. ____________________
   d. ____________________
   e. ____________________
   f. ____________________
   g. ____________________

3. Four responsibilities of the nurse when caring for a patient undergoing IV therapy are:
   a. ____________________
   b. ____________________
   c. ____________________
   d. ____________________

4. Signs of IV infiltration are: ____________________
   ____

5. Describe corrective actions to be taken for each of the following complications of IV therapy.
   a. infiltration ____________________
   ____
   b. phlebitis ____________________
   ____
   c. speed shock ____________________
   ____
   d. circulatory overload ____________________
   ____
   e. air embolus ____________________
   ____

6. Signs and symptoms of a blood transfusion reaction are
   ____
   ____
   ____

7. Describe actions to be taken if a transfusion reaction occurs.
   ____
   ____

8. The average adult needs ____________________ mL of fluids in a 24-hour period to replace fluids lost by elimination.

9. An intravenous solution of 5 percent dextrose in water provides __________ calories.

10. When selecting an IV solution, it should be inverted 2-3 times and inspected for ________________________.

11. When setting the rate of flow for an IV infusion, the ________________ must be checked for the tubing before calculating the flow rate.

12. The advantage of the IV piggyback system attached to the main IV infusion for medication administration is that ________________________________

13. The only intravenous fluid used in conjunction with blood administration is ________________.

14. Intermittent intravenous devices are used for patients who:
    a. ________________________________
    b. ________________________________

15. When an intermittent intravenous device is in place it must be ________________ regularly.

16. When infusing fluids by infusion pump, the pump should be checked for proper function at least every ________________.

17. The three types of short-term intravenous cannulas inserted into a peripheral vein are:
    a. ________________________________
    b. ________________________________
    c. ________________________________

18. A central venous catheter is positioned in the ________________________ or the right ________________________.

19. A PICC catheter is used when the type of IV therapy requires a ________________.

20. When a PICC or MLC is in place in an extremity, you must not ________________ on that arm.

21. A rule regarding subclavian central lines is that ________________________________ ________________________________.

22. When an infusion port is in place, only ________________________ needles are used to infuse solutions.

23. IV fluids for adults are best administered at a rate of ________________ mL/hour.

24. When the vein chosen for an IV site is not easily palpable, it may be necessary to ________________________________.

25. When choosing an IV insertion site, the rule is to pick the most ________________.

26. A medication that is **never** given as an IV bolus is ________________________.

APPLICATION OF THE NURSING PROCESS

Directions: Write a brief answer for each question.

1. Four assessment responsibilities of the nurse when the patient is undergoing intravenous therapy are:
    a. ________________________________
    b. ________________________________
    c. ________________________________
    d. ________________________________

2. Two very important assessments to make before starting the infusion of an IV medication are:
   a. ______________________________
   b. ______________________________

3. One nursing diagnosis that is appropriate for every patient who is receiving an intravenous infusion is ______________________________
   ______________________________.

4. An expected outcome for the patient who is receiving intravenous fluids because of NPO status would be ______________________________.

5. Implementation of intravenous therapy requires calculation of IV flow rates. Calculate the correct flow rate for the following IV orders:
   a. 1000 mL D_5RL at 125 mL/hr. Drop factor: 15 gtt/mL
      Correct flow rate: ______________ per minute
   b. 250 mL D_5W with 20 mEq potassium chloride over 3 hours. Drop factor: 60 gtt/mL
      Correct flow rate: ______________ per minute
   c. 1000 mL NS q 10 hours. Drop factor 15 gtt/mL
      Correct flow rate: ______________ per minute
   d. 1000 cc D_5W 1/2NS q 8 hours. Drop factor 10 gtt/mL
      Correct flow rate: ______________ per minute
   e. 500 cc D_5W at 80 cc/hr. Drop factor 10 gtt/mL
      Correct flow rate: ______________ per minute

6. Managing IV therapy means keeping the IV solution running. When at the bedside, you would observe:
   a. ______________________________
   b. ______________________________
   c. ______________________________
   d. ______________________________

7. Evaluation data that would indicate that intravenous fluid infusion is hydrating the patient would be
   ____
   ____

8. When a blood product is given by intravenous infusion, evaluation criteria indicating success of the transfusion would be ______________________________
   ______________________________.

MULTIPLE CHOICE

*Directions: Choose the **best** answer for each of the following questions.*

1. N.P. is to receive intravenous therapy for at least a week. If all of the following sites are suitable, which is the preferred site in this situation?
   1. the antecubital space
   2. the plantar aspect of the lower arm
   3. the dorsum of the hand
   4. above the wrist and below the elbow

2. The order for N.P. reads "D_5W 1000 cc to follow the container that is hanging presently." There are 50 mL left in the container hanging. You should
   1. hang the new container now before the old one runs dry.
   2. wait until another 25 mL have infused before hanging the new container.
   3. hang the new container when the remaining fluid has infused.
   4. hang the new container when there are 10 mL left in the container.

3. The next IV order for N.P. reads "1000 cc D_5W with 20 mEq of KCl to run over 10 hours." The drop factor is 10 gtt/mL. The correct flow rate per minute is
   1. 17 gtt/minute.
   2. 2 gtt/minute.
   3. 23 gtt/minute.
   4. 24 gtt/minute.

4. N.P. complains that the IV site is stinging. It is not reddened or warm to the touch. He has been up and about and the flow rate has increased from where it was set. You should first
   1. stop the infusion.
   2. take the vital signs.
   3. reset the drip rate.
   4. change the IV site.

5. N.P. will need intravenous therapy for at least a week. You would change the IV cannula every
   1. 24 hours.
   2. 48–72 hours.
   3. 12 hours.
   4. 4 days.

6. While checking on N.P., you see that his IV is not running. You should first
   1. lower the container to see if there is a blood return.
   2. discontinue the infusion and restart at a new IV site.
   3. undo the dressing and rotate the needle or cannula.
   4. attempt to aspirate a clot from the IV cannula.

7. N.P.'s IV is changed to an intermittent intravenous access for antibiotic administration. You go to hang a piggyback and the first thing you do is
   1. attach the tubing to the PRN device.
   2. flush the cannula with normal saline.
   3. change the IV site to the other hand.
   4. set the flow rate for the piggyback infusion.

8. After the piggyback infusion is finished, you would first
   1. flush the cannula with normal saline.
   2. attach the next piggyback medication tubing.
   3. disconnect the piggyback tubing.
   4. cleanse the port on the PRN device with alcohol.

9. S.C. is receiving TPN through a central line. His TPN solution is behind schedule when you come on duty. You would
   1. increase the flow rate to "catch up."
   2. leave the flow rate alone.
   3. notify the physician that the solution is behind schedule.
   4. adjust the flow rate to that which is ordered.

10. During the first several days of TPN administration, it is especially important to check S.C.'s
    1. urine output.
    2. mental status.
    3. electrolyte status.
    4. blood glucose level.

CRITICAL THINKING ACTIVITIES

1. Your elderly patient needs a peripheral IV started. Although his vein was difficult to stabilize, you attempted to insert the cannula. You were unsuccessful. What can you do to ensure the best chance of success with the next attempt?

2. Your patient's peripheral IV has stopped running. There is no redness, edema, or pain at the IV site. What steps would you take to assess and re-establish patency of the site?

3. You meet resistance when you try to flush your patient's PRN lock. What would you do?

MEETING CLINICAL OBJECTIVES

Directions: The following suggested activities will help you meet the stated clinical practice objectives for the chapter. Review your school's clinical objectives for the week and outline a plan of activities that will help you meet them. If unsure as to how to meet them, consult with your instructor at the beginning of the clinical day.

1. If a skill laboratory is available:
   a. practice changing IV fluid containers with a peer observing your technique. Practice until you are comfortable with the procedure.
   b. practice adding medications to an IV fluid container and calculating the flow rate. Have a peer observe the procedure.
   c. practice adjusting the flow rate with the roller clamp. Practice until you can smoothly and quickly adjust the rate.
2. For each assigned clinical patient who has an IV, calculate the flow rate from the order sheet.
3. Have a staff nurse or your instructor show you how to set up an IV infusion pump.
4. Go with a staff nurse whenever he or she goes to "troubleshoot" an infusion pump.
5. Seek opportunities to change IV solutions in the clinical setting by telling the nurses on the unit that you desire this experience and asking them to call you whenever a solution is to be changed while you are there. Remember to check the order yourself and to follow the five rights.
6. Observe other nurses starting IV lines in the clinical setting. Practice IV starts in the skill lab using an IV arm or seek this practice through the clinical facility education department.
7. Ask for experience in helping to monitor a patient receiving a blood product.

STEPS TOWARD BETTER COMMUNICATION

VOCABULARY BUILDING GLOSSARY

Term	Pronunciation	Definition
A. Individual Terms		
ascertain	as cer TAIN	make certain, find out for sure
chevron	CHEV ron	a wide "V" shape
discrepancy	dis CREP an cy	errors; things that do not match or fit
mimic	MIM ic	to look and act like
runaway	RUN a way	out of control, going too fast
taut	TAUT	tight, under tension
tonicity	to NI ci ty	state of tissue tone or tension; referring to body fluid pressure/ concentration
B. Phrases		
criss cross	CRISS cross	make an "X" shape
piggyback	PIG gy BACK	something riding (or following) on another larger, more powerful object (or idea) Example: A child riding on her father's shoulders
rule of thumb	RULE of THUMB	A general guideline that applies in most cases

COMPLETION

A. Directions: Fill in the blank(s) with the correct term(s) from the Vocabulary Building Glossary to complete the sentence.

1. Intravenous antibiotics are administered by __________________, where a small bag of medication is added to the main IV line.
2. When the patient complains of soreness at an IV site, you must do your best to __________________ what the problem is.
3. Proper documentation of each dose of medication administered prevents any __________________ between what was given and the charges from the pharmacy.
4. A __________________ concerning an IV that has stopped running is that you never irrigate the cannula as this might force a clot into the bloodstream.
5. A __________________ IV fluid may cause fluid overload and is especially dangerous for an infant or an older adult.

B. Directions: Replace the underlined general vocabulary word with a word from the Vocabulary Building Glossary.

1. She followed the guideline in placing the X's and V's and made sure there were no errors.
2. The little boy copied his sister and carried his doll on his shoulders.
3. The nerves of the mother of the out of control juvenile were under tension.

PRONUNCIATION OF DIFFICULT TERMS

Directions: Practice pronouncing the following words.

antineoplastic	AN ti NE o PLAS tic
autologous	au TOL o gous
osmolality	os mo LAL i ty
subclavian	sub CLA vi an

GRAMMAR POINTS

In order to clearly understand what patients and co-workers mean, learning the differences in past tenses is vitally important.

PAST TIME CLAUSES: MEANING AND ORDER

Dependent time clauses using *when, while, before*, and *after* were discussed in Chapter 33. They describe the relationship in time between two events. The past time clause helps us understand which event happened first and which happened second.

Both Verbs in Simple Past:

- If both verbs are in the simple past, the action in the when and after clause happened first. (It does not matter where the clause appears in the sentence.)

First Action	Second Action
When she received the IV,	her condition improved.
After her condition improved,	she went home.

First Action	Second Action
Her condition improved	**when she received the IV.**
She went home	**after her condition improved.**

- The action in a before clause happened second: (The order in the sentence does not matter.)

First Action	Second Action
He went home	**before his wound healed.**
His wound healed	**before he went home.**

Second Action	First Action
Before his wound healed,	he went home.

One Verb in Simple Past, One in Past Continuous/Progressive:

- In *when* or *while* sentences, when one verb is in the simple past and one is in the past continuous (was —ing), **the action in the past continuous always starts first and lasts longer**:

First Action	Second Action
The fluid was infusing correctly	**when I left the room.**
While the fluid was infusing correctly,	**I left the room.**

First Action	Second Action
When I left the room,	the fluid was infusing correctly.

- Both *while* and *when* can introduce a past continuous time clause that means *during the time.*

First Action	Second Action
The nurse assessed the patient	**while she was taking vital signs.**

Both Verbs in Past Continuous

- When both verbs are in the past continuous, the activities are happening at the same time (simultaneously) in *while* or *when* sentences:

First Action	Second Action
The nurse was assessing the IV site	**while she was taking vital signs.**
While the solution was infusing,	the patient was sleeping comfortably.

Directions: Underline the action that was happening first.

1. The nurse observed the patient while checking the IV.
2. She checked the level of fluid remaining in the bag before disconnecting it.
3. The intravenous solution was leaking out of the bag when the patient pushed the call button.
4. Before making the subcutaneous pocket, the surgeon entered the subclavian vessel.

Review the chapter highlights, answer the study questions, and complete the critical thinking activities at the end of the chapter in the textbook.

THIRTY-FIVE

Care of the Surgical Patient

TERMINOLOGY

A. MATCHING

Directions: Match the terms in column I with the definitions in column II.

Column I	Column II
1. ______ anesthesia	a. Voluntary
2. ______ autologous	b. To relieve pain or complication without curing
3. ______ elective	c. Care from decision to have surgery through the recovery period
4. ______ laser	d. Light amplification by the stimulated emission of radiation
5. ______ palliative	e. Loss of sensory perception
6. ______ perioperative care	f. Own; originating within an individual
7. ______ prosthesis	g. Artificial body part
8. ______ stasis	h. Stoppage of flow

B. COMPLETION

Directions: The following terms relate to complications of surgery. Briefly describe the complication.

1. Atelectasis ____

____

2. Dehiscence ____

____

3. Embolus ____

____

4. Evisceration ____

____

5. Hemorrhage ____

____

6. Hypostatic pneumonia ____

7. Aspiration pneumonia ____

8. Thrombosis ____

9. Thrombophlebitis ____

C. COMBINING

Directions: Combine the correct suffix with the correct stem to complete each sentence correctly. Consult Table 35-1 and the appendix "Medical Terminology" at the back of the textbook or use your medical dictionary.

-ectomy	mammo-
-oma	orchio-
-ostomy	fibr-
-otomy	col-
-plasty	cholecyst-
-pexy	thorac-

1. A ______________________ is the creation of an outlet from the colon.
2. A ______________________ is the cutting into the chest cavity.
3. A ______________________ is removal of the gallbladder.
4. An ______________________ is the fixation of an undescended testicle into the scrotum.
5. Removal of a ______________________ is the removal of a fatty tumor.
6. A ______________________ is often done after a mastectomy.

SHORT ANSWER

Directions: Write a brief answer for each question.

1. The three main reasons surgery is performed are to:
   a. ______________________
   b. ______________________
   c. ______________________
2. The four types of anesthesia and an example of the type of procedure for which they may be used are:
   a. ______________________
   b. ______________________
   c. ______________________
   d. ______________________

3. Six types of patients who would be considered at higher risk for surgery than others would be:
   a. ______
   b. ______
   c. ______
   d. ______
   e. ______
   f. ______

4. How could you help to prepare the patient psychologically for surgery?

   ______
   ______
   ______

5. Name two surgical innovations that have made surgery more precise and have reduced recovery time.
   a. ______
   ______
   b. ______
   ______

6. Tasks you would complete during the immediate preoperative period to assess that the patient is ready for surgery are:

   ______
   ______
   ______
   ______

7. L.M., a 76-year-old male, is scheduled for colon surgery in the morning. He tells you, "I hate the thought of being under anesthesia. I'm concerned that this cancer might be more serious than they think. I'm worried about my wife if I die. If I have to have a colostomy, how will I ever cope?" What would you choose as appropriate nursing diagnoses for L.M.?

   ______
   ______
   ______

8. Write one expected outcome based on your nursing diagnoses for the planning phase of your care for L.M. ______
   ______
   ______

9. Your preoperative nursing goals for the patient undergoing surgery would be:
   a. ______
   b. ______
   c. ______
   d. ______

10. Three tasks of the scrub nurse in the OR are:
    a. ______
    b. ______
    c. ______

11. Three tasks of the circulating nurse in the OR are:
    a. ______
    b. ______
    c. ______

12. The patient remains in the postanesthesia care unit (PACU) after surgery until:
____
____

TABLE ACTIVITY

Directions: For the following complications of surgery, fill in the one major sign or symptom of the complication.

Complication	Sign or Symptom
Atelectasis	
Pneumonia (hypostatic or aspiration)	
Paralytic ileus	
Thrombophlebitis	
Urinary retention	
Urinary tract infection	
Wound infection	
Pulmonary embolus	
Hemorrhage and shock	
Wound dehiscence	
Fluid imbalance	

SHORT ANSWER

Directions: Write a brief answer for each question.

1. Five points to cover for home care of the patient during discharge teaching include:
   a. ____
   b. ____
   c. ____
   d. ____
   e. ____

2. It is essential to send home ____ for the patient being discharged to home care.

3. General goals for the postsurgery patient might be:
   a. ____
   b. ____
   c. ____
   d. ____
   e. ____

APPLICATION OF THE NURSING PROCESS

Directions: Write a brief answer for each question.

Your assigned patient has just returned from the PACU after having a left thoracotomy. He has a chest tube to a disposable portable drainage unit with suction, a Foley catheter, an intravenous line, oxygen by cannula, a left lateral chest dressing, and is on pulse oximetry.

1. What specific assessments would you make as soon as you have received report and settled the patient in bed?

2. Your assessment reveals that the patient is in pain, has decreased breath sounds, cannot turn without assistance, and is very groggy from the anesthesia. Based on this information and the type of operation that was performed, what would be the nursing diagnoses for this patient?

3. Write an expected outcome for each nursing diagnosis:

4. What aspects of care for this patient would require some special planning, if any?

5. What interventions would you mark on your work organization sheet for specific times during the shift?

6. List interventions to be included on the plan of care for the nursing diagnosis related to lung status.

7. What evaluation data would you need to determine if the expected outcome for the nursing diagnosis related to lung status was being met?

8. Write three evaluation statements that would indicate that the expected outcome for the nursing diagnosis related to lung status was being met by these interventions.
   a. ______
   b. ______
   c. ______

MULTIPLE CHOICE

*Directions: Choose the **best** answer for each of the following questions.*

Situation: O.S. is scheduled for major abdominal surgery. You are in charge of her care preoperatively.

1. When teaching O.S. to cough, you would advise her to
   1. sit with her back away from the mattress or chair.
   2. perform coughing every 15 minutes postoperatively.
   3. bend over to cough more effectively.
   4. take four very deep breaths before coughing.
2. If O.S. states that she is having second thoughts and is not sure she wants to have the surgery, you would
   1. assure her that everything will go well.
   2. ask her husband to speak to her to reassure her.
   3. tear up the surgical consent she signed.
   4. notify the surgeon right away of the situation.
3. When teaching O.S. to perform the leg exercises, you would tell her that the purpose of the exercises is to
   1. ease the stiffness from being on the operating table.
   2. decrease pain from immobile extremities.
   3. increase venous return and decrease stasis.
   4. increase activity to help prevent atelectasis.
4. When the transport person comes to take the patient to surgery, it is *most* important that you
   1. assist with the transfer of the patient to the stretcher.
   2. verify the patient's I.D. number with the chart and transport slip.
   3. tell the family how to get to the surgical waiting room.
   4. list the patient off the unit on the computer.

Situation: In the operating room you observe the scrub nurse and the circulating nurse performing their functions.

5. You note that a grounding pad is placed beneath the patient. The purpose of the pad is to
   1. allow electricity to penetrate the patient's body.
   2. provide safety by dissipating electricity from the cautery.
   3. illuminate the interior body cavity in which the surgeon is operating or inspecting.
   4. keep the surgical team from receiving electrical shocks.

Situation: After the surgery, the patient is transferred to the PACU.

6. A major function of the nurse in the PACU is to
   1. assist the patient to maintain a patent airway.
   2. keep the family posted on the patient's condition.
   3. reposition the patient frequently to prevent stiff joints.
   4. stimulate the patient to hasten return of consciousness.

Situation: O.S. returns to your unit. You prepare to give her immediate postoperative care.

7. Once O.S. has aroused completely from general anesthesia, most fluid is initially provided by the intravenous route. Ice chips only are given by mouth because
   1. nausea persists for at least 24 hours.
   2. a great deal of IV fluid is given in surgery.
   3. GI motility is slowed by anesthesia.
   4. hunger is not a problem in the first 48 hours.
8. It is very important to monitor O.S.'s urine output because
   1. urinary tract infections are common at this stage.
   2. decreased urine output may be a sign of shock.
   3. a distended bladder is uncomfortable.
   4. swelling may block the ureters or urethra.

9. You carefully monitor O.S. for which of the following signs that might indicate internal hemorrhage and impending shock?
   1. falling blood pressure, rapid pulse, and anxiety
   2. copious, bloody drainage from the wound site
   3. abdominal distention and lack of bowel sounds
   4. increased amounts of blood-tinged urine

10. O.S. is being monitored by pulse oximeter. You know to
    1. adjust the nasal oxygen flow according to the readings.
    2. remove the oximeter probe when assisting the patient to cough.
    3. lower the room lights to obtain an accurate reading.
    4. report readings below 95% to the physician immediately.

CRITICAL THINKING ACTIVITIES

1. Prioritize the following list of preoperative activities for the morning of surgery.

______ Check the physician's orders.
______ Check for a signed surgical consent form.
______ Check that lab work is complete and on the chart.
______ Have the patient empty the bladder.
______ Check to see that preoperative medications ordered are available on the unit.
______ Complete the preoperative checklist.
______ Have the patient shower.
______ Prepare the unit for the postoperative return of the patient.
______ Give the preoperative medications.
______ Document the patient's readiness for the OR.
______ Transfer the patient to the OR.

2. What are the possible causes of a low urine output during the second postoperative day?
3. What actions would be necessary if your patient who had general anesthesia does not have any bowel sounds on the second postoperative day?

MEETING CLINICAL OBJECTIVES

Directions: The following suggested activities will help you meet the stated clinical practice objectives for the chapter. Review your school's clinical objectives for the week and outline a plan of activities that will help you meet them. If unsure as to how to meet them, consult with your instructor at the beginning of the clinical day.

1. Ask to observe in the OR for a clinical day or two.
2. Prepare a patient for surgery and complete the preoperative checklist.
3. Ask to accompany an assigned patient to surgery and observe the operation.
4. Accompany a nurse who is receiving a patient back from surgery to observe the immediate postoperative assessment and care.
5. Perform a postoperative assessment and immediate postoperative care.
6. Assist a patient to perform postoperative turning, breathing, coughing, and leg exercises.
7. Begin discharge instruction for a surgical patient including wound care, diet, activity and rest, elimination, pain control, and medications.

STEPS TOWARD BETTER COMMUNICATION

VOCABULARY BUILDING GLOSSARY

Term	Pronunciation	Definition
A. Individual Terms		
allay	al LAY	to calm, reduce fears
elective	e LEC tive	voluntary
groggy	GROG gy	unsteady and with an unclear mind
grounded	GROUND ed	made an electrical connection with the earth to reduce chance of shock
hamper	HAM per	to make something hard to do
kink	kink	a sharp bend in a hose or pipe
predisposes	PRE dis PO ses	makes vulnerable, makes something more likely to happen
prior	PRI or	before
sharps	sharps	needles, scalpel blades, razors, or sharp instruments
vigilant	VIG i lant	watchful
B. Phrases		
significant other	sig NIF i cant OTH er	important loved one or spouse
up and about	up and about	able to be out of bed and walk around

COMPLETION

Directions: Circle the correct word in each sentence below.

1. The nurse's discussion with the patient allayed/hampered his fears about the surgery.
2. It is important to place the used kinks/sharps in the biohazard container.
3. When checking the patient an hour after surgery, he was groggy/up and about.
4. The electric cautery pad is placed beneath the patient during surgery so that the patient is predisposes/grounded properly.
5. Sedative medication is administered elective/prior to most surgical procedures.

PRONUNCIATION OF DIFFICULT TERMS

Directions: Practice pronouncing the following words.

atelectasis	a te LEC ta sis
antiembolic	an ti em BOL ic
dehiscence	de HIS cence
evisceration	e VIS er A tion

hemorrhage	HEM orrh age
paralytic ileus	par a LIT ic IL e us
perioperative	per i OP er a tive
prosthesis	pros THE sis
thrombophlebitis	throm bo phle BI tis

COMMUNICATION EXERCISE

1. Prepare an appropriate answer for L.M.'s concerns in the Short Answer #7 exercise above.
2. When you have prioritized the preoperative activities in Critical Thinking Activity #1, write what you will say to the patient as you prepare him for surgery.
3. Write what you will say to L.M. as you perform discharge teaching necessary for his postoperative home self-care.

Review the chapter highlights, answer the study questions, and complete the critical thinking activities at the end of the chapter in the textbook.

THIRTY-SIX

Providing Wound Care and Treatment for Pressure Ulcers

TERMINOLOGY

A. COMPLETION

Directions: Fill in the blank(s) with the correct term(s) from the terms list in the chapter in the textbook to complete the sentence.

1. One sign of inflammation around a wound is ___________________.
2. When eschar is present ___________________ of the wound is necessary.
3. The abdominal incision is swollen, painful, reddened, and warm, indicating the possible presence of an ___________________.
4. Sometimes an ___________________ forms after surgery, firmly connecting two surfaces of tissue.
5. The ___________________ from the wound was clear and nonodorous.
6. The patient unfortunately developed a ___________________ between the rectum and vagina.
7. The presence of pus in a wound indicates an ___________________.
8. Dark, tough tissue around or within a wound is called ___________________ and must be debrided.
9. If cellular blood supply is disrupted, ___________________ may occur.
10. When healing occurs by primary intention, the edges of the wound ___________________ reducing the chance of infection.
11. The process of ___________________ protects wounds against bacterial invasion.
12. Wounds around joints require maintaining joint mobility in order to prevent ___________________.
13. When blood collects beneath the skin, a ___________________ forms.
14. ___________________ is an inflammation of the tissue surrounding the initial wound and is characterized by redness and induration.
15. When there is a flat hemorrhagic spot in the skin, it is termed ___________________.
16. Drainage that is ___________________ is red.
17. Drainage that contains both serum and blood is termed ___________________.
18. An abnormal passage between an internal organ and the outside of the body is a ___________________.
19. Wound exudate composed of serum and pus is called ___________________.

B. MATCHING

Directions: Match the terms in column I with the definitions in column II.

Column I		Column II
1. ______ adipose	a.	The skin
2. ______ binders	b.	Permanent, raised, enlarged scar
3. ______ fibrin	c.	Insoluble protein essential to clotting
4. ______ integument	d.	Monocyte that is phagocytic
5. ______ laceration	e.	Breakdown
6. ______ lysis	f.	Fatty
7. ______ macrophage	g.	Wide, elasticized, fabric bands used to decrease tension around a wound
8. ______ keloid		
9. ______ suture	h.	Material used to sew a wound together
	i.	A disruption in the skin or tissue

SHORT ANSWER

Directions: Write a brief answer for each question.

1. The cardinal signs of the inflammatory process are:
   a. ______
   b. ______
   c. ______
   d. ______
   e. ______

2. Schematically or verbally describe in brief the process by which wounds heal.
   ______
   ______
   ______

3. Give an example for each of the six factors that can affect wound healing.
   a. ______
   b. ______
   c. ______
   d. ______
   e. ______
   f. ______

4. Wound healing is slower in the elderly because
   ______
   ______
   ______

5. If internal hemorrhage is extensive, hypovolemic shock may occur with the following signs and symptoms:
   ______
   ______
   ______

6. The major purpose of a wound drain is to. ______
   ______.

7. Four signs and symptoms of a wound infection are:
   a. ______________________________
   b. ______________________________
   c. ______________________________
   d. ______________________________

8. If wound dehiscence and subsequent evisceration occurs, in order of priority for patient safety, you should
   ____
   ____
   ____

9. Local applications of heat are used to:
   a. ______________________________
   b. ______________________________
   c. ______________________________
   d. ______________________________
   e. ______________________________
   f. ______________________________

10. Heat works to reduce pain by ______________________________
    ______________________________.

11. Cold reduces pain by ______________________________
    ______________________________.

12. Cold helps decrease swelling by ______________________________
    ______________________________.

13. Shivering may occur during a cold treatment as a result of the body ______________
    ______________________________.

COMPLETION

Directions: Fill in the blank(s) with the correct word(s) from the chapter in the textbook to complete the sentence.

1. ____________________ is a localized protective response brought on by injury or destruction of tissues.
2. A wound with tissue loss heals by ____________________ intention.
3. An abdominal wound left open and then later closed heals by ____________________ intention.
4. If a ____________________ forms, it will restrict joint movement.
5. The microorganism most frequently present in wound infections is ____________________.
6. The best way to prevent wound infection is to maintain ____________________ when performing ____________________ care.
7. A yellow wound needs to be continually cleansed and should have a dressing that will ____________________ drainage and act to ____________________ the surface mechanically.
8. A drainage device is emptied at the end of each shift and the drainage is measured and entered on the ____________________ record.

9. The ____________________ side of a nonadherent dressing is applied to the wound.
10. Superficial wounds heal faster when kept ____________________.
11. ____________________ allow changing of the dressing without removing and reapplying tape.
12. Tape on a dressing should be placed ____________________ to body action in the wound location.

APPLICATION OF THE NURSING PROCESS

Directions: Write a brief answer for each question.

1. How would you assess a surgical wound? What parameters would you include?

____

____

____

2. What methods would you use to assess a nonsurgical wound?

____

____

____

3. What other data would you need to determine whether the patient might have a wound infection?

____

____

____

4. Your patient was involved in a bicycle accident. She has a 1 1/2" x 1" area of missing subcutaneous tissue on her left thigh. The area is reddened around it and the wound is weeping serosanguineous fluid with cream-colored exudate. Her temperature is 101.4° and her WBCs are 11,220µ. What would you list as the appropriate nursing diagnosis? What are the defining characteristics for this diagnosis?

____

____

____

5. Write an expected outcome for the above nursing diagnosis.

____

6. What interventions would you list on your nursing care plan for this nursing diagnosis?

____

____

____

____

____

____

7. What evaluation data would you need to determine if the expected outcome is being met?

____

____

____

MULTIPLE CHOICE

*Directions: Choose the **best** answer for each of the following questions.*

Situation: T.R. was transferred to your hospital after a fall in the LTC facility. He has fractured his hip. You want to do everything possible to prevent pressure ulcer formation while he is recuperating from his hip repair.

1. A factor that would increase T.R.'s risk of pressure ulcer formation is
   1. generalized edema.
   2. high fever.
   3. electrolyte imbalance.
   4. dry skin.
2. T.R. has an area over the sacrum that is reddened and the color does not subside when he is repositioned. It is prudent to
   1. cleanse the area with hydrogen peroxide and dress with a nonadherent dressing.
   2. massage the area with lotion several times a day.
   3. place a hydrocolloid dressing over the reddened area.
   4. protect the reddened area with a thin dressing such as Opsite or Tegaderm.
3. T.R. is incontinent the first day after his surgery. This is a risk factor for the development of skin breakdown and infection because of the added moisture and because
   1. greater pressure is exerted by a wet bed.
   2. shearing is more likely from wet sheets.
   3. the patient has to be repositioned for the bed to be changed.
   4. the moisture creates an environment suitable for the growth of microorganisms in a wound.
4. T.R. entered the hospital with an reddened area containing an open, abraded area over the left hip. He states that it is painful. This is a ______________________ pressure ulcer.
   1. Stage I
   2. Stage II
   3. Stage III
   4. Stage IV
5. You assist T.R. to specifically improve his healing ability by encouraging
   1. increased exercise and deep breathing to increase oxygen.
   2. proper nutrition with adequate protein and vitamin C.
   3. increasing fluid intake to at least 3000 mL per day.
   4. resting as much as possible and keeping the incisional area still.
6. When preparing to change the sterile dressing over the incision for T.R, it is important to remember to
   1. place a discard bag as close to the wound as possible.
   2. refrain from talking while the wound is uncovered.
   3. remove the old dressing before assembling the sterile supplies.
   4. remind him to remain very still during the procedure.
7. When working with his closed wound drainage system, if it becomes 2/3 full, you should
   1. recompress the device and let it fill some more.
   2. wait until it is full to empty it.
   3. replace the entire device with another one.
   4. empty it and recompress the device.

Situation: When providing hot and cold treatments for patients, several principles apply. The following questions apply to these principles and practices.

8. A systemic effect of cold therapy is
   1. alteration of the pulse rate.
   2. shunting of blood from the periphery to the central organs.
   3. speeding up metabolic processes such as digestion and tissue building.
   4. numbing of the area of application.

9. Moist heat has the physiological effect of
   1. constricting the blood vessels.
   2. drawing fluid to the site of application.
   3. numbing the area treated.
   4. dilating the blood vessels.

10. When teaching the patient how to apply a cold pack, you would say which of the following?
    1. "Wrap the pack in thick cloth before applying it to the skin.
    2. "Use the ice pack continuously for the first 24 hours."
    3. "Leave the pack in place for 20 minutes out of each hour for the first 24 hours."
    4. "Only use the ice pack for 10 minutes four times a day."

11. When applying an ice pack, it is necessary to
    1. use a light cover on the pack.
    2. use small ice cubes.
    3. fill the pack and refreeze it.
    4. cover the pack with plastic wrap.

12. Safety factors involved in using an aquathermia pad unit for a patient include
    1. securing the pad to the patient.
    2. using a thermometer to check the temperature of the pad.
    3. inspecting the plug and cord for cracks or fraying.
    4. instructing the patient not to lie on the pad for more than 15 minutes.

13. When giving a hot soak treatment, it is most important to
    1. soak only the affected area.
    2. test the temperature of the solution.
    3. position the patient comfortably.
    4. use only sterile equipment and solution.

Situation: O.P., a 28-year-old male, is a patient at your clinic. He states that had a minor accident with his motorcycle five days ago. He sustained several scrapes and wounds.

14. The wound on his calf has a pinkish-red center area that looks bumpy. This indicates that the wound is
    1. becoming infected.
    2. beginning to heal.
    3. needs to be debrided.
    4. is purulent.

15. When changing the dressing on his right arm, you see that the dressing has a moist yellow-red stain on it. You would chart this as ____________________ drainage.
    1. sanguineous
    2. purulent
    3. infected
    4. serosanguineous

CRITICAL THINKING ACTIVITIES

1. P.S. has an open wound on her right heel. It is 3 x 5 cm and has a blackened area in the center. It is reddened around the perimeter. How would you stage this pressure ulcer? How would you treat it?

2. List the equipment and supplies you would need to change a sterile dressing over a 4" abdominal incision that contains a Penrose wound drain.

3. B.W. has developed a cellulitis in the arm where he had an IV line. He is placed on antibiotics and told to use heat on it at home. How would you instruct B.W. to safely give his own heat treatments at home?

MEETING CLINICAL OBJECTIVES

Directions: The following suggested activities will help you meet the stated clinical practice objectives for the chapter. Review your school's clinical objectives for the week and outline a plan of activities that will help you meet them. If unsure as to how to meet them, consult with your instructor at the beginning of the clinical day.

1. Ask nurses on the units to which you are assigned to allow you to accompany them to see various types of wounds and observe dressing techniques.
2. Study the AHCPR Guideline booklet "Pressure Ulcers in Adults: Prediction and Prevention" to become more familiar with pressure ulcers and their care.
3. Practice sterile dressing changes in the skill lab or at home until you are comfortable and confident of your sterile technique.
4. Perform a wound irrigation.
5. Ask to be assigned to patients who have pressure ulcers for experience in providing care for these wounds.
6. Remove sutures or staples from a wound and apply Steri-Strips.
7. Give a heat treatment and a cold treatment to a patient and teach the patient how to do these treatments at home.
8. Question other nurses about ways to decrease the trauma of dressing changes on the skin of the elderly patient.
9. Seek assignment to patients who need sterile dressing changes.

STEPS TOWARD BETTER COMMUNICATION

VOCABULARY BUILDING GLOSSARY

Term	Pronunciation	Definition
A. Individual Terms		
adhere	ad HERE	to hold, stick to something
binder	BIND er	a wide band, usually cloth, to hold something together
cardinal	CARD i nal	the most important, primary
cessation	ces SA tion	a stopping
frayed	FRAY ed	worn with loose threads at the edge
friable	FRI a ble	easily crumbled, broken
gauze	Gauze	lightweight fabric with a loose, open mesh weave
hydrate	hy DRATE	keep moist or wet
immunocompromised	im mu no COM promised	poor immune response because of illness, drugs, poor physical condition
nonadherent	non ad HER ent	will not stick to another surface
nosocomial	no so CO mi al	originating in a hospital

numbing	NUM bing	lacking in feeling
obese	o BESE	excessively overweight
occlusive	oc CLU sive	obstructing
radiant	RA di ant	diverging from a center
regeneration	re gen e RA tion	the natural renewal, regrowth
sloughing	SLOUGH (sluf) ing	the shedding or dropping off of dead tissue

B. Phrases

frost bite (frost nip)	FROST bite	a condition in which body tissue is exposed to low temperatures and begins to freeze
shearing forces	SHEAR ing forces	two surfaces sliding across each other in opposite directions

COMPLETION

Directions: Fill in the blank(s) with the correct term(s) from the Vocabulary Building Glossary to complete the sentence.

1. Often, IV fluids are essential to ____________________ the patient.
2. The nurse must check for a ____________________ cord before plugging in a piece of electrical equipment.
3. The elderly often have very ____________________ skin.
4. Right lower quadrant pain is a ____________________ sign of appendicitis.
5. An open wound often requires a ____________________ type of dressing.
6. A lift sheet is used to turn a patient to prevent the consequences of ____________________ that occur if the patient is pulled across the sheets rather than lifted.
7. An abdominal ____________________ keeps a patient who has had major abdominal surgery more comfortable when out of bed.
8. It is a major nursing responsibility to prevent ____________________ infection in hospitalized patients.
9. A safety device when placed too tightly around a limb may result in ____________________ of the distal part of the extremity.
10. Safety devices that are placed improperly may cause a ____________________ of blood flow in the body part.

VOCABULARY EXERCISE

Directions: Which of the words in the Vocabulary Building Glossary have you seen or heard used in another way in everyday speech? Give some examples; i.e., cardinal = a red bird: There were three cardinals at my bird feeder this morning.

____

____

____

PRONUNCIATION OF DIFFICULT TERMS

Directions: Practice pronouncing the following words.

cellulitis	CELL u li tis
dehiscence	de HIS cence
ecchymosis	ec chy MO sis
erythema	er y THE ma
eschar	ES char(kar)
evisceration	E vis cer A tion
hypoallergenic	hy po al ler GEN ic
hypovolemic	hy po vo LE mic
purulent	PU ru lent
phagocytosis	pha go cy TO sis
sanguineous	san GUIN e ous
serosanguineous	ser o san GUIN e ous

The word debridement is given the French pronunciation "da BREED maw"

COMMUNICATION EXERCISE

1. Using the following as an example, explain to a patient or peer how to care for an abdominal wound at home.

   "When at home Ms. T., I want you to change the dressing every day. Wash your hands well before touching the dressing or the wound. You can use a pair of these clean disposable gloves each time you do the dressing change. I usually prepare the tape strips before I start. This tape can be torn easily. I just stick it on the side of the table or the counter where I can reach it. I do that before I put on the gloves. You may want to shower before you change the dressing. Just tape a piece of plastic over the dressing. Try not to let the shower water run directly over that area. This way if the dressing gets a bit wet, you will be changing it anyway. With the gloves on, remove the old dressing and put it into a sealable plastic bag for disposal. Inspect the wound for redness, tenderness around it, increased drainage, or separation of the edges. If these occur, report them to the doctor. Clean around the wound with gauze squares moistened with saline. Clean from the center of the wound outward. That way you don't bring bacteria into the wound area. You can prepare those ahead of time as I just did also. Pat the area dry and attach a new dressing just like the old one."

2. Write out how you would explain to a mother how to care for her child's wound at home. Have a peer or your instructor critique your instructions.

Review the chapter highlights, answer the study questions, and complete the critical thinking activities at the end of the chapter in the textbook.

THIRTY-SEVEN

Promoting Musculoskeletal Function

TERMINOLOGY

A. MATCHING

Directions: Match the terms in column I with the definitions in column II.

	Column I			Column II
1.	f	blanch	a.	Exertion of a pulling force
2.	c	cast	b.	Bandage for supporting a body part
3.	g	debilitating	c.	A stiff dressing used to immobilize a body part
4.	h	dorsum	d.	Moving
5.	i	hydrotherapy	e.	Artificial substitute for a body part
6.	j	immobilization	f.	To become pale
7.	d	kinetic	g.	Weakening
8.	K	paresthesia	h.	Back
9.	e	prosthesis	i.	Use of water to treat injury
10.	b	sling	j.	To prevent movement
11.	a	traction	k.	Tingling or burning sensation

B. COMPLETION

Directions: Fill in the blank(s) with the correct term(s) from the terms list in the chapter in the textbook to complete the sentence.

1. When a cast becomes too tight due to swelling of an extremity, the physician will bivalve it to relieve the pressure.
2. The young man had been in a diving accident and was quadriplegics, having no use of his arms or legs.
3. Often, while a patient is in leg traction, the doctor will order Isometric exercises to strengthen muscles and prevent atrophy.
4. The patient had paralysis of the legs after the accident and was paregalegic.
5. A traction bed often requires an over-the-bed Frame from which to hang the traction apparatus.

6. A __spice__ cast may be needed to immobilize a part of the trunk and one or both legs.

7. After the stroke, G.R. had right-sided __hemiparesis__ and could not walk unassisted.

8. The accident left I.B. with __hemiplegia__ and he had no use of his left arm or leg.

9. For skin traction, sometimes adhesive ______________ is used to attach the traction to the skin.

10. A __trapeze Bar__ hung over the bed is used so the patient in traction can reposition him- or herself.

SHORT ANSWER

Directions: Write a brief answer for each question.

1. In what ways does inactivity affect respiratory exchange and airway clearance?
   secretions can collect in lower airways leads to congestion and respiratory illness (provides medium for Bacteria growth/hypostatic pneum activity causes people to breath easier & encourage cleaning of airways

2. To perform a neurovascular assessment on an immobilized extremity, you would
   inspect area distal to injury (palpate skin temp) have pt. move area distal to injury - should be no discomfort. check sensation with paper clip - ask of feel of numbness or tingling (paresthesia), palpate pulse distal to injury, capillary refill to injury, question about degree of pain.

3. H.D. has just had a long leg cast applied. Describe the care of this cast during the drying period.
   Use palm or flat part of fingers when handling, pad sufficiently - add padding or changing position. It is critical the cast be protected from uneven pressure during the drying period because the shape or position can be changed

4. Describe the special features of each of the following specialty beds and the advantages of each.
   a. Air-fluidized bed have tiny silicone beads - warm air passes thru and act as a fluid that suspends pt. free from contact with an hard surface, Reduces occlusion of blood vessels & shearing of tissues, Reduces Body pain & Pressure ulcers for Bedridden pts.
   (used for Pressure ulcers, fresh grafts, flap repairs of injury)
   b. Low air-loss bed distributes air thru multiple cushions - low air flow controls moisture of the skin, segments of cushions can be deflated for pt. care. Head of Bed can be raised,
   c. Continuous lateral-rotation bed decrease incidence of lung collapse, nosocomial pneumonia facilitate normal flow of urine, reduces risk of deep vein thrombosis, pulmonary embolism by encouraging venous flow, skin breakdown reduced, built in scale, constant side to side motion keep
   d. CircOlectric bed used especially for burn pt. moves 360° arc allowing change of position for pt. Circular frame

5. Five pressure relief devices used to help prevent skin injury for immobilized patients are:
   a. foam & gel pads
   b. sheep-skin Pads
   c. heel & elbow protectors
   d. pulsating air pads
   e. water mattress

6. Four principles or guidelines for applying an elastic or roller bandage are:
   a. elevate the Limb & support it while applying the bangge
   b. Face Pt, & wrap the bandage from the distal to the proximal area
   c. apply even pressure by exerting equal tension throughout wrapping bandge
   d. overlap turns of the bandage equally, check color & sensation
   e. smooth Bandage removing wrinkles f. secure end of bandage with safety
   Remove Band. for Bathing

7. List one nursing action to prevent each of the following potential complications of immobility:
   a. Thrombus formation: circulatory status & Blood flow must be monitored on a regular Basis. Assess color, sensation & movement, Rom, Reposition every 2 hrs.
   b. Atelectasis: Deep Breathing excercises, frequent turning, ROM, excercises
   c. Constipation: increase fluid intake 3000 mL, increase fiber in diet
   d. Joint contracture: perform active or passive Rom excercises
   stool softeners & laxatives ordered as needed
   e. Renal stones: more fluids - fiber diet, R
   f. Skin breakdown: Turn pt. every 2 hrs, skin to be kept moist & dry
   keep linens smooth & clean
   g. Boredom: space visits from friends & family, chat w/ Pt. about things that interest them. (crossword puzzles) send notes & cards

8. How can you promote adequate nutrition for the immobilized elderly patient who is anorexic?
   Frequent small feedings, & bedtime nourishments may be used, having favorite foods brought in by family & friends

9. Traction is used to maintain parts of the body in extension and alignment.

✓ 10. When moving a patient in the bed, you must be careful to avoid a shearing injury to the skin.

11. Two main aspects of nursing care for the patient in traction are to keep the weights free & off the floor and to keep the patient in alignment.
    the end traction ropes

✓ 12. It is very important that the weight of traction be exerted when the patient is moved in the bed.

✓ 13. For traction to be maximally effective, the ropes must pull.

14. When traction is being used, it is important to maintain a balance between traction pull and countertraction force (wt. pulling against the wt. of traction)

15. Countertraction force is provided by the weight of the patient and the position of the bed.

16. Dents in a cast can lead to circulatory impairment and consequent pressure injuries

17. When a cast is to be applied, the patient is told to expect a feeling of heat, especially with a plaster of paris cast.

18. It is critical that the cast be protected from uneven pressure while drying.

19. When handling the cast while it is drying, use the palm & flat part of fingers rather than the fingertips.

20. When the patient has a spica cast, never use the Spreader Bar to help turn the patient.

21. When transferring a patient with a mechanical lift, never leave the person alone or attended.

22. Walkers are helpful to patients who are weak or tend to lose their Balance.

23. The height of the walker is correct if the person grasping the hand grips is standing upright with the elbow bent 15 - 30 degrees.

24. A very important point in teaching a patient to use crutches is to teach NOT to rest body wt. on axillary bar.

√ 25. Crutches need to be adjusted to the individual patient both in ________________ and from the ________________ to the ________________.

APPLICATION OF THE NURSING PROCESS

Directions: Write a brief answer for each question.

1. M.B. has been immobilized with a Thomas splint with Pearson attachment on her left leg after she fractured it in an automobile accident. Your beginning-of-shift assessment of M.B. would include

____

____

____

____

2. Your nursing diagnosis related to M.B.'s main problem would be

____.

3. Another nursing diagnosis for every patient who is immobilized by traction is

____.

4. One expected outcome for the nursing diagnosis in #2 would be

____.

5. Three nursing interventions to prevent boredom for M.B. while she is immobilized are:
   a. ____
   b. ____
   c. ____

6. How would you evaluate the effectiveness of the traction and immobilization treatment for M.B.?

____

____

7. Write two evaluation statements that would assist in evaluating whether M.B. was meeting the expected outcome in #4.
   a. ____
   b. ____

MULTIPLE CHOICE

*Directions: Choose the **best** answer for each of the following questions.*

1. C.E. was injured in an industrial accident and has suffered a fractured left leg and left wrist. His wrist is treated with a cast and the leg is placed in skeletal traction. Because of immobilization of his leg, C.E. is at risk for
   1. respiratory depression.
   2. venous thrombosis.
   3. generalized edema.
   4. foot drop.

2. C.E. is to be encouraged to deep breathe, cough, and use his incentive spirometer to prevent
   1. pulmonary embolus.
   2. bronchoconstriction.
   3. hypostatic pneumonia.
   4. delayed healing.

3. Another aspect of caring for C.E. while in skeletal traction is to
   1. use aseptic technique for pin care.
   2. exercise the leg in traction passively.
   3. remove the traction while showering him.
   4. lift the weights to remove pressure while moving him.

4. To make C.E.'s bed while he is in skeletal traction you would
   1. roll him from one side to the other.
   2. make the bed from top to bottom.
   3. only change the top sheet.
   4. move him to a stretcher while making the bed.

5. C.E., although right handed, will have self-care deficits while he is recovering. He will especially need assistance with
   1. toileting.
   2. eating.
   3. combing his hair.
   4. drinking from a cup.

6. J.T., eight years old, has fractured his leg. It is placed in a cast. When instructing his mother about repositioning the new cast, you tell her to
   1. lift the leg with a sling to move it.
   2. have J.T. move the cast.
   3. use the flat palm of the hand to lift the cast.
   4. wait until thc cast is completely dry.

7. While assessing J.T., an indication that swelling is occurring and the cast is becoming too tight would be
   1. the cast is hot to the touch.
   2. the area distal is a dusky color and cold.
   3. capillary refill distally is 10–15 seconds.
   4. the patient complains of discomfort.

8. It is discovered that J.T. sprained his wrist when he broke his leg. An elastic bandage wrap is ordered. You would be sure to
   1. pull the bandage tightly around the extremity.
   2. elevate the extremity before beginning to wrap it.
   3. wrap the bandage very lightly around the extremity.
   4. use a circular technique from the wrist up the arm.

9. J.T. is given some exercises to do while his leg is healing. The purpose of the exercises is to
   1. help the bone heal.
   2. prevent boredom.
   3. increase circulation.
   4. prevent loss of muscle tone.

10. J.T.'s cast is dry and he is started on crutch walking. You explain that when going up stairs he is to
    1. first move the crutches up onto the stair.
    2. move the good leg up onto the stair and then the crutches and the bad leg.
    3. move the bad leg and one crutch onto the stair and then move the other leg and crutch.
    4. move the good leg and opposite crutch up onto the stair and then move the bad leg and other crutch up.

CRITICAL THINKING ACTIVITIES

1. L.K., age 46, is going to be immobilized for several weeks while his injuries heal. Design an activity program to help prevent boredom and depression.
2. How would you handle the situation if your new amputee states that she has no interest in learning to wrap her stump properly?
3. How would you explain to an elderly patient who has had a stroke and has hemiparesis how using a walker can both protect her safety and provide more independence for her?

MEETING CLINICAL OBJECTIVES

Directions: The following suggested activities will help you meet the stated clinical practice objectives for the chapter. Review your school's clinical objectives for the week and outline a plan of activities that will help you meet them. If unsure as to how to meet them, consult with your instructor at the beginning of the clinical day.

1. Actively seek assignment to patients with problems of immobility so that experience is gained in caring for patients with casts, traction, prostheses, paralysis, and so forth.
2. Whenever there is a special bed in use on the unit, ask the staff nurse to explain its use and any special nursing care or problems associated with the bed's use.
3. Observe a physical therapist adjusting crutches for a patient and when teaching crutch walking.
4. Practice transferring a person with hemiparesis into and out of a wheelchair safely and smoothly. Have a peer role play the patient.
5. Ask a staff nurse to teach you to use a mechanical lift if one is available on your unit.
6. Any time someone asks for help in transferring a patient to or from a stretcher, if possible, go and assist so that you learn all the tricks of performing this procedure efficiently and safely. Observe exactly where a slide or roller board is placed or how a lift sheet is utilized.
7. Apply an elastic bandage to a patient's extremity.

STEPS TOWARD BETTER COMMUNICATION

VOCABULARY BUILDING GLOSSARY

Term	Pronunciation	Definition
A. Individual Terms		
buoyancy	BUOY an cy	ability to float
debilitating	de BIL i TA ting	making weak
diminished	de MIN ished	made less, decreased
diversionary	di VER sion ar y	distracting, to put attention in another place
disintegrate	dis IN te grate	to fall apart; break into small pieces
gait	GAIT	the way a person walks
groundless	GROUND less	without basis in fact; with no reason
kinetic	ki NET ic	moving
longitudinally	lon gi TUD in al ly	along the length of something
regress	re GRESS	to go back; return to an earlier state
trapeze	tra PEZE	a horizontal bar hung by ropes (often used as a swing for acrobats)
B. Phrases		
oscillating saw	OS cil la ting saw	an electrical saw that goes back and forth, not around
pen pal	PEN pal	a person you know only through letters; someone you write to regularly
work things through	work things through	to think and talk about a problem or feelings, and come to a resolution

COMPLETION

Directions: Fill in the blank(s) with the correct term(s) from the Vocabulary Building Glossary to complete the sentence.

1. The nurse tried to plan some grounaless activities for the boy in traction who stated he was very bored and was really hurting.
2. The leg was swelling and the cast was becoming tight, so the cast was bivalved longitudnally down the leg.
3. The six-year-old with the fractured leg in skeletal traction began to regress and started wetting the bed.
4. After several weeks, the area around the toes of the walking cast began to dverse and it had to be replaced.
5. The nurse used a diagram to help teach the patient the proper gait to use when crutch walking.
6. The motor vehicle accident and resulting fractures and injuries ended up being very debilitatmg for the patient.

VOCABULARY EXERCISE

These words may be used as a verb or a noun.

	Verb	Noun
hamper	to make difficult	a basket or container for food or clothing
dictate	to tell someone what to do, say, or write	a rule or regulation
stress	to emphasize, or consider important	anxiety; mental or physical strain caused by pressure

Directions: Use each word above in a sentence first as a noun and then as a verb.

1. a. (Noun) Place dirty laundry in hamper
   b. (Verb) Teach hampered students activities.
2. a. (Noun) The dictate of the classroom behavior was followed
   b. (Verb) He dictated everything with pleasure
3. a. (Noun) The stress was overwhelming
   b. (Verb) I stress the importance of this assignment

PRONUNCIATION OF DIFFICULT TERMS

Directions: Practice pronouncing the following words.

atelectasis	a te lec ta sis
hemiplegia	hem i PLE gi a
hemiparesis	HEM i par E sis
paraplegic	par a PLE gic
prosthesis	pros THE sis
quadriplegic	QUAD ri PLE gic

COMMUNICATION EXERCISE

Directions: Practice these questions for neurovascular assessment with a peer.

Do you feel any tingling or numbness?

Where does it hurt? Describe the pain—is it sharp, or dull, constant or intermittent? When does it hurt? How much does it hurt?

CULTURAL POINTS

In the United States today, a great deal of emphasis is placed on rehabilitation. Amputees are fitted with prostheses with the goal of enabling them to return to as normal a life a possible. People who use wheelchairs may participate in sports such as basketball, and the Americans with Disabilities Act (ADA) makes more buildings, job sites, and outdoor areas accessible to them. Amputees have run across the country and climbed mountains. These are exceptional people, but they show that they can succeed in spite of the physical difficulties they have. Their success may have more to do with their own attitudes and how people treat them than their actual physical status. This is something to remember as you deal with patients.

How are people with physical limitations treated in your native country? Are they encouraged to return to normal life and given training and assistance? Many countries may not have the finances to remove all physical barriers, but are there social and emotional barriers still in place?

Have you known a person with such a disability? Have you ever talked with him or her about it? What are the problems the person faces? What is his or her philosophy in dealing with the problem?

To raise your own awareness of the difficulties a person with physical limitations might face, even temporarily while in a cast or wheelchair, pay attention for one day or even a morning. Notice what might be difficult for you if you were on crutches, in a wheelchair, had only use of one hand, or were unable to see clearly. Could you navigate stairs, step off the curb, reach your car, push the elevator button, use the soft-drink machine, open the door, cross the street, leave your house? How would it affect what you could and could not do? How would it change your life?

Review the chapter highlights, answer the study questions, and complete the critical thinking activities at the end of the chapter in the textbook.

THIRTY-EIGHT

Common Physical Care Problems of the Elderly

TERMINOLOGY

A. MATCHING

Directions: Match the terms in column I with the definitions in column II.

Column I

1. __g__ beta-carotene
2. __F__ cataracts
3. __B__ dysphagia
4. __e__ glaucoma
5. __h__ presbycusis
6. __d__ presbyopia
7. __I__ polypharmacy
8. __A__ postural hypotension
9. __C__ visual accommodation
10. __J__ over-the-counter

Column II

a. Unusually low blood pressure when standing
b. Difficulty swallowing
c. Ability to focus on far and near objects
d. Age-related decreased ability to focus on near objects
e. Excess fluid in eye that exerts pressure on the optic nerve
f. Clouding of the lens of the eye
g. Substance found in orange vegetables and fruits and dark green, leafy vegetables
h. Inability to hear high-pitched sounds and spoken words
i. Use of multiple medications
j. Drugs that can be purchased at the pharmacy without a prescription

B. COMPLETION

Directions: Fill in the blank(s) with the correct term(s) from the terms list in the chapter in the textbook to complete the sentence.

1. At the onset of menopause, many women take ________________ to decrease the unpleasant symptoms.
2. Often, urinary incontinence can be corrected by __Bladder Retrain__ and without surgery.
3. A disease that often robs the elderly of their vision is __glaucoma__.

4. One technique used in bladder retraining is PRompted Voiding where the patient is assisted to void just before times when incontinence has been known to occur.

5. When an elderly, inactive person experiences a change in bowel pattern that includes passage of small amounts of liquid stool, Fecal capation should be suspected.

SHORT ANSWER

Directions: Write a brief answer for each question.

1. Five age-related common physical care problems of the elderly to be considered when assessing an elderly patient are:
   a. ______
   b. ______
   c. ______
   d. ______
   e. ______

2. Describe how chronic urinary incontinence might affect a person both physically and psychologically.
   ______
   ______
   ______

3. Three ways to promote mobility in the elderly are:
   a. ______
   b. ______
   c. ______

4. Four ways to prevent falls in the home are:
   a. ______
   b. ______
   c. ______
   d. ______

5. Identify four factors affecting the elderly that may lead to an alteration in nutrition.
   a. ______
   b. ______
   c. ______
   d. ______

6. List four techniques that will facilitate communication and safety for the patient with a sensory deficit.
   a. ______
   b. ______
   c. ______
   d. ______

7. Identify five reasons the older adult is prone to the problem of polypharmacy.
   a. ______
   b. ______
   c. ______
   d. ______
   e. ______

8. Describe how a chronic respiratory disease can affect an elderly person's mobility.

____

____

9. Describe the ways in which decreased activity on the part of an elderly person may affect his or her mobility.

____

____

____

10. List the five factors you consider the most important for safety in the home for an elderly person.
   a. _______________
   b. _______________
   c. _______________
   d. _______________
   e. _______________

11. Diseases that interfere with _______________ or _______________ contribute to activity intolerance and immobility.

12. Four accessible activities that can promote mobility in the elderly are
   a. _______________, b. _______________, c. _______________, and
   d. _______________.

13. To protect against osteoporosis, all adults should engage in _______________ exercise and take in sufficient _______________.

14. One factor to consider in promoting mobility among the elderly is that most would rather risk _______________ than be placed in a _______________.

15. Approximately one __________ of people over 65 years old and _______________ of those over 80 fall each year.

16. With each additional _______________ taken, the risk of falls is increased.

17. Elderly patients need to be moved slowly out of bed to prevent possible _______________.

18. When an elderly person who lives alone is discharged home, it is wise to make a referral for a home health team member to assess the home for _______________.

19. If an elderly person has some difficulty with balance, the person should be told not to reach for objects _______________ level.

20. When incontinence occurs, the _______________ should be sought.

21. For the person who does experience urinary incontinence, odor can be reduced by encouraging the person to _______________ to dilute the urine.

22. The ill older adult who is on bed rest, receiving pain medication, and not eating a normal diet is at high risk for _______________.

23. The primary dietary guidelines for the elderly are to reduce the _______________ and _______________ intake and to increase _______________ in the diet.

24. Three visual changes that occur with aging because of decreased blood supply to the retina are:
   a. _______________
   b. _______________
   c. _______________

25. When a patient has considerable visual deficit, it is important to identify yourself when __________________ or __________________ the room.

26. For the person with a visual deficit, it is also important to refrain from __________________ personal belongings without permission or explanation.

27. Hearing deficits are usually intensified by the presence of __________________.

28. The problem of polypharmacy often occurs because the older adult with multiple health problems sees multiple __________________.

29. The goal of prompted voiding is to ____ ____.

30. The percentage of the daily calories that should be protein in the diet of the person over age 51 is __________________.

TABLE ACTIVITY

Directions: Use a separate sheet of paper to list three contributing factors for each physical care problem of the elderly.

Physical Care Problem	Contributing Factors
Impaired mobility	
Alteration in elimination	
Alteration in nutrition	
Sensory deficit—vision	
Sensory deficit—hearing	
Polypharmacy	

MULTIPLE CHOICE

*Directions: Choose the **best** answer for each of the following questions.*

1. S.T., age 78, has a stasis ulcer on her right leg. As her home health nurse you visit to change her dressing. During the visit you perform other assessments. Since S.T. is mostly immobile because she needs to keep the right leg elevated and because she is taking pain medication, it is especially important to assess her
   1. mental status.
   2. urinary status.
   3. bowel status.
   4. heart status.

2. When asked if she is taking her antibiotics for the infection in her leg, S.T. replies, "Yes, but I have so many pills, I'm not sure I'm taking them at the right times." What would be a good method to assist S.T. to take her pills correctly?
   1. Have a neighbor come in and give her the pills at different times during the day.
   2. Set up a seven-day medicine planner for her that you can refill during your nursing visits.
   3. Have her daughter call and remind her when to take her pills.
   4. Write out a list of the medications and the times that each is to be taken.

3. When listing S.T.'s medications, you find that she has two very similar blood pressure medications prescribed by different doctors. To remedy the problem of polypharmacy you would recommend that she
   1. give each doctor she sees a list of her medications.
   2. make certain that she knows exactly what each prescription is supposed to treat.
   3. obtain all her prescription medications from one pharmacy.
   4. ask her daughter to monitor her prescriptions for her.
4. S.T. indicates she is not eating much as it is difficult to cook. A nursing intervention that is appropriate in this case is
   1. ask her best friend to prepare meals for her.
   2. ask her daughter to bring her several microwave meals.
   3. suggest using supplements such as Ensure to maintain her nutrition.
   4. ask the social worker to set up Meals on Wheels service for her.
5. Which one of the following chronic conditions that S.T. also has may become worse due to her decreased mobility?
   1. asthma
   2. hypertension
   3. hypothyroidism
   4. osteoarthritis
6. F.S., an alert, well-groomed, 82-year-old resident of the long-term care facility has been experiencing bladder incontinence since she had pneumonia. She seems quite depressed and you suspect that this development has seriously affected her
   1. self-esteem.
   2. attitude toward others.
   3. personality.
   4. mental acuity.
7. The first thing that should be done when beginning a bladder retraining program for F.S. is
   1. planning scheduled toileting times.
   2. decreasing her fluid intake.
   3. tracking when incontinence occurs.
   4. placing her in adult diapers.
8. When considering a teaching session for F.S. about the bladder retraining program, you would plan to
   1. eliminate outside noise and distractions.
   2. use printed materials to explain the process.
   3. quickly present the material so as not to cause fatigue.
   4. speak distinctly in a very loud voice.
9. F.S. also has been having some difficulty with constipation from decreased appetite and antibiotic therapy. To assist her with this problem, you would encourage her to
   1. increase roughage with fresh fruits and vegetables.
   2. take a laxative each night at bedtime.
   3. attempt to evacuate the bowels after breakfast.
   4. choose more breads and pastas at meals.
10. F.S. has moderate macular degeneration. To decrease the possibility of falls at night, you would
    1. keep a very bright light burning in her room.
    2. ask her to call for assistance to the bathroom.
    3. keep her cane within reach of the bed.
    4. have an attendant stay with her at night.
11. A drug that may be used to arrest osteoporosis in the elderly is
    1. aspirin
    2. Motrin
    3. Fosamax
    4. prednisone
12. A leading cause of hospitalization and placement in long-term care is
    1. cardiac disease.
    2. diabetes.
    3. hip fracture.
    4. pneumonia.

13. A medicine that may contribute to falls in the elderly is
    1. Thorazine.
    2. Miacalcin.
    3. Flonase.
    4. ampicillin.

14. A common physical care problem in the elderly that has been reported to cost billions for nursing home care is
    1. chronic obstructive pulmonary disease (COPD).
    2. urinary incontinence.
    3. hip fracture.
    4. immobility.

15. An herbal approach to reduce prostate swelling is
    1. saw palmetto.
    2. St. John's wort.
    3. evening primrose.
    4. ginkgo biloba.

16. Patients with dysphagia should be put in which position for 45–60 minutes following eating?
    1. semi-Fowler's
    2. high Fowler's
    3. supine
    4. Sims'

17. Glaucoma is a common eye disorder that is characterized by
    1. a clouding of the lens.
    2. inability to focus on near objects.
    3. an accumulation of excess fluid inside the eye.
    4. a yellowing of the sclera.

18. Antioxidants that may help protect against macular degeneration include
    1. calcium and vitamin C.
    2. calcium and vitamin D.
    3. vitamin C and vitamin B.
    4. vitamin C and vitamin E.

19. Presbycusis is characterized by the inability to hear
    1. low-frequency sounds.
    2. high-frequency sounds.
    3. mid-frequency sounds.
    4. vowel sounds.

20. Strategies to increase compliance in self-medication administration include all *except*
    1. the use of color-coded medication bottles.
    2. periodically counting the remaining pills.
    3. an alarm clock.
    4. cueing with daily events.

CRITICAL THINKING ACTIVITIES

1. Your home care patient is having a difficult time obtaining adequate nutrition. She has family two hours away, but lives alone. She has limited mobility, but can walk short distances. How would you go about assisting her to obtain better nutrition?
2. Perform a safety assessment of an elder relative or friend's home. What hazards did you find?
3. Describe ways you might assist an elderly adult who has a visual deficit stay independent.

MEETING CLINICAL OBJECTIVES

Directions: The following suggested activities will help you meet the stated clinical practice objectives for the chapter. Review your school's clinical objectives for the week and outline a plan of activities that will help you meet them. If unsure as to how to meet them, consult with your instructor at the beginning of the clinical day.

1. Work with an elderly patient on a bladder retraining program.
2. Develop a teaching plan to assist the elderly patient who has a small appetite increase his or her nutritional intake with appropriate foods.
3. Assess each elderly patient assigned for signs of polypharmacy.

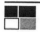

STEPS TOWARD BETTER COMMUNICATION

VOCABULARY BUILDING GLOSSARY

Term	Pronunciation	Definition
A. Individual Terms		
address (verb)	ad DRESS	to deal with; to treat a problem
chore	CHORE	work, a routine job to be done that is not fun
clutter	CLUT ter	objects scattered around, not neat
cueing	CUE ing	giving a reminder
engaged	en GAGEd	turned on, put into active use
enhance	en HANCE	to improve, to add to in order to make better
imperative	im PER a tive	necessary; urgent
inclement	in CLEM ent	refers to bad or severe conditions, especially weather
odoriferous	o dor IF er ous	smelly; having a strong odor
prudently	PRU dent ly	carefully; with good judgment
B. Phrase		
coupled with	COUP led with	together with; joined with

COMPLETION

A. Directions: Fill in the blank(s) with the correct term(s) from the Vocabulary Building Glossary to complete the sentence.

1. It was difficult for D.R. to __________________ the problem of the high cost of the new prescription since she is on a fixed income.
2. It is __________________ to stop S.P. from driving, as he has suffered a stroke and becomes confused easily.
3. Signs were posted at the entrance to the dining room of the assisted living facility for __________________ the residents as to the day, date, and season.
4. Having lots of __________________ such as old boxes and magazines stacked all over tends to lead to accidents in the home of the older adult.
5. Having someone with whom to eat meals can greatly __________________ both the appetite and quality of living of the older adult.
6. The older adult who remains __________________ in the community by doing volunteer work tends to be healthier.

B. Directions: Substitute words from the Vocabulary Building Glossary above for the underlined words in the paragraph below.

<u>Together with</u> the mud from the <u>bad</u> weather we were having, cleaning up the <u>mess</u> was quite a <u>job</u>. <u>With good judgment</u>, I <u>took care of</u> the problem by <u>using</u> help to clean up the <u>smelly</u> mess. The situation was <u>improved</u> by <u>reminding</u> my helper that it was <u>necessary</u> to finish early.

PRONUNCIATION OF DIFFICULT TERMS

Directions: Practice pronouncing the following words.

dysphagia	dys PHA gi a
orthostatic hypotension	OR tho STAT ic HY po TEN sion
presbycusis	pres by CU sis
presbyopia	pres by O pi a
rehabilitative	RE ha BIL i ta tive

COMMUNICATION EXERCISE

1. Write out the questions you would ask a patient to get information about current prescriptions, over-the-counter drugs, and any vitamins and herbal preparations being taken (See textbook chapter 38). Practice asking the questions with a partner.
2. Write an explanation you would give a patient about how to use a medication reminder system you have developed. Practice it with a partner who will play the role of the patient and ask questions for clarification.
3. With a partner, write a short dialogue in which you assess an elderly patient's activity, nutrition, medications, and elimination habits during a home visit with the patient. Write your questions and the patient's possible responses.

Review the chapter highlights, answer the study questions, and complete the critical thinking activities at the end of the chapter in the textbook.

THIRTY-NINE

Common Psychosocial Care Problems of the Elderly

TERMINOLOGY

A. MATCHING

Directions: Match the terms in column I with the definitions in column II.

Column I

1. __D__ behavior modification
2. __h__ delirium
3. __C__ dementia
4. __A__ depression
5. __e__ electroconvulsive therapy (ECT)
6. __B__ nocturnal delirium
7. __F__ reminiscence
8. __g__ resocialization

Column II

a. A morbid sadness, dejection, or melancholy
b. Increase in symptoms of confusion or agitation as sunlight fades
c. Permanent impairment of memory, intellectual functioning, and ability to problem solve
d. Intervention used to change agitated behavior by giving positive feedback for desired behaviors and negative feedback for undesired behaviors
e. Electric shock to the brain in an effort to change symptoms of severe depression
f. Re-examine the past to promote socialization and mental stimulation
g. Encourage active socialization patterns with a group
h. Acute confusional state that can occur as a result of an underlying biologic or psychologic cause

B. COMPLETION

Directions: Fill in the blank(s) with the correct term(s) from the terms list in the chapter in the textbook to complete the sentence.

1. The lapses in memory that occur as people get older are termed ____________________.
2. Making lists of things is one way to cope with ____________________.
3. Stimulating the senses while introducing factual information is used during ____________________ therapy.

4. The ______________________ are one class of antidepressants that have proven helpful in treating depression in the elderly.
5. Sharing family photos is a technique used for ______________________ therapy.

IDENTIFICATION

Directions: Identify the condition for which each of the following symptoms/signs occurs. Use "delirium," "dementia," or "depression." Symptoms/signs may occur with more than one condition.

1. Resolves with treatment ______________________
2. Impaired memory for recent events ______________________
3. Sparse, repetitive speech ______________________
4. Sudden onset ______________________
5. Despair, worry ______________________
6. Coherent speech ______________________
7. Poor prognosis ______________________
8. Inability to perform activities of daily living (ADLs) ______________________
9. Changes in sleep-wake cycle ______________________
10. Self-neglect ______________________
11. Intact remote memory ______________________
12. Decreased ability to concentrate ______________________

SHORT ANSWER

Directions: Write a brief answer for each question.

1. Identify four principles of nursing care for the patient with cognitive impairment.
   a. ______________________
   b. ______________________
   c. ______________________
   d. ______________________
2. Explain the interrelationship of alcohol abuse, suicide, and depression in the elderly patient.
   ____
   ____
   ____
   ____
3. List five crimes commonly occurring to the elderly along with one intervention that could possibly prevent the crime.
   a. ______________________
   ____
   b. ______________________
   ____
   c. ______________________
   ____
   d. ______________________
   ____
   e. ______________________
   ____

4. Identify the four main categories of elder abuse with an example for each one.
   a. ______________________________
   b. ______________________________
   c. ______________________________
   d. ______________________________

5. Identify two future psychosocial issues for the elderly population.
   a. ______________________________
   b. ______________________________

6. When assessing significant changes in mental functioning in an elderly person, you should ______________________________
____
____

7. When assessing an elderly person, you should exercise ____________ and allow enough time for the person to ____________.

8. Five factors that can contribute to an altered mental state in the elderly are:
   a. ______________________________
   b. ______________________________
   c. ______________________________
   d. ______________________________
   e. ______________________________

9. Signs of confusion include ______________________________
____
______________________________.

10. Dementia is characterized by a slow, insidious onset that affects ______________________________
______________________________.

11. When a plan of care with therapy to decrease confusion and disorientation is implemented, it is very important that ______________________________.

12. The desired effects of drugs when used for patients with dementia are to ______________________________
______________________________.

13. Family support is essential when one member is suffering from dementia because the family members are subject to ______________________________
____
____

14. Families who are caring for a member with dementia should be encouraged to take advantage of ____________ opportunities in their community.

15. Three characteristics for each stage of Alzheimer's disease are:
   a. Early stage: ______________________________
   ____
   b. Middle stage: ______________________________
   ____
   c. Late stage: ______________________________
   ____

16. Aggressive behavior may also occur as a self-protective response to ______________________________.

17. When agitation and hostility become a problem, physical restraints are only used
____.

18. For the patient with paranoia, developing ____________________ is the most important goal to accomplish.

19. Identify three interventions to decrease wandering.
    a. ____________________
    b. ____________________
    c. ____________________

20. The underlying principle for developing interventions for the patient experiencing "sun-down syndrome" is to ____________________.

21. Three strategies to improve nutritional status of the patient with dementia are:
    a. ____________________
    b. ____________________
    c. ____________________

22. Signs of depression in the elderly may be slightly different and could include:
____
____

23. Alcoholism should be considered if the elderly person has some of the following signs and symptoms:
____
____
____

24. It is especially important to protect the depressed patient from self-injury after ____________________ has been initiated.

25. Signs of potential suicide are
____
____.

TABLE ACTIVITY

Directions: Fill in the following table with the cause, signs and symptoms, methods of diagnosis, and treatment for Alzheimer's disease.

	Alzheimer's Disease
Cause	
Signs and Symptoms	
Diagnosis	
Treatment	

MULTIPLE CHOICE

*Directions: Choose the **best** answer to each of the following questions.*

1. B.R., a 79-year-old female, lives with her son. She has come into the clinic for the second time with bruises and abrasions she claims came from a fall. She seems unkempt and says she has difficulty grooming and dressing because of the severe arthritis in her hands. She is very thin. You know that in order to assess her for elder abuse it is necessary to first
   1. confront her with the facts.
   2. establish a confidential, trusting relationship.
   3. remove her from her current living situation.
   4. say you do not believe the injuries are from a fall.

2. If there seems to be a likelihood of elder abuse involved in B.R.'s injuries, you know
   1. definite proof is necessary before calling the authorities.
   2. it must be corroborated by a third person.
   3. legally, it must be reported to the authorities.
   4. nothing can be done if B.R. denies abuse occurred.

3. Sometimes elder abuse can be avoided by
   1. admonishing the elder to "do as she is told."
   2. making weekly visits to the home.
   3. obtaining help for the caregiver with daily care.
   4. medicating the elder to improve behavior.

4. N.D., your neighbor, shares with you that two of his elderly friends have been victims of telemarketing crime lately. He asks for advice on how to avoid this. You tell him
   1. refrain from answering the phone in the evening.
   2. not to put his telephone number on forms requesting it.
   3. give only a false credit card number to a phone solicitor.
   4. not to order anything over the telephone; ask for written information.

5. P.C., age 82, is displaying signs of confusion. Before assuming that her confusion is related to mental causes, you should
   1. question her family about a cause.
   2. obtain an order for an antidepressant.
   3. check her fluid and electrolyte status.
   4. perform a mental status exam.

6. P.C.'s confusion is worsening. Reality orientation is part of her therapy. Which one of the following would be part of reality orientation?
   1. displaying memory aids such as a clock and calendar
   2. singing favorite songs with a group
   3. relating a favorite past experience to the group
   4. helping serve refreshments after an activity

7. P.C.'s confusion becomes worse at about 5:00 PM. One intervention that may help decrease her confusion is to
   1. institute creative therapy activities in the late afternoon.
   2. reduce stimulation in the environment.
   3. reward positive behaviors.
   4. use a security vest to keep her in the chair.

8. G.A., age 80, drinks a lot of alcohol. He is on several medications for his heart disease and hypertension. One danger of alcoholism—in addition to interaction with medication—is
   1. loss of income.
   2. increased anxiety.
   3. loss of insurance.
   4. inadequate nutrition.

9. When assessing G.A., in addition to determining his alcohol pattern, you should look for signs of
   1. underlying depression.
   2. paranoia.
   3. spousal abuse.
   4. mental deficiency.

10. If G.A. shows signs of both alcohol abuse and depression, it is *most* important to assess for
   1. social isolation.
   2. suicidal intent.
   3. accident potential.
   4. gastrointestinal bleeding.

11. Delirium in the elderly is often characterized by a(n)
   1. gradual onset.
   2. rapid onset.
   3. poor prognosis.
   4. intact remote memory.

12. A psychosocial approach for confusion/disorientation that re-examines the past to promote socialization and mental stimulation is
   1. validation therapy.
   2. remotivation therapy.
   3. reminiscence.
   4. resocialization.

13. Early-stage Alzheimer's disease is characterized by all of the following *except*
   1. mild short-term memory loss.
   2. suspicion.
   3. difficulty learning new things.
   4. mild depression.

14. Complaints of vague aches and pains, fatigue, and "just not feeling good" may be indicative of what condition in the elderly?
   1. delirium
   2. confusion
   3. depression
   4. dementia

15. Intentionally withholding medication from an elder would be considered
   1. physical abuse.
   2. social abuse.
   3. psychological abuse.
   4. neglect.

16. Clues to alcoholism may include all of the following *except*
   1. mental alertness.
   2. insomnia.
   3. gastritis.
   4. anemia.

17. Three conditions that are interrelated and have similar risk factors associated with loss are
   1. alcohol abuse, suicide, and dementia.
   2. drug abuse, suicide, and delirium.
   3. alcohol abuse, suicide, and depression.
   4. alcohol abuse, depression, and elder abuse.

18. A primary nursing intervention for a depressed patient *after* he or she has initiated antidepressive therapy is
   1. protection for other people.
   2. avoidance of contact with other depressed patients.
   3. protection from self-injury.
   4. avoidance of overly concerned family members.

19. Elder abuse is often related to
   1. caregiver stress and unresolved family conflicts.
   2. caregiver stress and economic problems.
   3. belligerent elder behaviors.
   4. uneducated caregivers.

20. An organization that is instrumental in helping elders achieve the goal of increasing healthy life after age 65 is the
    1. UAW.
    2. AARP.
    3. Salvation Army.
    4. NOW.

CRITICAL THINKING ACTIVITIES

1. It has been two years since V.E.'s husband died. She has not been able to shake her depression and has become more withdrawn in the past month. She comes to the clinic for monitoring of her diabetes. What plan could you devise to assist B.E. to deal with her depression?
2. You suspect that J.P. is being abused by the grandson with whom he lives. Identify signs that might contribute to your suspicion. How would you approach J.P. about this issue?
3. What three things do you feel should be done to address the challenges that will face the elderly in another ten years?

MEETING CLINICAL OBJECTIVES

Directions: The following suggested activities will help you meet the stated clinical practice objectives for the chapter. Review your school's clinical objectives for the week and outline a plan of activities that will help you meet them. If unsure as to how to meet them, consult with your instructor at the beginning of the clinical day.

1. Assess each elderly patient assigned for signs of depression.
2. Formulate a teaching plan for the elderly members of a church group regarding ways to avoid crimes against the elderly. Include specific measures.
3. Your patient is in the middle stage of Alzheimer's disease. Write a care plan to deal with her cognitive impairment and need for assistance with ADLs.

STEPS TOWARD BETTER COMMUNICATION

VOCABULARY BUILDING GLOSSARY

Term	Pronunciation	Definition
A. Individual Terms		
adaptation	a dap TA tion	change to function in a new way; adjustment
advocacy	AD vo ca cy	supporting or working for a person or an issue
condescending	CON de SCEND ing	having a self-important or superior attitude
distraction	di STRAC tion	turning the attention to something else
implications	im pli CA tions	suggestions
inflicted	in FLIC ted	forced upon someone
insidious	in SID i ous	something bad or harmful that is not easily seen

manifestation	man i FES TA tion	an example; a sign
pose	POSE	to present or put forward
retaliation	re TAL i A tion	doing something bad to someone because of what they did; striking back
scams	SCAMS	schemes or plans to make money by deceiving people
symptomatic	symp to MA tic	based on symptoms
undetected	un de TEC ted	not seen or discovered
unkempt	un KEMPT	messy; deficient in order and neatness

B. Phrases

go to sleep for the last time	go to SLEEP for the LAST time	to die in one's sleep
one-stop-shopping	one-stop-shop ping	everything needed is available at one place
out to get them	out to GET them	threatening them; intending harm or danger
solely attributable to	SOLE ly at TRIB-u ta ble to	caused only by one thing
the graying of America	the GRAY ing of a MER i ca	the increasing number of older people in the United States (because of better health care)
white collar crime	WHITE COL lar crime	criminal acts through a business or office involving paper or money schemes; not physical crime like taking a purse, or breaking into a house

COMPLETION

Directions: Underline the words from the Vocabulary Building Glossary in the following sentences, and fill in the blanks correctly with one of the words below.

advocacy/ condescending /implication /unkempt /pose

1. The scams inflicted on the ________________ woman were undetected.
2. ________________ for respite care is very welcome for caregivers.
3. Retaliation may be symptomatic when a caregiver is angry and can ________________ an insidious danger to a patient.
4. A ________________ attitude is sometimes a manifestation of low self-esteem.
5. The use of distraction and adaptation is an ________________ that the nurse understand how to deal with the patient's outburst.

WORD ATTACK SKILLS

Directions: Look at these words composed of a stem and suffix.

adaptation
distraction
implication
manifestation
retaliation

-ation—is a suffix added to a verb to create a noun. The meaning of the noun is an action or process connected with the verb.

Verb	Meaning	Noun	Meaning
adapt	to change to fit the situation	adaptation	a change to suit the situation
distract	to put attention on something else	distraction	an action that puts the attention on something else
imply	to suggest indirectly	implication	an indirect suggestion
manifest	to exhibit, to show	manifestation	a sign showing or displaying something
retaliate	to respond to an action with another similar action	retaliation	a direct response to an action with a similar action

PRONUNCIATION OF DIFFICULT TERMS

Directions: Practice pronouncing the following words and phrases with a peer.

benign senescent forgetfulness	be NIGN se NES cent for GET ful ness
electroconvulsive therapy	e LEC tro con VUL sive ther a py
remotivation therapy	re mo ti VA tion THER a py
resocialization therapy	re SO cial i ZA tion THER a py
reminiscense	rem i NIS cense
selective serotonin reuptake inhibitors	se LEC tive ser o TON in re UP take in HIB i tors

COMMUNICATION EXERCISE

Dealing with the possibility of elder abuse is a sensitive issue. The following is an example of how this issue might be approached with the patient mentioned in Critical Thinking Exercise #2 above.

Nurse: How do you like living with your grandson, J.P.?

J.P.: I guess it's O.K.

Nurse: Young people don't always understand what it is like to be older. Sometimes they become impatient with older people.

J.P.: You can say that again.

Nurse: Has that happened to you?

J.P.: He is always wanting me to hurry, and he asks another question before I can get out an answer to his first one. I move rather slowly, and that irritates him too.

Nurse: I noticed these marks on your upper arm, J.P. Do you know how those happened?

J.P.: I'm not sure. Sometimes he will grab my arm and pull me along when he is a hurry to get to the car.

Nurse: Are there other ways in which he becomes impatient with you?

J.P.: I stumbled and fell one day when he kind of had a hold of me and was dragging me into the house. I don't think he meant to hurt me.

Nurse: I'll talk to him about giving you time to do things, J.P. I don't want you to get really hurt.

Directions: Write a dialogue explaining to a family the effects of alcohol on medications and the chronic health conditions (hypertension and gastritis) of their father. Be ready to answer their questions and objections and denials. Compare your dialogue with your partner's, combine the two dialogues into one, and practice the dialogue together.

CULTURAL POINTS

Does your native country or cultural community have any of the problems of the elderly that are described in this chapter? If not, why do you think it is different? If you do, how are they handled? Have you seen any of these problems in your own family? What about your grandparents? If they had any of these problems, how were they cared for and what were the family and society attitudes about the problems? Would things be different today? Talk about these questions in a group, preferably with people from different cultures. Compare your attitudes. What similarities and differences do you find? Notes for discussion:

Review the chapter highlights, answer the study questions, and complete the critical thinking activities at the end of the chapter in the textbook.

Performance Checklists

SKILL 14-1 POSTMORTEM CARE

Student: Diane Pepperdine

Date: 2-5-03

		Satisfactory	Unsatisfactory
1.	Carries out Standard Steps A, B, C, D, and E as need indicates.	☐	☐
2.	Prepares equipment and provides privacy.	☑	☐
3.	Washes hands and dons gloves.	☑	☐
4.	Positions body supine, in proper alignment, with head slightly elevated.	☑	☐
5.	Replaces dentures as appropriate, closes mouth and secures it.	☑	☐
6.	Removes jewelry and clothing and prepares items to be returned to family.	☑	☐
7.	Cleans body appropriately and combs hair.	☑	☐
8.	Removes or secures all tubes and lines, and changes dressings.	☑	☐
9.	Dresses body in clean gown and straightens room.	☑	☐
10.	Allows viewing time for family; remains in room to offer emotional support.	☑	☐
11.	Follows agency procedure for tagging body and preparing it in a shroud.	☑	☐
12.	Removes gloves and washes hands.	☑	☐
13.	Transports the body to the morgue.	☑	☐
14.	Documents the procedure.	☑	☐

Pass ☑
Fail ☐

Comments:

Instructor: [illegible signature]

SKILL 15-2 USING PERSONAL PROTECTIVE EQUIPMENT: GOWN AND MASK

Student: ____________________

Date: ____________________

		Satisfactory	Unsatisfactory
1.	Correctly puts on gown.	❑	❑
2.	Places mask to cover nose and mouth and secures it correctly.	❑	❑
3.	Dons protective eyewear.	❑	❑
4.	Dons shoe covering and head cover if indicated.	❑	❑
5.	Dons non-sterile gloves and pulls gloves over gown cuffs.	❑	❑
6.	Removes PPEs in correct order.	❑	❑
7.	Correctly disposes of PPEs without contaminating self.	❑	❑
8.	Washes the hands.	❑	❑

Pass ❑
Fail ❑

Comments:

Instructor: ____________________

SKILL 16-1 PERFORMING A SURGICAL HAND SCRUB

Student: ____________________

Date: ____________________

		Satisfactory	Unsatisfactory
1.	Removes jewelry.	❑	❑
2.	Adjusts water to correct temperature and force.	❑	❑
3.	Wets hands and arms from above elbows to fingertips, keeping hands higher than elbows.	❑	❑
4.	Applies soaping agent or uses soap impregnated brush or sponge pad. Works up a lather.	❑	❑
5.	Cleans nails on each hand while holding the scrub brush/pad in other hand.	❑	❑
6.	Starts scrubbing at fingertips with a circular motion scrubs each finger, between fingers, palm and back of hand using light to moderate friction; scrubs wrist and up the arm to 2" above the elbow.	❑	❑
7.	Scrubs each arm for approximately 2–2½ minutes. Times the scrub by the clock.	❑	❑
8.	Rinses each hand and arm thoroughly keeping the hands pointed up and allowing water to run from the fingertips down off of the elbow area.	❑	❑
9.	Turns off water using foot or knee control.	❑	❑
10.	Dries hands with a sterile towel without contaminating sterile field or scrubbed hands.	❑	❑
11.	Drops used towel into proper receptacle.	❑	❑

Pass ❑
Fail ❑

Comments:

Instructor: ____________________

SKILL 16-2 OPENING STERILE PACKS AND PREPARING A STERILE FIELD

Student: ______________________________

Date: ______________________________

		Satisfactory	Unsatisfactory
1.	Carries out Standard Steps A, B, C, D, and E as indicated for the procedure.	❑	❑
2.	Clears a working surface.	❑	❑
3.	Removes outer wrap.	❑	❑
4.	Opens pack with proper aseptic technique.	❑	❑
5.	Arranges items on the sterile field.	❑	❑
6.	Performs procedure.	❑	❑
7.	Carries out Standard Steps X, Y, and Z.	❑	❑

Pass ❑
Fail ❑

Comments:

Instructor: ______________________

SKILL 16-3 STERILE GLOVING AND UNGLOVING

Student: ____________________

Date: ____________________

		Satisfactory	Unsatisfactory
1.	Obtains pair of sterile gloves of correct size; washes hands.	❑	❑
2.	Peels open outer wrapper and positions inner glove package on flat surface.	❑	❑
3.	Opens the inner glove package exposing the gloves without contaminating them.	❑	❑
4.	Picks up the first glove by the folded over cuff.	❑	❑
5.	Inserts hand into glove without touching the outside of the glove to any part of the skin or other unsterile object; keeps hands above waist level.	❑	❑
6.	Picks up the second glove by placing gloved fingers under the cuff slips hand into the glove being careful not to allow bare skin to touch the other gloved hand.	❑	❑
7.	Slides cuffs over the wrists; adjusts the fingers inside the gloves.	❑	❑
Ungloving			
8.	Grasps the outside surface of one glove at the top of the palm and pulls glove off while rolling it inside out.	❑	❑
9.	Holds removed glove in palm of other hand; slips bare fingers under the cuff of the remaining glove and slides the glove down over the hand, rolling it inside-out as it is removed.	❑	❑
10.	Disposes of the contaminated gloves.	❑	❑
11.	Washes the hands.	❑	❑

Pass ❑
Fail ❑

Comments:

Instructor: ____________________

SKILL 18-4 SHAMPOOING HAIR

Student: ______________________________

Date: ______________________________

		Satisfactory	Unsatisfactory
1.	Carries out Standard Steps A, B, C, D, and E as need indicates.	❑	❑
2.	Raises the bed, lowers the near side rail, and moves patient to near side of bed.	❑	❑
3.	Drapes the patient.	❑	❑
4.	Brushes or combs tangles from hair.	❑	❑
5.	Positions shampoo tray and places drainage receptacle beneath spout of tray.	❑	❑
6.	Obtains warm water in pitcher maintaining patient safety.	❑	❑
7.	Moistens hair and applies shampoo.	❑	❑
8.	Works shampoo into hair massaging scalp thoroughly.	❑	❑
9.	Rinses hair.	❑	❑
10.	Repeats shampoo process if needed.	❑	❑
11.	Applies conditioner if needed; rinses thoroughly.	❑	❑
12.	Wraps head in towel, dries face and shoulders .	❑	❑
13.	Removes shampoo tray and drainage receptacle.	❑	❑
14.	Towel-dries hair or uses hair dryer.	❑	❑
15.	Repositions patient for comfort.	❑	❑
16.	Finishes arranging hair.	❑	❑
17.	Lowers bed, raises rail, and restores unit.	❑	❑
18.	Cleans and stores equipment.	❑	❑
19.	Documents the procedure.	❑	❑

Pass ❑
Fail ❑

Comments:

Instructor: ______________________

SKILL 19-3 APPLYING A PROTECTIVE DEVICE

Student: ______________________________

Date: ______________________________

		Satisfactory	Unsatisfactory
1.	Carries out Standard Steps A, B, C, D, and E as need indicates.	❑	❑
2.	Explains the purpose and need for the device to the patient and family.	❑	❑
3.	Applies the security device correctly.	❑	❑
4.	Checks for correct application.	❑	❑
5.	Secures device correctly with a half-bow knot.		
6.	Verbalizes need to check on patient at specific intervals.	❑	❑
7.	Verbalizes need to remove device and exercise joints and muscles every 2 hours.	❑	❑
8.	Documents reason for use of restraint, other measures attempted, and correct application of device.	❑	❑
9.	Carries out Standard Steps X, Y, and Z.	❑	❑

Pass ❑
Fail ❑

Comments:

Instructor: ______________________

SKILL 23-1 OBTAINING BLOOD SAMPLES WITH A VACUTAINER SYSTEM

Student: ______________________________

Date: ______________________________

		Satisfactory	Unsatisfactory
1.	Carries out Standard Steps A, B, C, D, and E as need indicates.	❑	❑
2.	Washes hands and dons latex gloves.	❑	❑
3.	Selects an appropriate venipuncture site and positions the tourniquet; has patient form a fist with the hand.	❑	❑
4.	Cleanses the area thoroughly.	❑	❑
5.	Punctures the site and gathers needed blood samples.	❑	❑
6.	Releases the tourniquet.	❑	❑
7.	Withdraws the needle and applies a dry gauze pad and pressure to the site.	❑	❑
8.	When bleeding has stopped, applies an adhesive bandage.	❑	❑
9.	Disposes of used equipment properly; removes gloves and washes hands.	❑	❑
10.	Places labels on tubes and prepares them for transport to the laboratory with the requisition slips.	❑	❑
11.	Documents the procedure.	❑	❑

Pass ❑
Fail ❑

Comments:

Instructor: ______________________

SKILL 23-2 PERFORMING CAPILLARY BLOOD TESTS: BLOOD GLUCOSE OR HEMOGLOBIN

Student: ____________________

Date: ____________________

		Satisfactory	Unsatisfactory
1.	Carries out Standard Steps A, B, C, D, and E as need indicates.	❑	❑
2.	Prepares the hand and finger for the test.	❑	❑
3.	Washes hands and puts on gloves.	❑	❑
4.	Prepares the fingerstick site.	❑	❑
5.	Turns on the machine and prepares the lancet.	❑	❑
6.	Checks that the machine is set properly.	❑	❑
For Glucometer (Follows Directions for Type of Machine)			
7.	Inserts a test strip into the machine.	❑	❑
8.	Performs the fingerstick.	❑	❑
9.	Correctly obtains drop of blood.	❑	❑
10.	Places drop of blood on test strip.	❑	❑
11.	Applies cotton ball or gauze to finger to stop bleeding.	❑	❑
12.	Notes the reading on the screen and documents it.	❑	❑
For Hemoglobin Test			
13.	After step 6, performs the fingerstick, wipes away the first drop of blood with gauze pad; gathers second drop in capillary collection device.	❑	❑
14.	Gently wipes the flat back side of the test stick on the clean gauze pad.	❑	❑
15.	Places cotton ball or gauze firmly against puncture site to stop bleeding.	❑	❑
16.	Places capillary collection device in the machine.	❑	❑
17.	Reads and documents the result.	❑	❑
For Both Tests			
18.	Turns off the machine and properly disposes of used equipment.	❑	❑
19.	Applies bandage to puncture site as needed.	❑	❑
20.	Removes gloves and washes hands.	❑	❑

Pass ❑
Fail ❑

Comments:

Instructor: ____________________

SKILL 23-3 PERFORMING A URINE DIPSTICK TEST

Student: ______________________________

Date: ______________________________

		Satisfactory	Unsatisfactory
1.	Carries out Standard Steps A, B, C, D, and E as need indicates.	❑	❑
2.	Fills out report slip with patient information.	❑	❑
3.	Obtains a urine specimen.	❑	❑
4.	Washes hands and dons gloves.	❑	❑
5.	Wets a dipstick correctly.	❑	❑
6.	Times and reads the series of tests accurately.	❑	❑
7.	Notes the test results on the report slip.	❑	❑
8.	Disposes of urine and used equipment appropriately.	❑	❑
9.	Removes gloves and washes hands.	❑	❑
10.	Delivers the report slip to the person who ordered the test.	❑	❑

Pass ❑
Fail ❑

Comments:

Instructor: ______________________________

SKILL 23-4 ASSISTING WITH A PELVIC EXAMINATION AND PAP TEST (SMEAR)

Student: ______________________________

Date: ______________________________

		Satisfactory	Unsatisfactory
1.	Carries out Standard Steps A, B, C, D, and E as need indicates.	❑	❑
2.	Labels slide with patient's name and date.	❑	❑
3.	Fills out requisition slip.	❑	❑
4.	Sets up the table and equipment.	❑	❑
5.	Readies patient and positions on table with appropriate draping.	❑	❑
6.	Passes equipment to examiner.	❑	❑
7.	Dons gloves and applies fixative to the slide.	❑	❑
8.	Removes gloves and washes hands.	❑	❑
9.	Assists patient after examination to arise from the table.	❑	❑
10.	Prepares slide for laboratory and sends to lab.	❑	❑
11.	Restores the examination room and disposes of used equipment and supplies properly.	❑	❑
12.	Documents procedure as necessary.	❑	❑

Pass ❑
Fail ❑

Comments:

Instructor: ______________________

SKILL 26-2 INSERTING AN NASOGASTRIC TUBE

Student: ____________________

Date: ____________________

		Satisfactory	Unsatisfactory
1.	Carries out Standard steps A, B, C, D, and E as indicated.	❏	❏
2.	Checks airflow through the nostril.	❏	❏
3.	Positions patient with HOB at 30–90 degrees.	❏	❏
4.	Provides basin, tissues, and water with straw for patient as appropriate.	❏	❏
5.	Puts on gloves.	❏	❏
6.	Measures distance to insert tube correctly.	❏	❏
7.	Prepares tube for insertion.	❏	❏
8.	Inserts tube correctly.	❏	❏
9.	Verifies correct placement of tube.	❏	❏
10.	Secures tube to patient.	❏	❏
11.	Attaches tube to suction at proper setting.	❏	❏
12.	Positions tube in most functional position.	❏	❏
13.	Removes gloves and washes hands.	❏	❏
14.	Makes patient comfortable and restores unit.	❏	❏
15.	Assesses tube function.	❏	❏
16.	Documents procedure.	❏	❏

Pass ❏
Fail ❏

Comments:

Instructor: ____________________

SKILL 26-3 ADMINISTERING A NASOGASTRIC/DUODENAL TUBE FEEDING OR FEEDING VIA A PEG TUBE

Student: ______________________________

Date: ______________________________

		Satisfactory	Unsatisfactory
1.	Carries out the Standard Steps A, B, C, D, and E as indicated.	❑	❑
2.	Elevates HOB to 30–90 degrees.	❑	❑
3.	Puts on gloves.	❑	❑
4.	Prepares feeding.	❑	❑
5.	Attaches syringe and verifies tube placement.	❑	❑
6.	Checks for residual feeding for gastrostomy tube.	❑	❑
7.	Pinches off tube and pours formula into syringe or hooks up gavage bag; regulates flow correctly.	❑	❑
8.	Prevents air from entering the tube.	❑	❑
9.	For continuous feeding: sets up feeding pump and sets rate correctly.	❑	❑
10.	Follows formula with 1–2 ounces water to clear the tube.	❑	❑
11.	Removes syringe or connecting tubing and clamps the tube for intermittent feeding.		
12.	Washes equipment appropriately.	❑	❑
13.	Removes gloves and washes hands.		
14.	Monitors lab values and weight daily.	❑	❑
15.	Documents the procedure.	❑	❑
16.	Carries out Standard Steps X, Y, and Z.	❑	❑

Pass ❑
Fail ❑

Comments:

Instructor: ______________________

SKILL 26-4 USING A FEEDING PUMP

Student: ______________________________

Date: ______________________________

		Satisfactory	Unsatisfactory
1.	Checks the order for type and amount of feeding.	❑	❑
2.	Carries out the Standard Steps.	❑	❑
3.	Washes hands and puts on gloves.	❑	❑
4.	Elevates head of bed to at least 30 degrees. Keeps bed elevated.	❑	❑
5.	Sets up feeding pump and tubing.	❑	❑
6.	Verifies tube's placement location.	❑	❑
7.	Primes tubing and attaches it to NG or PEG tube.	❑	❑
8.	Sets flow rate and turns on pump.	❑	❑
9.	Observes infusion for several minutes.	❑	❑
10.	Removes gloves and washes hands.	❑	❑
11.	Assesses patient for signs of complications periodically.	❑	❑
12.	Checks stomach residual every 4 hours.	❑	❑
13.	Documents tube status, stomach residual, and feeding.	❑	❑

Pass ❑
Fail ❑

Comments:

Instructor: ______________________

SKILL 27-1 ADMINISTERING THE HEIMLICH MANEUVER

Student: ______________________________

Date: ______________________________

		Satisfactory	Unsatisfactory
1.	Verifies that person is choking.	❑	❑
2.	Positions self to deliver appropriate thrusts.	❑	❑
3.	Places hands in correct position.	❑	❑
4.	Repeats thrust sequence until foreign body is expelled or person becomes unconscious.	❑	❑
	For Unconscious Person		
5.	Calls for help.	❑	❑
6.	Positions person on ground.	❑	❑
7.	Positions hands correctly for thrusts.	❑	❑
8.	Delivers thrusts.	❑	❑
9.	Checks mouth for debris.	❑	❑
10.	Opens airway and attempts to ventilate.	❑	❑
11.	Repeats sequence as needed.	❑	❑
	For Infant (Conscious)		
12.	Positions infant with head lower than trunk straddling arm; supports chest and jaw.	❑	❑
13.	Delivers five back blows correctly.	❑	❑
14.	Turns infant and delivers chest thrusts.	❑	❑
15.	Repeats sequence until object is dislodged.	❑	❑
	For Unconscious Infant		
16.	Places infant on hard surface and attempts to visualize object; removes with a finger.	❑	❑
17.	Opens airway and attempts to ventilate.	❑	❑
18.	If unable to ventilate, repositions head and attempts to ventilate again.	❑	❑
19.	If unable to ventilate, repositions infant for back blow and chest thrust sequence.	❑	❑
20.	Performs tongue-jaw lift after each sequence to attempt visualization of object in mouth; removes object.	❑	❑
21.	Activates EMS if obstruction not relieved within 1 minute.	❑	❑

Pass ❐
Fail ❐

Comments:

Instructor: ______________________

SKILL 27-2 CARDIOPULMONARY RESUSCITATION

Student: ______________________________

Date: ______________________________

		Satisfactory	Unsatisfactory
1.	Shakes victim and shouts.	❑	❑
2.	Positions victim supine and opens airway.	❑	❑
3.	Looks, listens, and feels for air movement.	❑	❑
4.	Calls for help.	❑	❑
5.	Forms seal and delivers 2 quick, short breaths.	❑	❑
6.	Repositions head and attempts ventilation again if first breath is unsuccessful.	❑	❑
7.	Performs Heimlich maneuver if needed.	❑	❑
8.	Checks carotid pulse.	❑	❑
9.	Positions hands on sternum correctly.	❑	❑
10.	Performs chest compressions correctly.	❑	❑
11.	Opens airway and delivers 2 breaths at appropriate intervals.	❑	❑
12.	Checks carotid pulse every minute.	❑	❑
13.	Continues rescue breathing or CPR sequence as needed until relieved or unable to continue.	❑	❑

Pass ❑
Fail ❑

Comments:

Instructor: ______________________

SKILL 28-2 APPLYING A CONDOM CATHETER

Student: ______________________________

Date: ______________________________

		Satisfactory	Unsatisfactory
1.	Carries out Standard Steps A, B, C, D, and E as need indicates.	❑	❑
2.	Washes and dries genital area; trims pubic hair as necessary.	❑	❑
3.	Applies condom catheter and smooths out adhesive surface for good adherence.	❑	❑
4.	Leaves a 1-1/2 in. space at tip of penis.	❑	❑
5.	Connects the condom catheter to a drainage tube.	❑	❑
6.	Attaches drainage bag.	❑	❑
7.	Checks to see that catheter has not become twisted, preventing urine flow.	❑	❑
8.	Carries out Standard Steps X, Y, and Z.	❑	❑

Pass ❐
Fail ❐

Comments:

Instructor: ______________________

SKILL 28-5 PERFORMING INTERMITTENT BLADDER IRRIGATION AND INSTILLATION

Student: ______________________________

Date: ______________________________

		Satisfactory	Unsatisfactory
1.	Carries out Standard Steps A, B, C, D, and E as need indicates.	❑	❑
2.	Positions and drapes patient.	❑	❑
3.	Opens irrigation tray and positions it appropriately while maintaining sterile technique.	❑	❑
4.	Pours irrigation solution or prepares solution for instillation.	❑	❑
5.	Determines amount of urine in drainage bag.	❑	❑
6.	Dons sterile gloves correctly.	❑	❑
7.	Clamps connecting tubing or disconnects tubing from catheter maintaining aseptic technique.	❑	❑
8.	Draws up solution and instills it into the catheter port.	❑	❑
9.	Uses 30–50 cc of solution for each irrigation; instills total amount of fluid ordered.	❑	❑
10.	Allows fluid to flow back after appropriate period of time.	❑	❑
11.	For irrigation, continues to irrigate 3–4 times.	❑	❑
12.	Withdraws syringe and cleanses the port with a fresh antiseptic swab.	❑	❑
13.	Cleans up used supplies.	❑	❑
14.	Carries out Standard Steps X, Y, and Z.	❑	❑

Pass ❑
Fail ❑

Comments:

Instructor: ______________________

SKILL 30-1 OPERATING A TRANSCUTANEOUS ELECTRICAL NERVE STIMULATOR (TENS) UNIT

Student: ______________________________

Date: ______________________________

		Satisfactory	Unsatisfactory
1.	Carries out Standard Steps A, B, C, D, and E as need indicates.	❑	❑
2.	Correctly applies the electrodes to the skin.	❑	❑
3.	Attaches the electrodes to the stimulator unit.	❑	❑
4.	Turns on TENS unit.	❑	❑
5.	Explains sensations that should be felt.	❑	❑
6.	Explains how to increase and decrease the amplitude of the TENS unit.	❑	❑
7.	Turns off unit and removes electrodes when treatment has ended.	❑	❑
8.	Assists in cleaning the skin and rearranging clothing.	❑	❑
9.	Assesses how patient tolerated the procedure.	❑	❑
10.	Document the treatment and results.	❑	❑

Pass ❑
Fail ❑

Comments:

Instructor: ______________________

SKILL 30-2 SETTING UP (OR MONITORING) A PATIENT-CONTROLLED ANALGESIA (PCA) PUMP

Student: ______________________________

Date: ______________________________

		Satisfactory	Unsatisfactory
1.	Carries out Standard Steps A, B, C, D, and E as need indicates.	❑	❑
2.	Assembles the equipment.	❑	❑
3.	Starts an IV if one does not exist.	❑	❑
4.	Assembles the PCA ordered medication vial and tubing.	❑	❑
5.	Flushes air from system.	❑	❑
6.	Connects the primed IV set and PCA tubing.	❑	❑
7.	Inserts vial into PCA pump correctly.	❑	❑
8.	Plugs the PCA pump into a power source.	❑	❑
9.	Sets the PCA pump according to ordered parameters.	❑	❑
10.	Opens all slide clamps.	❑	❑
11.	Reviews for patient how to use the pump.	❑	❑
12.	Assesses the patient frequently for ability to use the pump and for effectiveness and side effects of the medication.	❑	❑
13.	Documents use of pump, effectiveness, and any side effects.	❑	❑

Pass ❑
Fail ❑

Comments:

Instructor: ______________________

SKILL 32-1 ADMINISTERING ORAL MEDICATIONS

Student: ______________________________

Date: ______________________________

		Satisfactory	Unsatisfactory
1.	Carries out Standard Steps A, B, C, D, and E as need indicates.	❑	❑
2.	Verifies that MAR orders have been compared with physician's orders.	❑	❑
3.	Takes medication cart to patient's room.	❑	❑
4.	Verifies patient is ready to receive medications.	❑	❑
5.	Performs first check of medications to be given cross-checking the drug name, dosage, route ordered, date and time to be given, and expiration date of the drug.	❑	❑
6.	Performs a second check of each medication.	❑	❑
7.	Verbalizes signs and symptoms of adverse effects and any special precautions for each medication to be given.	❑	❑
8.	Pours liquid medications correctly.	❑	❑
9.	Identifies the patient by checking the I.D. band, comparing name and hospital number to information imprinted on MAR or card.	❑	❑
10.	Checks each medication a third time and tells the patient what the medication is for.	❑	❑
11.	Pours water for use of patient in taking the medications.	❑	❑
12.	Positions patient properly and assesses vital signs as indicated.	❑	❑
13.	Administers medications, observing patient taking them.	❑	❑
14.	Documents medication doses taken.	❑	❑
15.	Repeats the process for the next patient.	❑	❑
16.	Returns the unit-dose cart and supplies to the central area.	❑	❑

Pass ❑
Fail ❑

Comments:

Instructor: ______________________

SKILL 32-2 INSTILLING EYE MEDICATIONS

Student: ______________________________

Date: ______________________________

		Satisfactory	Unsatisfactory
1.	Carries out Standard Steps A, B, C, D and E as need indicates. (Checks medication; washes hands thoroughly.)	❑	❑
2.	Positions patient properly for procedure.	❑	❑
3.	Exposes the conjunctival sac and instills correct number of drops of medication, or amount of ointment, into the sac.	❑	❑
4.	Occludes lacrimal duct for 1–2 minutes.	❑	❑
5.	Cautions patient not to clamp eye tightly shut.	❑	❑
6.	For ointment, has patient roll eye around.	❑	❑
7.	Cleanses excess medication off of eyelid.	❑	❑
8.	Carries out Standard Steps X, Y, and Z.	❑	❑

Pass ❑
Fail ❑

Comments:

Instructor: ______________________

SKILL 32-3 ADMINISTERING TOPICAL SKIN MEDICATIONS

Student: ____________________

Date: ____________________

		Satisfactory	Unsatisfactory
1.	Carries out Standard Steps A, B, C, D, and E as need indicates. (Checks medications three times.)	❑	❑
	To Apply Lotion		
2.	Prepares work surface and shakes lotion.	❑	❑
3.	Moistens gauze or cotton balls using aseptic technique.	❑	❑
4.	Applies the liquid to the affected area by patting.	❑	❑
5.	Discards gauze or cotton balls correctly, recaps medicine.	❑	❑
	For Application of Cream or Ointment		
6.	Applies the medication with a gloved finger or a tongue blade correctly.	❑	❑
7.	Applies dressing if ordered.	❑	❑
	For Antianginal Ointment		
8.	Measures correct amount of ointment using paper measuring guide.	❑	❑
9.	Applies paper to the patient's skin distributing the ointment beneath the paper gently.	❑	❑
10.	Removes all old ointment from previous site.	❑	❑
11.	Washes hands after removing gloves.	❑	❑
12.	Carries out Standard Steps X, Y, and Z.	❑	❑

Pass ❑
Fail ❑

Comments:

Instructor: ____________________

SKILL 32-4 ADMINISTERING MEDICATION THROUGH A FEEDING TUBE

Student: ______________________________

Date: ______________________________

		Satisfactory	Unsatisfactory
1.	Carries out Standard Steps A, B, C, D, and E as need indicates.	❑	❑
2.	Checks each medication three times and assesses all necessary parameters.	❑	❑
3.	Crushes medications that can be safely crushed and administered; mixes each medication with 5–15 mL of warm water.	❑	❑
4.	Correctly identifies the patient.	❑	❑
5.	Correctly positions the patient.	❑	❑
6.	Dons gloves and prepares tube for medication administration.	❑	❑
7.	Administers each medication with at least 10 mL of water between them.	❑	❑
8.	Irrigates with 15–30 mL of water after last medication.	❑	❑
9.	Clamps or plugs tube for 30 minutes before reattaching to suction or restarts feeding at appropriate time.	❑	❑
10.	Leaves HOB up for 30–60 minutes.	❑	❑
11.	Cleans up equipment, removes gloves, and washes hands.	❑	❑
12.	Restores the unit.	❑	❑
13.	Documents procedure.	❑	❑

Pass ❑
Fail ❑

Comments:

Instructor: ______________________

SKILL 33-1 ADMINISTERING AN INTRADERMAL INJECTION

Student: ______________________________

Date: ______________________________

		Satisfactory	Unsatisfactory
1.	Carries out Standard Steps A, B, C, D, and E as need indicates.	❑	❑
2.	Checks the medication with the MAR using the five rights.	❑	❑
3.	Draws up the medication correctly.	❑	❑
4.	Rechecks the medication using the five rights.	❑	❑
5.	Properly identifies the patient.	❑	❑
6.	Dons gloves and cleanses the injection area.	❑	❑
7.	Gives injection and forms bleb.	❑	❑
8.	Carries out Standard Steps X, Y, and Z.	❑	❑

Pass ❑
Fail ❑

Comments:

Instructor: ______________________________

SKILL 33-2 ADMINISTERING A SUBCUTANEOUS INJECTION

Student: ________________________________

Date: ________________________________

		Satisfactory	Unsatisfactory
1.	Carries out Standard Steps A, B, C, D, and E as need indicates.	❑	❑
2.	Prepares the medication following the five rights.	❑	❑
3.	Properly identifies the patient.	❑	❑
4.	Dons gloves and selects appropriate site.	❑	❑
5.	Cleanses site and administers injection correctly.	❑	❑
6.	Removes needle quickly and massages site if appropriate.	❑	❑
7.	Carries out Standard Steps X, Y, and Z.	❑	❑

Pass ❐
Fail ❐

Comments:

Instructor: ____________________

SKILL 33-3 ADMINISTERING AN INTRAMUSCULAR INJECTION

Student: ______________________________

Date: ______________________________

		Satisfactory	Unsatisfactory
1.	Carries out Standard Steps A, B, C, D, and E as need indicates.	❑	❑
2.	Verifies the medication with the MAR using the five rights.	❑	❑
3.	Draws up the medication correctly.	❑	❑
4.	Rechecks the medication using the five rights.	❑	❑
5.	Properly identifies the patient.	❑	❑
6.	Chooses appropriate location and utilizes correct landmarks for site.	❑	❑
7.	Dons gloves, cleanses area, and gives injection correctly.	❑	❑
8.	Removes needle quickly and massages area.	❑	❑
9.	Carries out Standard Steps X, Y, and Z.	❑	❑

Pass ❒
Fail ❒

Comments:

Instructor: ______________________

SKILL 34-1 STARTING THE PRIMARY INTRAVENOUS SOLUTION

Student: ______________________________

Date: ______________________________

		Satisfactory	Unsatisfactory
1.	Carries out Standard Steps A, B, C, D, and E as need indicates.	❑	❑
2.	Checks the IV solution with the order.	❑	❑
3.	Checks solution for sterility and expiration date.	❑	❑
4.	Attaches IV administration set efficiently without contaminating it.	❑	❑
5.	Clears tubing of air without wasting solution.	❑	❑
6.	Places time tape label on container and marks it correctly.	❑	❑
7.	Re-verifies IV solution and additives, if any, with MAR.	❑	❑
8.	Verifies patient identity correctly.	❑	❑
9.	Chooses appropriate IV site for infusion.	❑	❑
10.	Prepares the IV site properly.	❑	❑
11.	Dons gloves and inserts IV cannula or needle.	❑	❑
12.	Removes tourniquet and attaches IV tubing; begins infusion.	❑	❑
13.	Observes for any problems with infusion.	❑	❑
14.	Applies a sterile dressing to IV site; secures tubing to the patient.	❑	❑
15.	Regulates IV flow as ordered.	❑	❑
16.	Carries out Standard Steps X, Y, and Z.	❑	❑

Pass ❑
Fail ❑

Comments:

Instructor: ______________________________

SKILL 34-2 ADDING A NEW SOLUTION TO THE INTRAVENOUS INFUSION

Student: ______________________________

Date: ______________________________

		Satisfactory	Unsatisfactory
1.	Carries out Standard Steps A, B, C, D, and E as need indicates.	❑	❑
2.	Checks the solution for sterility and expiration date.	❑	❑
3.	Compares label with order.	❑	❑
4.	Places a time tape on the solution.	❑	❑
5.	Properly identifies patient before adding solution.	❑	❑
6.	Removes IV tubing from completed bag and spikes new bag of IV solution.	❑	❑
7.	Removes air bubbles that occurred in tubing.	❑	❑
8.	Readjusts flow rate to prescribed rate.	❑	❑
9.	Disposes of empty container.	❑	❑
10.	Records the added fluid on the parenteral infusion record.	❑	❑
11.	Carries out Standard Steps X, Y, and Z.	❑	❑

Pass ❑
Fail ❑

Comments:

Instructor: ______________________

SKILL 34-3 ADMINISTERING INTRAVENOUS PIGGYBACK MEDICATION

Student: ______________________________

Date: ______________________________

		Satisfactory	Unsatisfactory
1.	Carries out Standard Steps A, B, C, D, and E as need indicates.	❑	❑
2.	Checks medication with MAR and assesses for allergies.	❑	❑
3.	Calculates flow rate if not indicated on label.	❑	❑
4.	Hooks up the IVPB administration set to the small bag or bottle.	❑	❑
5.	Clears the tubing of air.	❑	❑
6.	Re-verifies the drug and dosage with MAR; follows five rights.	❑	❑
7.	Properly identifies patient and re-verifies allergies.	❑	❑
8.	Connects IVPB properly.	❑	❑
9.	Adjust the flow rate to correct flow.	❑	❑
10.	Monitors the patient for adverse reaction.	❑	❑
11.	Documents the IVPB on the MAR.	❑	❑
12.	Disposes of equipment when IVPB infusion is complete.	❑	❑
13.	Carries out Standard Steps X, Y, and Z.	❑	❑

Pass ❒
Fail ❒

Comments:

Instructor: ______________________

SKILL 34-4 ADMINISTERING MEDICATION VIA A PRN LOCK

Student: ______________________________

Date: ______________________________

		Satisfactory	Unsatisfactory
1.	Carries out Standard Steps A, B, C, D, and E as need indicates.	❑	❑
2.	Selects an appropriate site for insertion.	❑	❑
3.	Dons gloves and inserts IV cannula with cap or PRN lock.	❑	❑
4.	Flushes with 2 mL of normal saline.	❑	❑
5.	Secures the lock with a transparent dressing or other sterile dressing.	❑	❑
6.	Prepares the IV medication correctly, checking the medication with the order and following the five rights.	❑	❑
7.	Cleanses the injection cap of the lock before inserting a needle.	❑	❑
8.	Properly identifies patient and re-verifies allergies.	❑	❑
9.	Verifies drug with MAR one more time.	❑	❑
10.	Properly injects the medication into the PRN lock.	❑	❑
11.	Flushes the lock with 2 mL of normal saline.	❑	❑
12.	Documents medication administration and insertion of PRN lock.	❑	❑
13.	Carries out Standard Steps X, Y, and Z.	❑	❑

Pass ❑

Fail ❑

Comments:

Instructor: ______________________

SKILL 34-5 ADMINISTRATION OF MEDICATION WITH A VOLUME-CONTROLLED SET

Student: ____________________

Date: ____________________

		Satisfactory	Unsatisfactory
1.	Carries out Standard Steps A, B, C, D, and E as need indicates.	❑	❑
2.	Checks the medication with the MAR order.	❑	❑
3.	Prepares the medication and draws it up in a syringe.	❑	❑
4.	Properly identifies the patient; re-verifies the medication with the MAR.	❑	❑
5.	Cleanses the injection cap on the burette and adds the medication to the correct amount of IV solution.	❑	❑
6.	Labels the burette and mixes the medication and solution.	❑	❑
7.	Opens lower clamp and adjusts the rate of flow.	❑	❑
8.	As soon as burette empties, reopens top clamp to continue the IV infusion.	❑	❑
9.	Documents medication administration.	❑	❑
10.	Carries out Standard Steps X, Y, and Z.	❑	❑

Pass ❑
Fail ❑

Comments:

Instructor: ____________________

SKILL 34-6 ADMINISTRATION OF BLOOD PRODUCTS

Student: ______________________________

Date: ______________________________

		Satisfactory	Unsatisfactory
1.	Carries out Standard Steps A, B, C, D, and E as need indicates.	❑	❑
2.	Verifies size of IV catheter in place.	❑	❑
3.	Obtains blood using proper procedure.	❑	❑
4.	Double checks the blood with another nurse.	❑	❑
5.	Attaches the "Y" administration set and sets up normal saline solution.	❑	❑
6.	Spikes the blood component bag correctly.	❑	❑
7.	Properly identifies the patient and checks the blood identification bracelet with the transfusion record numbers.	❑	❑
8.	Dons gloves and connects the blood component to the administration set.	❑	❑
9.	Obtains baseline vital signs.	❑	❑
10.	Primes administration set with normal saline.	❑	❑
11.	Begins the blood administration, remains with patient for first 5 minutes, and checks the patient every 15 minutes for first half hour.	❑	❑
12.	Monitors vital signs every 30 minutes.	❑	❑
13.	Flushes line with normal saline at end of infusion.	❑	❑
14.	Carries out Standard Steps X, Y, and Z.	❑	❑

Pass ❒
Fail ❒

Comments:

Instructor: ______________________

SKILL 35-1 PERFORMING A SURGICAL PREP

Student: ______________________________

Date: ______________________________

		Satisfactory	Unsatisfactory
1.	Carries out Standard Steps A, B, C, D, and E as indicated.	❑	❑
2.	Trims hair close to the skin before clipping or using depilatory or antibacterial soap.	❑	❑
OR			
3.	Dons gloves.	❑	❑
4.	Works up a soapy lather.	❑	❑
5.	Holds skin taut while shaving.	❑	❑
6.	Washes off all loose hair.	❑	❑
7.	Strokes with razor in same direction as hair growth.	❑	❑
8.	Scrubs from center outward.	❑	❑
9.	Rinses and dries area.	❑	❑
10.	Removes and discards gloves.	❑	❑
11.	Carries out Standard Steps X, Y, and Z.	❑	❑

Pass ❒
Fail ❒

Comments:

Instructor: ______________________________

SKILL 35-2 APPLYING ANTIEMBOLISM STOCKINGS

Student: ______________________________

Date: ______________________________

		Satisfactory	Unsatisfactory
1.	Carries out Standard Steps A, B, C, D, and E as indicated.	❑	❑
2.	Measures leg correctly for type of stocking ordered.	❑	❑
3.	Prepares legs for application of stockings.	❑	❑
4.	Applies each stocking correctly.	❑	❑
5.	Smooths out any wrinkles.	❑	❑
6.	Carries out Standard Steps X, Y, and Z.	❑	❑

Pass ❑
Fail ❑

Comments:

Instructor: ______________________

SKILL 37-1 CAST CARE

Student: ______________________________

Date: ______________________________

		Satisfactory	Unsatisfactory
1.	Carries out Standard Steps A, B, C, D, and E as need indicates.	❑	❑
2.	Examines cast for any dents.	❑	❑
3.	Examines cast for areas where blood has seeped through, circles them and notes date and time. Reports excessive increase in seepage.	❑	❑
4.	Checks cast for sharp edges and tightness.	❑	❑
5.	Pads or covers any rough edges.	❑	❑
6.	Notifies MD or cast technician of any areas which are too tight or any skin damage from rough or tight areas.	❑	❑
7.	Elevates extremity with cast so hand or foot is at the level of the heart.	❑	❑
8.	Places the bed in slight Trendelenburg position during the first day or two for body casts, unless contraindicated by the patient's condition or physician orders.	❑	❑
9.	Turns the patient at intervals so that all surfaces of the cast are exposed to air to facilitate even drying.	❑	❑
10.	Instructs the patient in the dangers of using objects to scratch under the cast.	❑	❑
11.	Smells the open edges of the cast to assess for odor which may indicate infection under the cast		
12.	Carries out Standard Steps X, Y, and Z.	❑	❑

Pass ❑
Fail ❑

Comments:

Instructor: ______________________

SKILL 37-2 CARE OF THE PATIENT IN TRACTION

Student: ____________________

Date: ____________________

		Satisfactory	Unsatisfactory
1.	Carries out Standard Steps A, B, C, D, and E as need indicates.	❑	❑
2.	Checks order for desired amount of weight for traction.	❑	❑
3.	Assesses traction apparatus for correct function.	❑	❑
4.	Assesses skin, distal circulation, and sensation.	❑	❑
5.	Realigns patient in bed as needed.	❑	❑
6.	Performs pin or tong care as ordered or according to agency protocol.	❑	❑
7.	Carries out Standard Steps X, Y, and Z.	❑	❑

Pass ❑
Fail ❑

Comments:

Instructor: ____________________